STRABISMUS:
A DECISION MAKING APPROACH

STRABISMUS: A DECISION MAKING APPROACH

Gunter K. von Noorden, M.D.

Professor of Ophthalmology and Pediatrics
Baylor College of Medicine, Houston, Texas

Eugene M. Helveston, M.D.

Professor of Ophthalmology
Indiana University School of Medicine
Indianapolis, Indiana

FIRST EDITION

with 95 illustrations

Mosby

St. Louis Baltimore Berlin Boston Carlsbad Chicago London Madrid
Naples New York Philadelphia Sydney Tokyo Toronto

Mosby

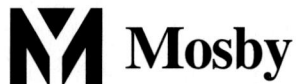

Dedicated to Publishing Excellence

Editor: Laurel Craven
Developmental Editor: Dana Battaglia
Project Manager: Linda Clarke
Manufacturing Supervisor: Kathy Grone

Printed in the United States of America
Composition by Top Graphics
Printing/binding by Maple Vail Book Mfg. Group, York

Mosby–Year Book, Inc.
11830 Westline Industrial Drive
St. Louis, Missouri 63146

Library of Congress Cataloging in Publication Data

International Standard Book Number
0-8151-4048-7

94 95 96 97 98 / 9 8 7 6 5 4 3 2 1

FOREWORD

Clinical problem solving is a highly complex process of deductive medical reasoning. The first step is to aggregate findings derived from history taking and the clinical examination into a logical hierarchy. The inexperienced student is overwhelmed by the excessive amount of information generated by an exhaustive, nonfocused history and physical examination. The seasoned diagnostician is able to search for a specific sign or finding based on the key issue. The identification of a distinctive or pathognomonic sign enables the clinician to generate a concise list of conditions potentially responsible for that particular sign. The ideal strategy is to select a distinctive sign with the shortest probable cause list. Equipped with a working differential diagnosis, the skilled clinician next uses a series of questions or comparisons to form probability estimates, ideally built around binomial "yes/no" or "present/absent" logic. Experience and clinical instinct generate the proper questions in a logical sequence. The process may either lead directly to the correct diagnosis or identify a series of other diagnostic procedures or laboratory studies by which to pursue the diagnosis. Algorithms or decision trees are simple, effective methods to express this method of problem solving.

In this masterful text, the authors depict their mental strategies in decision making in strabismus through a series of algorithms, crafted from years of experience in the diagnosis and management of virtually every variety of problem encounter. Whereas most textbooks on strabismus and other clinical topics in ophthalmology are organized by disease or organ system, the authors construct the distinct findings and signs in ocular motility and other related disorders into a system for decision making. They have mastered complex cognitive processes to generate probability estimates of likely responsible conditions. They know the proper questions and the most efficient sequence in which to ask them. As a result, the student is not only able to follow the plan to make the correct decision but to learn the methodology of utilizing distinctive signs in problem solving. In addition to the algorithmic approach for reaching a clinical diagnosis, the authors provide the preferred medical or surgical treatment for the various conditions, based also on answers to critically posed questions related to degrees of severity and adjunctive findings. Their approach to decision making in strabismus is simple, direct, and precise. Their ability to define and depict the process of deductive reasoning has produced a treasure for clinicians, inexperienced and seasoned alike, for all time.

Dan B. Jones, M.D.

PREFACE

The multitude of complex and often subtle symptoms and signs in strabismus present a unique clinical challenge. Even after the correct diagnosis has been established, the physician has to make additional selections from the multiple available treatment options. The authors, who for many years have specialized in the study, treatment, and teaching of ocular motility disorders, realize that the process underlying diagnostic problem solving or treatment decisions depends largely on mental access to past experience with similar or even identical clinical situations. However, what may be a split second decision with numerous and often subconscious mental shortcuts for the expert can present a confounding problem for the less experienced, who may never have seen a similar case and may easily become sidetracked and confused in the maze of diagnostic and therapeutic possibilities.

Orderly and practical approaches to diagnostic, differential diagnostic, and treatment decision making for common and less common forms of strabismus are provided in this book. After establishing some basic facts about the underlying condition—for instance the direction of the deviation or the nature of the patient's initial complaint (*shaded box*)—the required tests (*rounded boxes*), the diagnostic possibilities, test results and clinical findings (*rectangular boxes*) are explored. At the bottom of the flowchart, after excluding possible alternatives, the reader will find the diagnosis or treatment options (*heavily outlined rectangular boxes*). Different entry systems and cross-referencing are widely used to aid both the neophyte and the more experienced reader who recognizes

the problem correctly but wishes to explore it in all its ramifications.

The descriptive text is kept intentionally brief and contains numbered references to the algorithm on the page opposite, to other algorithms in this book, and to the literature, especially to our texts, to which this manual is meant to serve as a companion.

We hope that this book will bridge the gap between the available textbooks and atlases of strabismus and the actual clinical problem-solving process in an office setting. It is primarily addressed to residents, general ophthalmologists, optometrists, and orthoptists, but we hope that even the pediatric ophthalmologist may find this material occasionally helpful.

The senior author acknowledges being inspired to undertake this project by the algorithmic approach to clinical problem solving championed by Dr. Dan B. Jones during Grand Rounds at the Cullen Eye Institute.

We thank Cynthia Avila, C.O. for meticulous proofreading of the manuscript and Drs. Derek Sprunger and David Plager for their helpful suggestions.

Gunter K. von Noorden
Eugene M. Helveston

CONTENTS

2. DIAGNOSTIC AND TREATMENT DECISIONS

1

Preliminaries

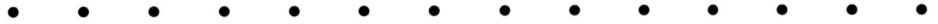

• • • • • • • • • • • • • • • • •

1.01 Equipment for Examination of the Patient With Strabismus

The equipment requirements for examination of the patient with strabismus are few, but those elements required are essential. This starts with a quiet examination lane, preferably of 6 M length and with a light source that can be dimmed. A comfortable, adjustable chair is needed for the patient, who may be seated either alone or on the parent's lap. The examiner also needs an adjustable chair with freely movable coasters. The examiner may wear the traditional white coat or other, possibly less "threatening" attire. Both authors wear the traditional garb. The equipment list should include the following items:

- Loose prisms, from $\frac{1}{2}^\Delta$ to 30^Δ
- One horizontal and one vertical plastic prism bar (1^Δ to 25^Δ)
- Rotary prism
- Opaque occluder
- A variety of small near fixation targets, silent or noise-producing and animated, with capabilities of maintaining attention and stimulating accommodation
- Animated distance fixation targets
- A trial lens set with plus cylinders and prisms (to fit in a trial frame)
- Adult and pediatric trial frames
- Red and white Maddox rods
- Stereo test (Titmus, Randot, Lang, TNO)
- Handheld fixation light
- Pinhole
- Worth 4-dot test and red-green spectacles
- Bagolini lenses
- Halberg clips
- Retinoscope
- Refraction lens bar with convex and concave lenses
- Portable biomicroscope
- Direct and indirect ophthalmoscopes
- Hertel exophthalmometer
- Visual acuity chart (B-VAT is strongly recommended)
- Near vision cards
- Optokinetic drum or tape
- Fine-tooth forceps for passive ductions and estimation of generated muscle force

- Afterimage tester (modified handheld camera flash)
- Reading comprehension charts and words lists

  - Major amblyoscope*
  - Deviometer
  - Hess or Lees' screen
  - Spielmann translucent occluders
  - Contrast sensitivity acuity chart
  - Neutral density filters
  - Visuscope or similar device to test fixation pattern
  - Perimeter to determine field of single binocular vision

This equipment list is relatively small and, for the most part, inexpensive. The "first-line" instruments should be available to anyone who evaluates a patient with strabismus. The "second-line" equipment (shown indented) is for special documentation, research, and for medicolegal purposes. Some items of "second-line" equipment represent the personal preference of an individual examiner. In addition to this equipment, a systematic recording scheme should be used. In most cases this includes a printed data collection sheet.[23 p.359] Drops for dilating the pupil and obtaining cycloplegia include cyclopentolate 1%, phenylephrine hydrochloride 10% and 2.5%, tropicamide 1%, and Cyclomydril. Drops used for anesthetizing the conjunctiva include proparacaine hydrochloride, tetracaine hydrochloride, lidocaine hydrochloride 4%, and cocaine 4%. We prefer to use lidocaine. Fresnel press-on prisms in powers ranging from 1^Δ to 40^Δ should be available, as well as +1.00, +2.00, and +3.00 diopter spherical lenses.

---

* A major amblyoscope is essential equipment for a practice with an orthoptist. When an orthoptist is not available, fusional amplitudes can be measured with the rotary prism or the horizontal prism bar.

1.02   History

(1) Family photographs are often very helpful to document the age of onset. Parents often report that the eyes have crossed continuously since birth. However, it has been shown that even infantile esotropia occurs infrequently at birth.[22]

(2) This information provides an important clue in strabismic infants because amblyopia is absent in alternating strabismus. Strong preference for fixation with the same eye, on the other hand, implies strabismic amblyopia in the nonpreferred eye.

(3) **See 1.33.**

(4) For example, a history of a bump on the head, a fall, or one of the usual febrile childhood diseases preceding the onset of strabismus is usually insignificant. However, acute strabismus, usually esotropia, **(see 2.10)** in an older child always requires a careful evaluation to rule out neurologic abnormalities.

(5) Intermittent strabismus indicates that fusion is present part of the time. The prognosis for recovery of normal binocular vision is better in such cases.

(6) Closure of one eye in bright sunlight and reports of light sensitivity are commonly encountered in patients with intermittent exodeviations. Although this symptom occurs also in esotropic and normal subjects, its presence should alert the examiner to search for intermittent exotropia. It is caused by a decreased binocular photophobia threshold.[72] Any complaint about photophobia requires a search for nonstrabismic causes, such as hypopigmentation of the eye or corneal or conjunctival disease.

(7) **See 1.32.**

(8) A history of malignant hyperthermia, familial hepatic porphyria, suxamethonium sensitivity, or allergic reactions to dilating drops requires special precautions because of serious, even fatal anesthetic complications.

(9) Low birth weight suggests the possibility of retinopathy of prematurity with pseudostrabismus from ectopia of the macula. Myasthenia gravis, although infrequent in childhood, may mimic almost any type of strabismus, and reports of easy fatigability should be further investigated for myasthenia.

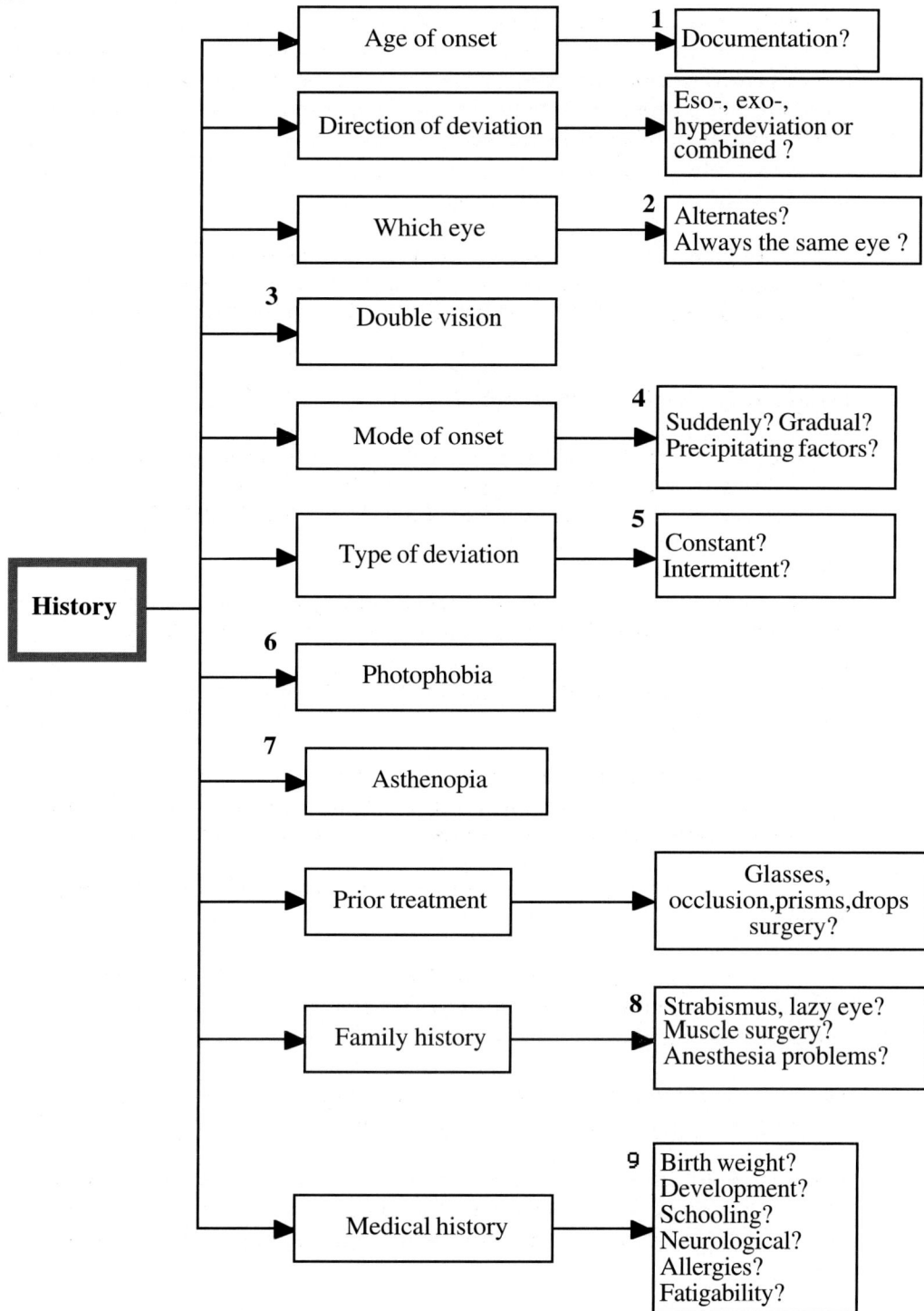

1.02

```
                          ┌──────────────────┐      1  ┌──────────────────┐
                  ┌──────▶│   Age of onset   │───────▶│  Documentation?  │
                  │       └──────────────────┘         └──────────────────┘
                  │                                      ┌──────────────────┐
                  │       ┌──────────────────┐          │ Eso-, exo-,      │
                  ├──────▶│Direction of      │─────────▶│ hyperdeviation or│
                  │       │deviation         │          │ combined ?       │
                  │       └──────────────────┘          └──────────────────┘
                  │       ┌──────────────────┐      2  ┌──────────────────┐
                  ├──────▶│   Which eye      │───────▶│ Alternates?      │
                  │       └──────────────────┘         │ Always the same  │
                  │                                     │ eye ?            │
                  │    3  ┌──────────────────┐          └──────────────────┘
                  ├──────▶│  Double vision   │
                  │       └──────────────────┘
                  │       ┌──────────────────┐      4  ┌──────────────────┐
                  ├──────▶│  Mode of onset   │───────▶│ Suddenly? Gradual?│
                  │       └──────────────────┘         │ Precipitating     │
                  │                                     │ factors?          │
                  │       ┌──────────────────┐      5  └──────────────────┘
┌──────────┐      ├──────▶│Type of deviation │───────▶┌──────────────────┐
│ History  │──────┤       └──────────────────┘         │ Constant?        │
└──────────┘      │    6  ┌──────────────────┐          │ Intermittent?    │
                  ├──────▶│  Photophobia     │          └──────────────────┘
                  │       └──────────────────┘
                  │    7  ┌──────────────────┐
                  ├──────▶│   Asthenopia     │
                  │       └──────────────────┘
                  │       ┌──────────────────┐          ┌──────────────────┐
                  ├──────▶│ Prior treatment  │─────────▶│ Glasses,         │
                  │       └──────────────────┘          │ occlusion,prisms,│
                  │                                      │ drops surgery?   │
                  │       ┌──────────────────┐      8  └──────────────────┘
                  ├──────▶│ Family history   │───────▶┌──────────────────┐
                  │       └──────────────────┘         │ Strabismus, lazy  │
                  │                                     │ eye? Muscle       │
                  │                                     │ surgery?          │
                  │                                     │ Anesthesia        │
                  │                                     │ problems?         │
                  │                                     └──────────────────┘
                  │       ┌──────────────────┐      9  ┌──────────────────┐
                  └──────▶│ Medical history  │───────▶│ Birth weight?     │
                          └──────────────────┘         │ Development?      │
                                                       │ Schooling?        │
                                                       │ Neurological?     │
                                                       │ Allergies?        │
                                                       │ Fatigability?     │
                                                       └──────────────────┘
```

1.03   **Inspection of Patient**

(1) During the initial discussion with the parents when the history is obtained, the examiner should observe the child inconspicuously. Valuable information can be gained without directing full attention to the child, who may be apprehensive. If a child is approached too vigorously, cooperation could be lost before the actual examination has even started.

(2) **See 1.38.**

(3) Although **A** and **V** patterns are not consistently associated with mongoloid or antimongoloid lid fissures, the presence of such anomalies should always alert the examiner to search for horizontal strabismus in upward and downward gaze.[47]

(4) **See 1.25, 1.26, 1.27, 1.28, and 1.29.**

(5) Acquired exophthalmos may signal Graves' disease, and long-standing exophthalmos may be associated with congenital craniofacial anomalies. Enophthalmos may be associated with Duane syndrome **(see 2.50, 2.51, and 2.52)** or an old blowout fracture **(see 2.54).**

(6) A complete N III paralysis with aberrant regeneration may be accompanied by lagophthalmos **(see 2.36),** as is severe Graves' disease **(see 2.55).**

(7) Plagiocephaly and superior oblique muscle paralysis may be associated with facial asymmetry.

(8) Closure of one eye is caused by lowered binocular thresholds to photophobia. It may occur in the absence of any ocular motility disorder but more frequently in association with strabismus, especially intermittent exotropia.[72]

(9) Prominent epicanthal folds can impart the impression of esotropia (pseudostrabismus).

(10) Generally, alternating strabismus is incompatible with amblyopia. Observation of free alternation in young children or infants provides the examiner with this most important clue at the beginning of the examination.

(11) A strong unilateral fixation preference should alert the examiner to suspect reduced visual acuity (amblyopia, organic causes) of the nonfixating eye.

(12) A variable angle of strabismus occurs frequently in association with an uncorrected refractive error (refractive accommodative esotropia) **(see 2.07),** anisometropia, or in association with the nystagmus compensation syndrome **(see 2.34).**

(13) **See 2.33, 2.34, and 2.35.**

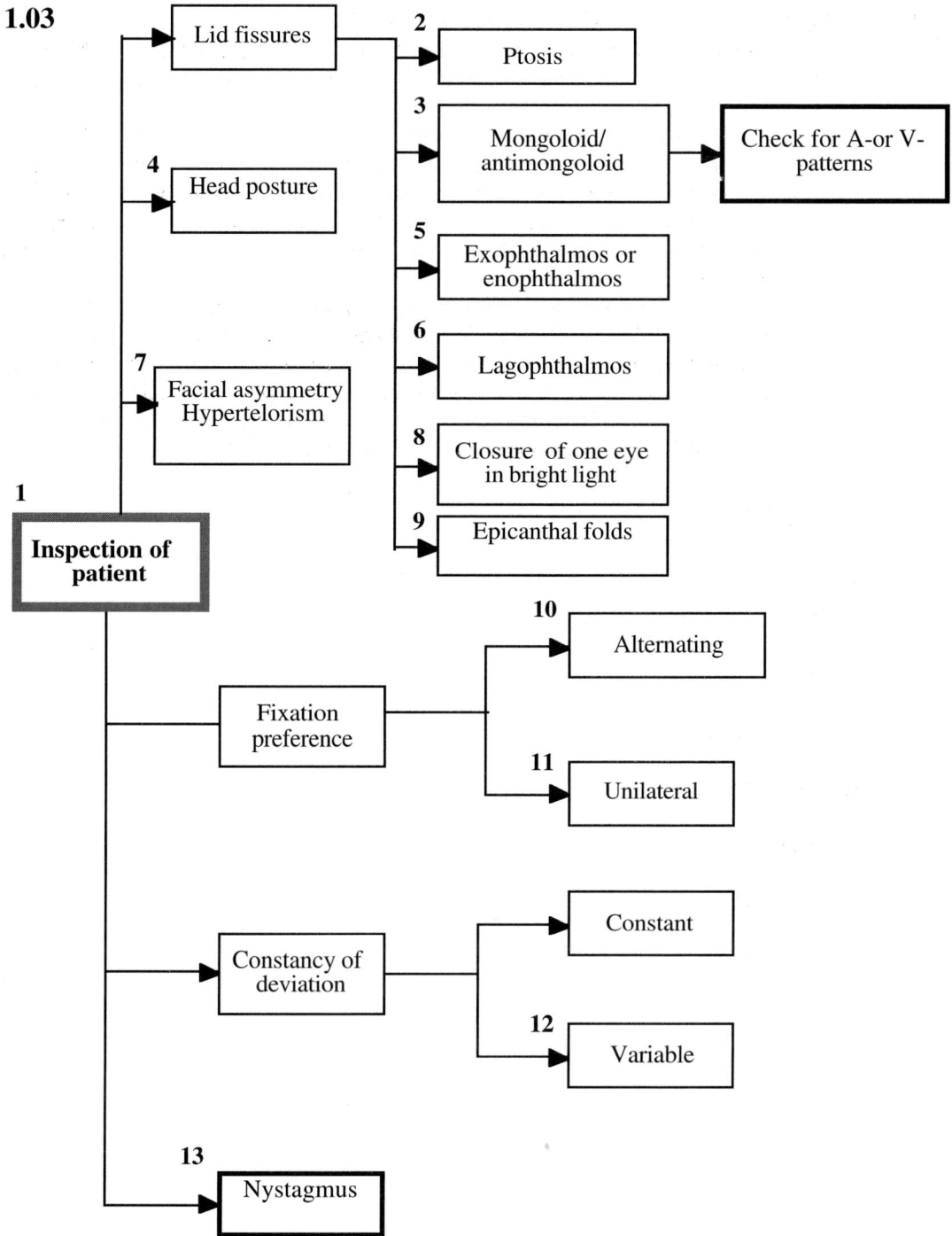

1.03

```
Lid fissures ──2──► Ptosis
             ──3──► Mongoloid/antimongoloid ──► Check for A-or V-patterns
4 Head posture
             ──5──► Exophthalmos or enophthalmos
             ──6──► Lagophthalmos
7 Facial asymmetry Hypertelorism
             ──8──► Closure of one eye in bright light
             ──9──► Epicanthal folds

1 Inspection of patient

Fixation preference ──10──► Alternating
                    ──11──► Unilateral

Constancy of deviation ──► Constant
                       ──12──► Variable

13 Nystagmus
```

1.04   Sequence of Motility Examination

One of the difficult challenges confronting the examiner of a patient with strabismus is to establish the proper order in which the various tests should be performed. Two guiding factors are as follows: (1) start with the least threatening test so as not to upset the younger patient, and (2) use the least dissociating tests at the beginning and progress to the more dissociating tests. For example: Measure stereo acuity before dissociating the eyes with the alternate prism and cover test. The doll's head maneuver in younger children, forced duction testing, and estimation of the generated muscle force in older children and adults are best left until the end of the examination.

The hierarchy of the strabismus examination is shown in the algorithm. History taking, observation, and the various tests are done in descending order.

Not all tests apply to all patients, either because they are not pertinent to the diagnosis or they are impossible to perform. Use of a printed motility examination form laid out essentially according to the flow of this scheme assists in performing an orderly and effective motility examination.[23 p.359]

(1) **See 1.03.**

(2) **See 1.02.**

(3) **See 1.05, 1.06, and 1.07.**

(4) **See 1.09 and 1.10.**

(5) **See 1.15 and 1.16.**

(6) **See 1.36.**

(7) **See 1.37.**

(8) **See 1.24.**

(9) **See 1.30.**

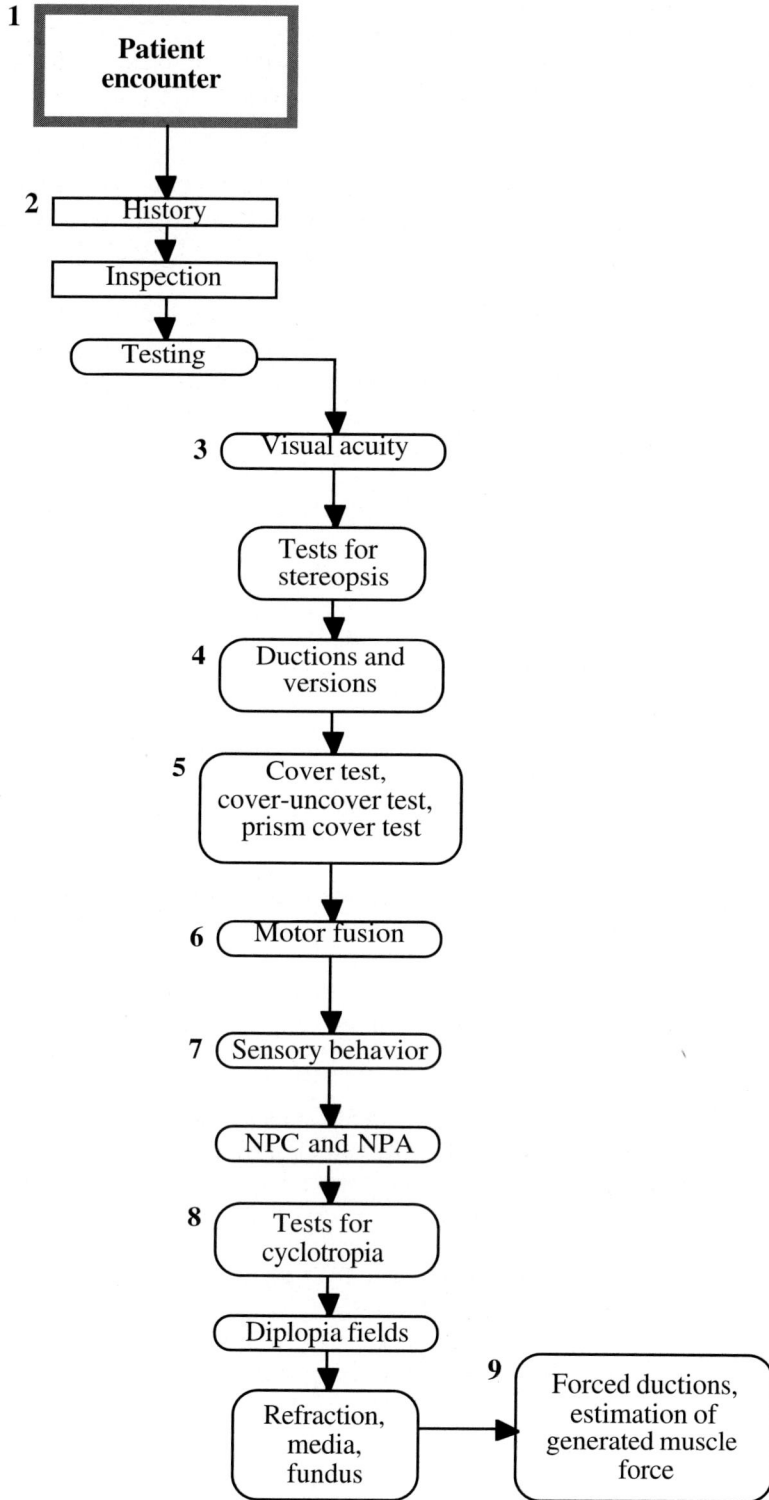

1.04

1
Patient encounter

2 History

Inspection

Testing

3 Visual acuity

Tests for stereopsis

4 Ductions and versions

5 Cover test, cover-uncover test, prism cover test

6 Motor fusion

7 Sensory behavior

NPC and NPA

8 Tests for cyclotropia

Diplopia fields

Refraction, media, fundus

9 Forced ductions, estimation of generated muscle force

1.05 **Does This Baby See?**

(1) This fundamental question should be asked at the beginning of the examination. A sequence of tests is necessary if this question cannot be answered satisfactorily.

(2) Evaluation starts with simple observation. The infant may be cradled in the parent's arms, or the examiner may gently hold the child facing him or her. If the room light is subdued, the infant is more likely to open his or her eyes.

(3) The examiner should establish eye contact with the infant and once this is accomplished, interpret the response. In most cases the infant will smile when eye contact is made. At this point, an assessment is made of the fixation, which is either steady or unsteady. Nystagmoid searching eye movements should be distinguished from true nystagmus.

(4) The examiner then moves his or her head from side to side, observing whether the infant's eyes follow this stimulus. It is important to use nonauditory stimuli.

(5) The examiner then rotates the child rapidly but smoothly to one side and then to the other. When this movement ceases, normal infants have one or two beats of nystagmus and then resume steady fixation. Infants with poor vision have prolonged postrotatory nystagmus that persists for several beats.

(6) The pupillary light reaction indicates an intact anterior visual loop (retina-optic nerve-pupillomotor nerves).[24 p.4]

(7) The optokinetic nystagmus (OKN) response tests resolution visual acuity and evaluates the intactness of the posterior visual loop (occipital cortex–brain stem–extraocular muscles).[24 p.4]

(8) The forced preferential looking test is a technique for quantifying recognition visual acuity.[14] This technique has limited practical clinical application.

(9) The electroretinogram (ERG) test is a measure of retinal function. It is an important diagnostic step in confirming Leber's congenital amaurosis and retinitis pigmentosa. However, subnormal visual acuity can be compatible with a normal ERG and vice versa.

(10) Visual evoked potential (VEP) registers the cortical response to retinal stimulation. The stimulus is either a light flash or a checkerboard with black and white blocks. Quantification is difficult, and this test is rarely used in a clinical setting to establish the presence of vision in an infant.[40]

1.05

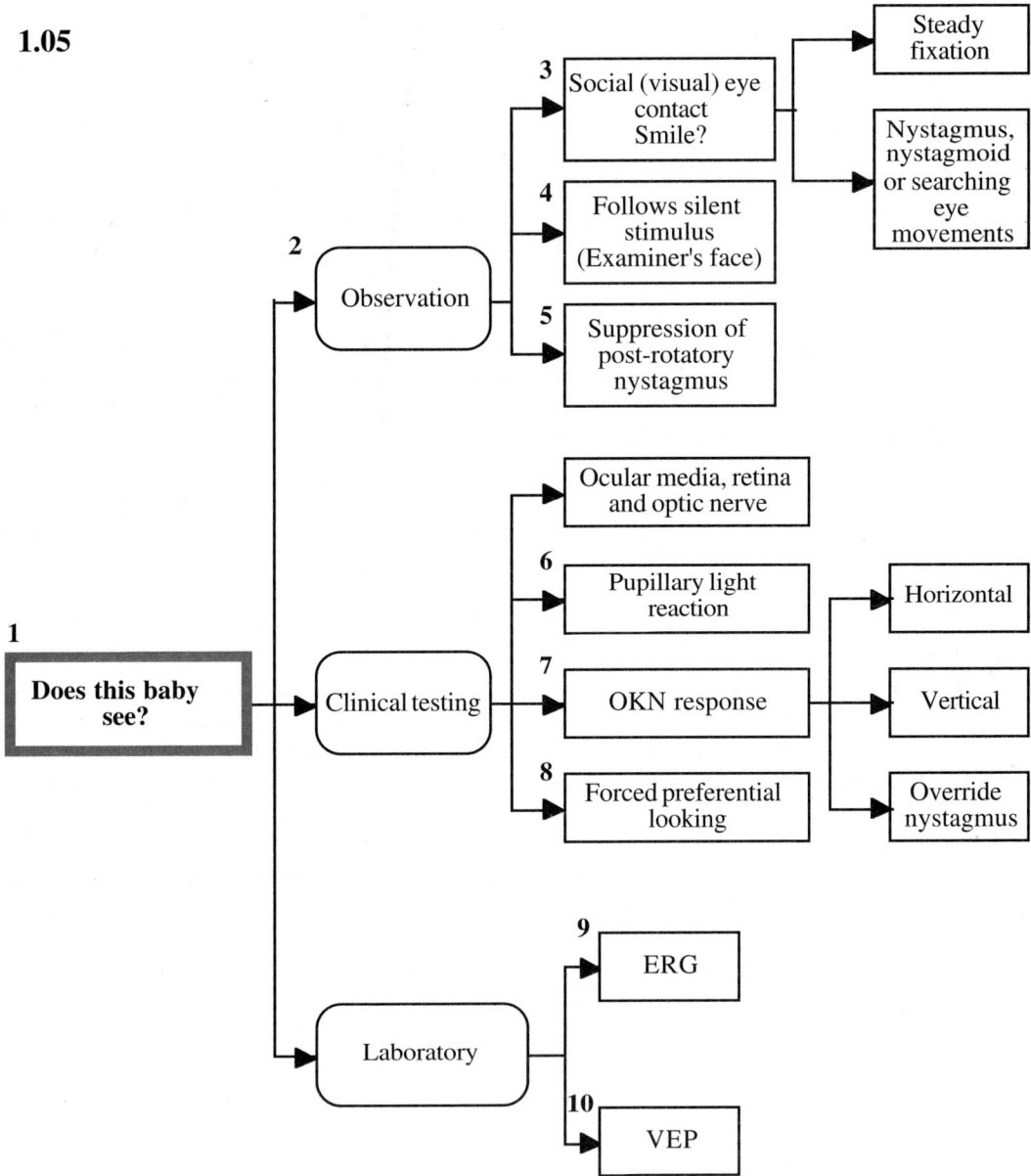

1.06   **Visual Acuity: Methods of Examination**

(1) Visual acuity when tested with both eyes open produces the highest acuity.

(2) Monocular acuity is reduced in cases with latent nystagmus. Monocular acuity may be equal to but is never better than binocular acuity.

(3) Grating acuity is less selective because it only requires that the patient distinguishes vertical stripes from a dull gray background of equal luminance. The forced preferential looking test (FPL) uses grating patterns.[3,14]

(4) Recognition acuity requires the patient to identify the object and tell the examiner what he or she sees, such as an A, E, or T. In terms of Snellen acuity, 20/20 vision is the ability to identify at a distance of 20 feet objects that subtend 5 minutes of arc with components of 1 minute of arc at 20 feet.

(5) Use of a pinhole or creation of a pinhole effect by the patient squinting improves visual acuity in the presence of an uncorrected refractive error, or in some cases when a media opacity is present.

(6) The visual evoked potential (VEP) test is done with either white flash or formed stimuli, usually stripes or a checkerboard pattern (sweep VEP). This test merely determines whether visual stimuli are being received at the visual cortex. This test is usually done to rule in (or rule out) cortical visual impairment. Recently sweep VEP has been used in an attempt to quantify "cortical visual acuity," and VEP binocular summation has been used as a measure of binocularity.[40]

(7) Full line resolution acuity at the distance fixation is the most sensitive measure of visual acuity in cases of refractive error. Other measures including glare sensitivity are helpful in cases of media opacity.

(8) In cases of functional amblyopia, visual acuity is usually improved one or more lines if single optotypes are used because of the crowding phenomenon.[57 p.216]

(9) Near acuity is always equal to or better than distance acuity, except in cases of uncorrected presbyopia, which may be either involutional or premature. Near vision should be measured at 14 inches with graded optotypes or sentences to compare with distance acuity. Near acuity may be tested at a shorter distance or with magnification to determine a patient's functional capacity for near work.

(10) In cases of null point nystagmus, vision improves when the patient assumes a compensatory head posture that places the eyes into a gaze position in which the nystagmus is reduced or absent.

1.06

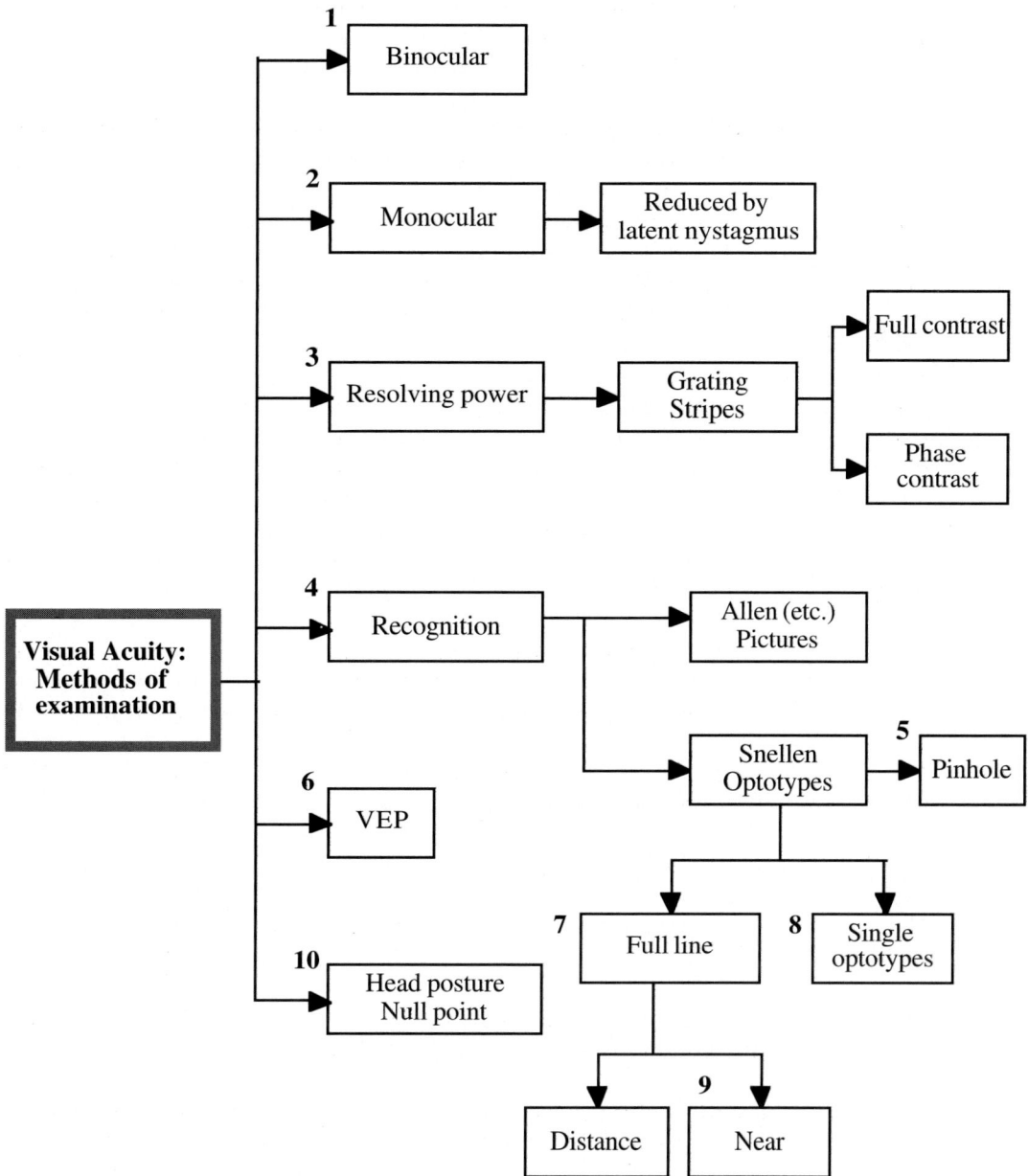

1.07   **Visual Acuity Testing in Infants**

(1) Quantitative visual acuity testing of infants is difficult, if not impossible, in an office environment, and it is usually unnecessary. Of greater importance is whether there is a difference in visual acuity between the two eyes.

(2) This technique is based on the fact that an infant's attention is attracted more by patterned stimuli than by a homogenous surface, provided the pattern is above the visual acuity threshold. The infant's eye or head movements in response to the appearance of the striped stimulus is interpreted as "seeing" the target. To adapt this time-consuming method to a clinical setting, acuity cards have been designed that contain grating patterns of varying spatial frequencies.[14,37] The usefulness of this method as an office procedure is still being evaluated.

(3) The fixation behavior is assessed by observation of the eyes while the patient fixates on a visual object or a fixation light. Searching, unsteady, or nystagmoid fixation movements and inability to pursue a moving visual target indicate poor vision. The examiner notes whether the child alternates, prefers fixation with one eye, or can hold fixation well with either eye. For instance, refusal of the child to have the right eye covered while not objecting to having the left eye covered is interpreted as evidence for reduced visual acuity in the left eye.

(4) OKN responses depend on visual acuity, attention, and intact motor responses. At best, this test provides information regarding whether vision is present. OKN testing has not been adapted successfully for quantitative testing.[24 p.4]

(5) If a patient with strabismus shows random alternating fixation, it is justified to conclude that visual acuity is equal in both eyes.

(6) Fixation preference for one eye usually indicates reduced vision in the non-preferred eye. However, this conclusion cannot be automatically made because some patients have normal and equal visual acuity in each eye despite a strong fixation preference.

(7) In cases of fixation preference, subtle differences in the steadiness of fixation and the ability to maintain fixation through a blink are noted.

(8) Alternation and fixation preference are difficult to judge in the absence of strabismus. In such instances a vertical strabismus is induced by holding a 10^Δ base-up or base-down before one eye.[75] A vertical prism held in front of one eye produces vertical dissociation, thereby allowing detection of fixation preference when no or only very small horizontal deviation is found.[75]

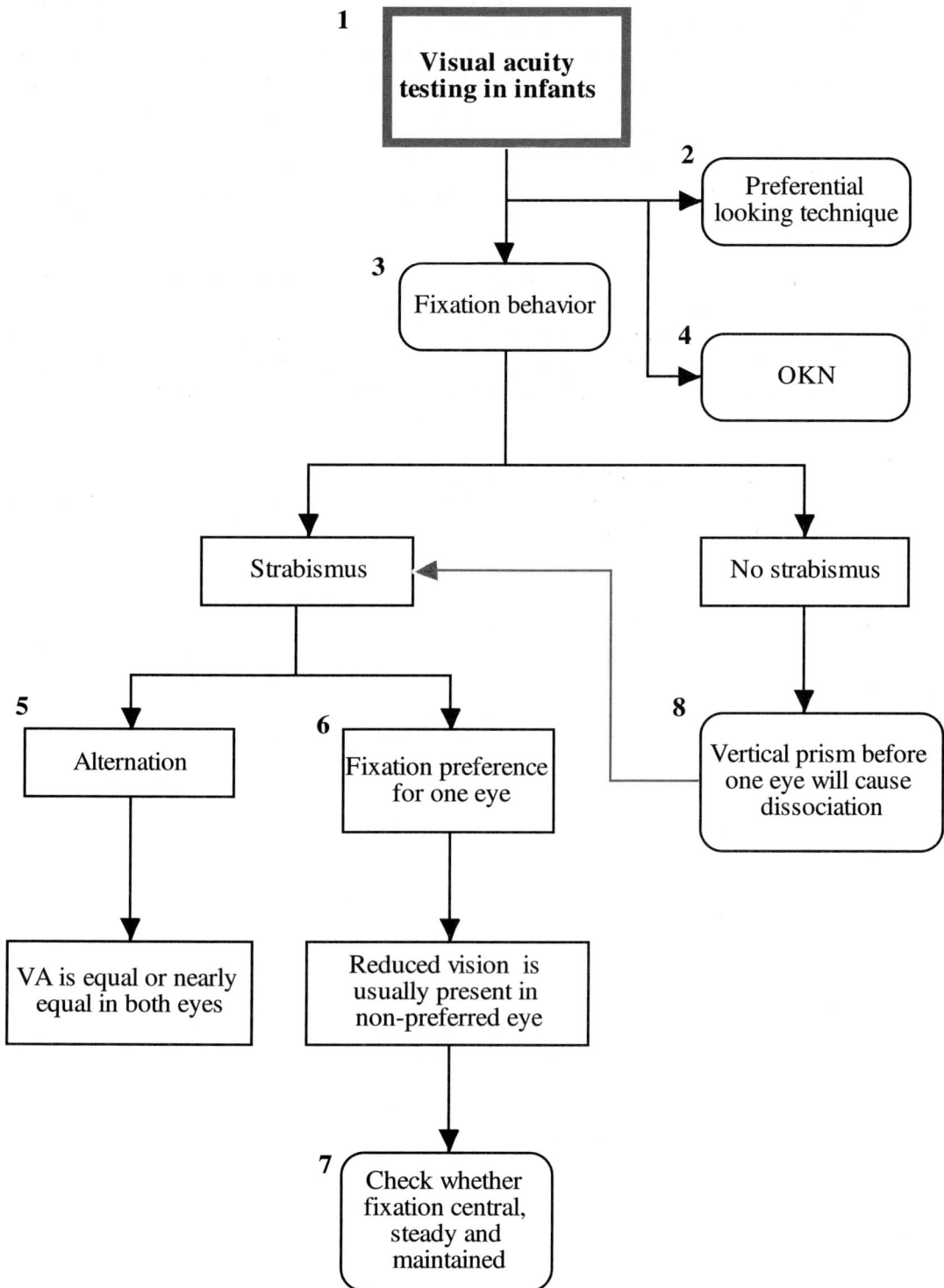

1.07

1 **Visual acuity testing in infants**

2 Preferential looking technique

3 Fixation behavior

4 OKN

Strabismus

No strabismus

5 Alternation

6 Fixation preference for one eye

8 Vertical prism before one eye will cause dissociation

VA is equal or nearly equal in both eyes

Reduced vision is usually present in non-preferred eye

7 Check whether fixation central, steady and maintained

1.08 Primary versus Secondary Deviation

(1) The determination of the fixation preference in the diagnostic workup of a patient with paretic or paralytic strabismus is essential. Such testing detects the offending eye and influences treatment decisions. It follows that in paralytic strabismus the deviation should be measured while the patient fixates with either eye.

(2) The primary deviation is always smaller than the secondary deviation because no excessive innervation is required when the patient fixates with the sound eye.[57 p.367]

(3) When the paretic or paralyzed eye is used for fixation, excessive innervation is required to move and maintain the eye in primary position. According to Hering's law of equal innervation[57 p.367] the same amount of innervation flows simultaneously to the yoke muscle in the sound eye, and the angle of strabismus is larger when the patient uses the paretic eye for fixation than when the patient fixates with the sound eye.

(4) Maximal innervation is required to move the eye into or toward the field of action of a paralyzed muscle. According to Hering's law, the deviation is maximal in this gaze position.

1.08

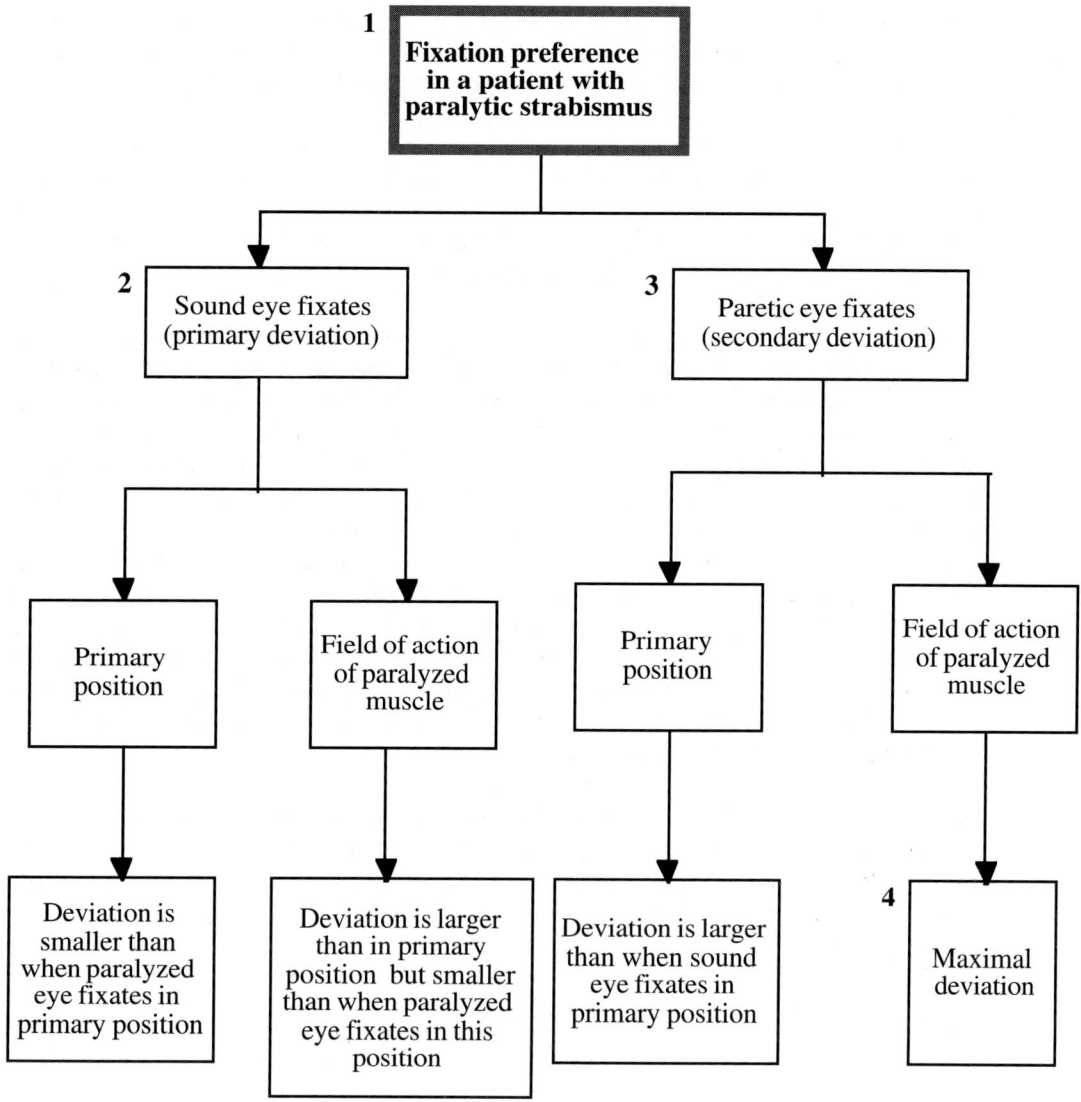

1.09   **Evaluation of Monocular Movements (Ductions)**

(1) The state of ocular motility of each eye is tested separately while the fellow eye is covered. These movements are called *ductions*, in contrast to *versions*, which refer to the movement of both eyes together and into the same direction. During examination of the ductions the patient fixates on a muscle light or other fixation target that is held by the examiner in the eight positions corresponding to the principal field of action of each muscle or muscle group.[23 p.369; 56 p.18]

(2) Normal ductions rule out mechanical restriction of ocular motility but do not exclude the possibility of paresis of an extraocular muscle. In the presence of a paresis the eye may move normally into the paretic field of gaze because of maximal innervation of the paretic muscle. A paresis is more likely to be detected by testing the versions **(see 1.10)** than by examining the ductions.

(3) A brisk saccade can be observed readily by asking the patient to switch fixation abruptly from the field opposite into the diagnostic gaze position. For example, in a patient with limitation of *abduction* of the right eye, saccadic velocity in the right lateral rectus is measured by asking the patient to switch fixation abruptly from far left gaze to far right gaze. The speed of the saccade is estimated as brisk (normal) or "floating" (paralysis). Saccadic velocity is quantified with electrooculography (EOG), a method not readily available in an office environment. A brisk saccade may occur even in the presence of a mechanical restriction from scarring, etc. In such cases, the eye moves rapidly until the movement is suddenly blocked by the mechanical leash effect. A brisk saccade is associated with normal generated muscle force. The muscle force may be estimated with a forceps[23 p.257; 49,57 p.375] or measured with a strain gauge that stabilizes the eye during an attempted duction. The tug on the forceps indicates the muscle force generated during the duction movement.

(4) In a paralysis of long duration, the unopposed antagonistic muscle may lose its elasticity and contracture may result. In such cases there is a positive forced duction test result, a floating saccade, and a reduced tug on the stabilizing forceps during estimation of the generated muscle force.

1.09

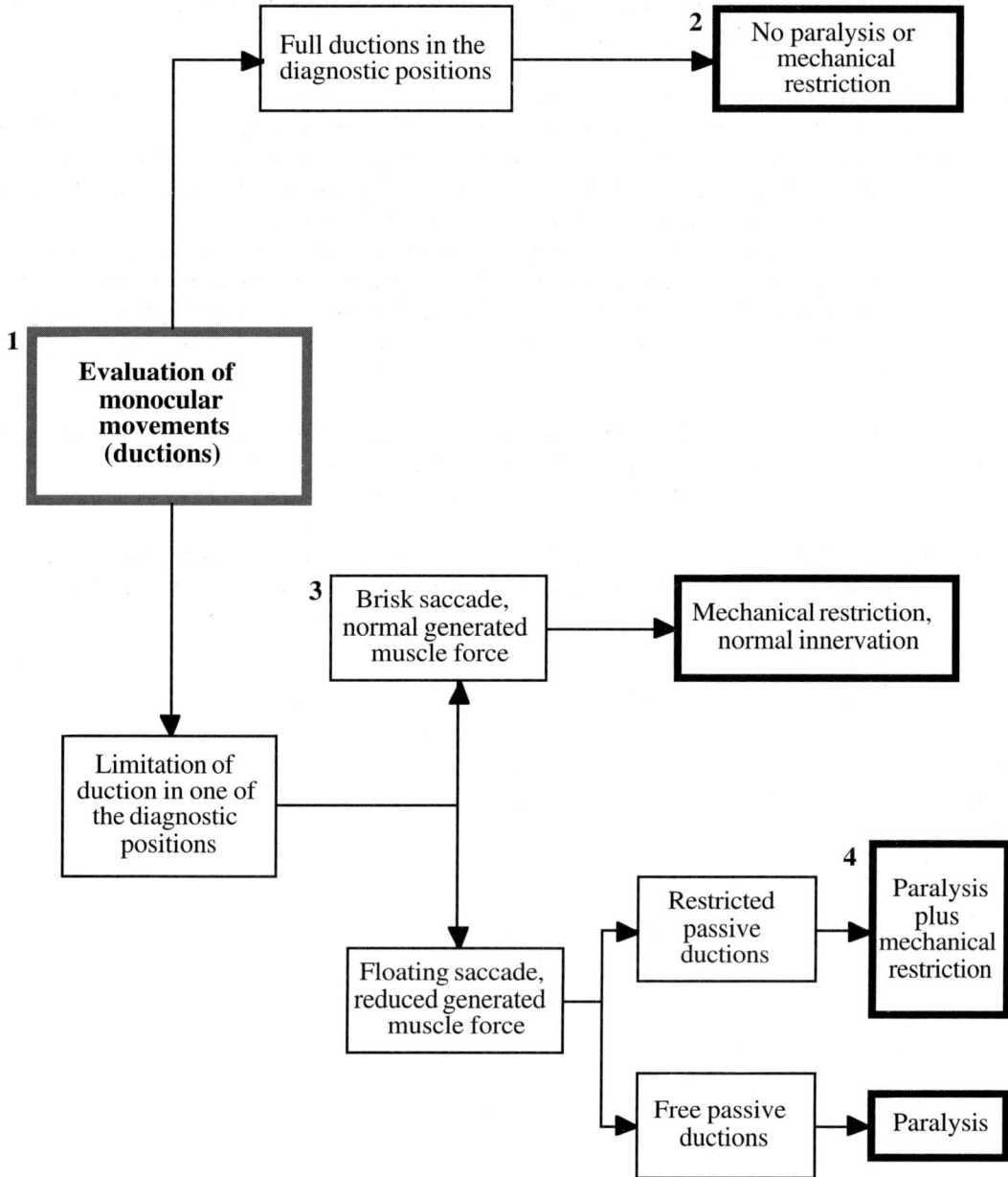

1.10   **Evaluation of Binocular Movements (Versions)**

(1) The ocular excursions are observed while both eyes are open and follow a fixation target, usually a hand light, into peripheral gaze positions (diagnostic positions of gaze). There are nine diagnostic positions in which ocular motility should be evaluated. Each position corresponds to the primary action of one muscle in each eye (yoke muscles).[23 p.373; 56 p.18] In primary position multiple muscles are involved in maintaining the eye in that position.

(2) During examination of the versions, the examiner must note whether both eyes move fully and simultaneously or whether there is limitation or excessive movement of the nonfixating eye in a particular gaze position. Overaction of a muscle is usually the result of underaction from paralysis, paresis, or mechanical restriction of its yoke in the fellow eye (secondary deviation) and occurs because maximal innervation flows to the paretic muscle(s) of the fixating eye. According to Hering's law[57 p.367] the same innervation flows to the yoke muscle in the fellow eye, where it causes apparent overaction of that muscle. Less frequently, apparent overaction is primary in nature—no weakness of the yoke muscle can be identified.

(3) Examination of the lateroversions may show that in certain conditions the eyes do not move in the same plane and that there is upshoot or downshoot of the adducted eye or abducted eye **(see 2.17, 2.18, 2.19, and 2.20).**

(4) Excursions of the eyes straight up or down from the primary position are almost exclusively accomplished by the vertical rectus muscles. The contribution of the oblique muscles to these eye movements is negligible.

1.10

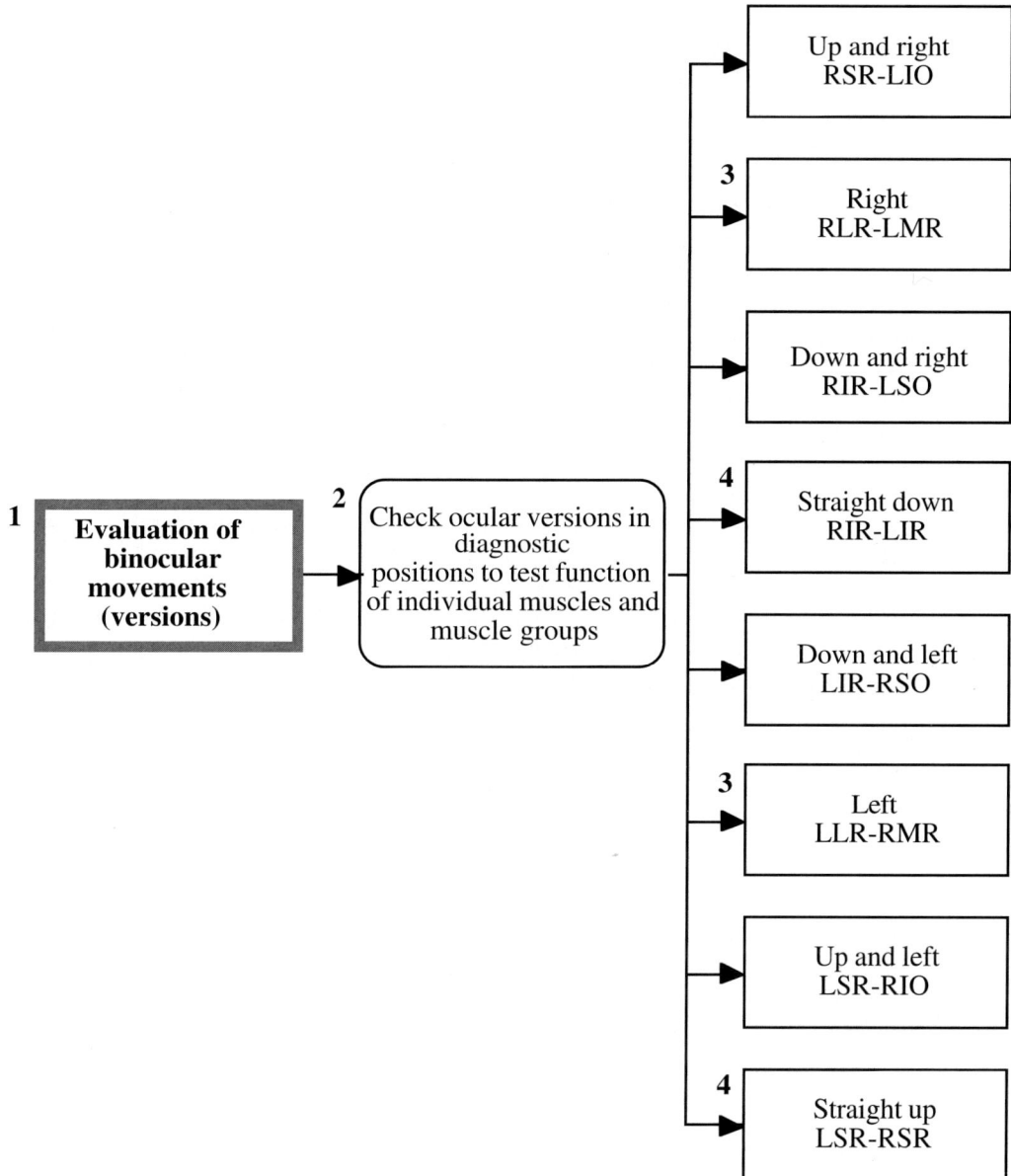

1.11   Uniiaterally Reduced Vision Associated With Orthotropia

(1) A functional (reversible) amblyopia may be superimposed on structural defects such as anomalies of the fundus or optic nerve that cause the initial reduction of visual acuity. Bangerter[2] coined the term *relative amblyopia* for that part of the visual acuity defect that may be reversed by occlusion treatment; it has been shown that improvement is possible in several conditions,[34] including abnormalities of the optic nerve[33] and amblyopia associated with juvenile glaucoma.[35]

(2) The exact amblyopiogenic degree of anisometropia is not known. Many authors believe that a spherical equivalent of 1.50 diopters or more is significant, although there are patients with higher degrees of anisometropia in whom amblyopia does not develop and some patients with less anisometropia who have anisometropic amblyopia. In doubtful cases it is best to prescribe the full anisometropic refractive error difference, which is always well tolerated by children. It is necessary to reduce the *spherical* correction equally when a spherical reduction becomes necessary, that is, to enhance tolerance of glasses, while maintaining the beneficial effect of anisometropic correction.

(3) When anisometropic amblyopia is suspected, the examiner should always try spectacles for the patient before occlusion therapy is considered. Visual acuity frequently improves after the glasses have been worn for a few weeks although no improvement was noted when the corrective lenses were first placed in the trial frame. This rule follows the concept that only one therapeutic modality at a time should be introduced.

(4) If visual acuity remains reduced despite proper spectacle correction of the refractive error, occlusion therapy for the amblyopia should be instituted **(see 2.03).** Anisometropic amblyopia is often associated with microtropia "with identity."[57] p.309

(5) Microtropia may occur in a primary or, more frequently, in a secondary form, that is, as an end stage of surgical treatment of essential infantile esotropia **(see 2.11)** or in association with anisometropic amblyopia.

(6) **See 2.01.**

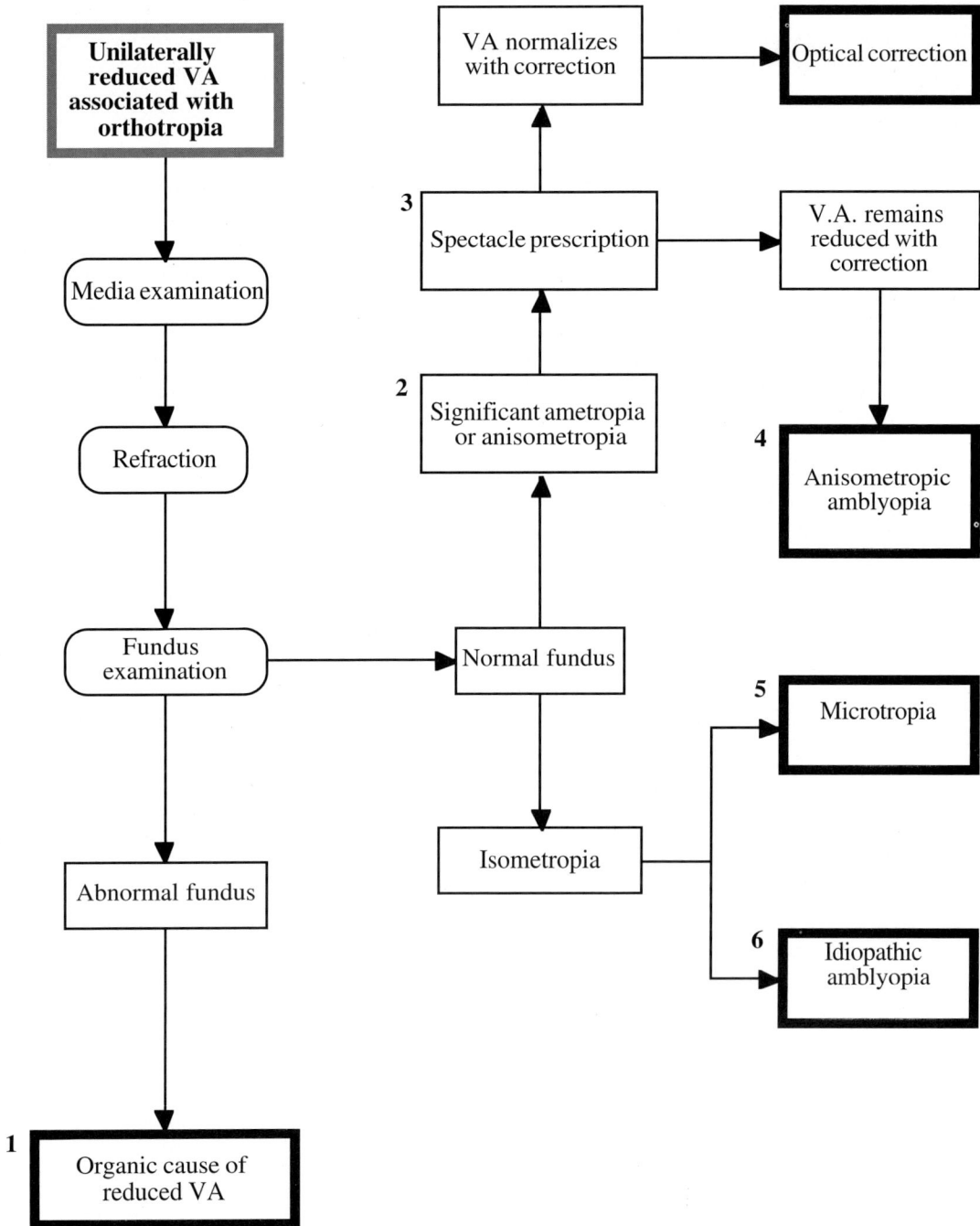

1.11

Unilaterally reduced VA associated with orthotropia

Media examination

Refraction

Fundus examination

Abnormal fundus

1 Organic cause of reduced VA

Normal fundus

Isometropia

2 Significant ametropia or anisometropia

3 Spectacle prescription

VA normalizes with correction

Optical correction

V.A. remains reduced with correction

4 Anisometropic amblyopia

5 Microtropia

6 Idiopathic amblyopia

1.12   Unilateral Decrease of Visual Acuity Associated With Heterotropia

(1-4) See comments on previous figure.

(5) **See 2.02.**

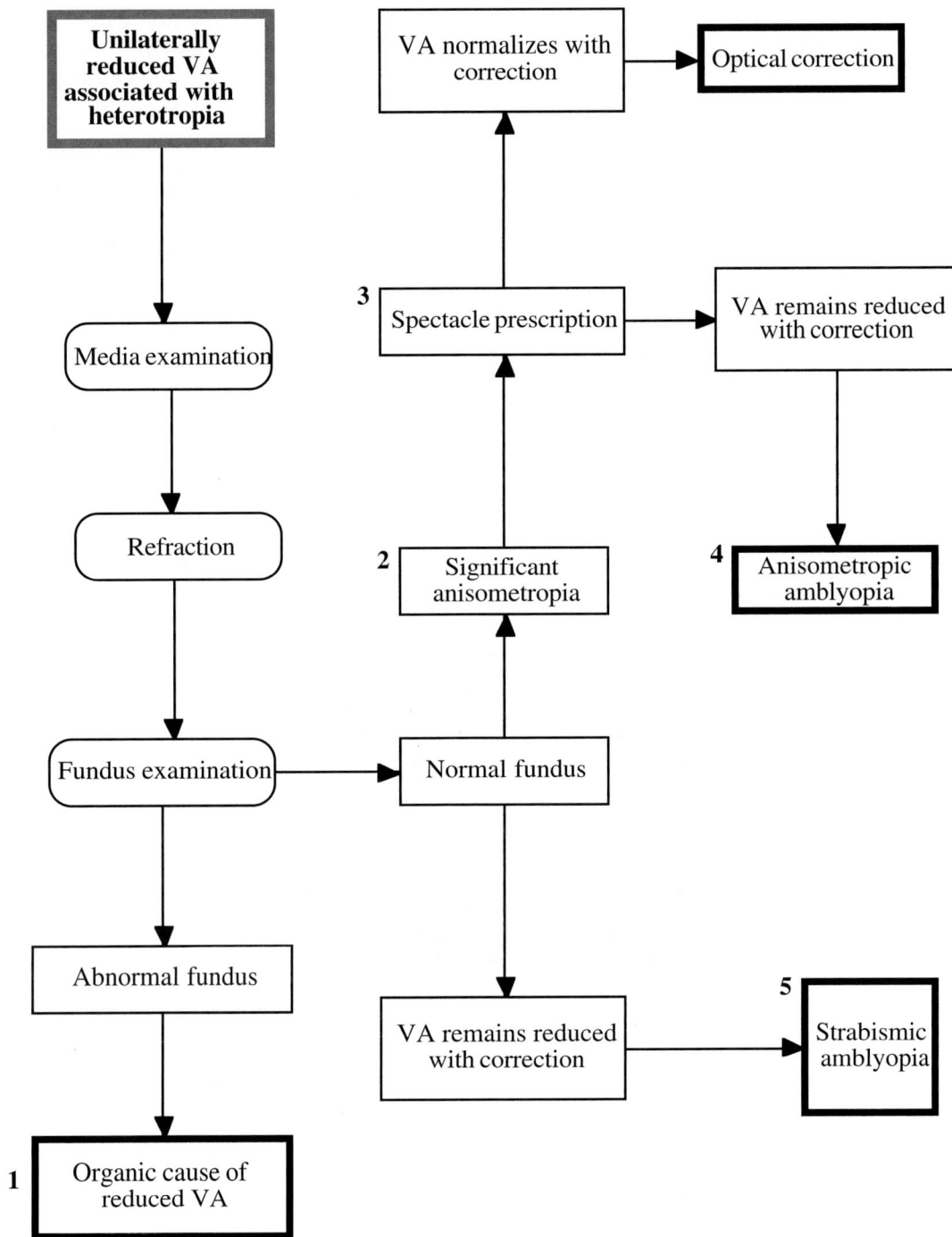

1.12

```
┌─────────────────┐
│  Unilaterally   │          ┌──────────────────┐         ┌──────────────────────┐
│  reduced VA     │          │ VA normalizes with│────────▶│  Optical correction  │
│  associated with│          │    correction     │         └──────────────────────┘
│  heterotropia   │          └──────────────────┘
└─────────────────┘                   ▲
        │                             │
        ▼                   3 ┌──────────────────┐         ┌──────────────────────┐
┌─────────────────┐           │ Spectacle        │────────▶│ VA remains reduced   │
│ Media examination│          │ prescription     │         │   with correction    │
└─────────────────┘           └──────────────────┘         └──────────────────────┘
        │                             ▲                                │
        ▼                   2 ┌──────────────────┐      4  ┌──────────────────────┐
┌─────────────────┐           │ Significant      │         │  Anisometropic       │
│   Refraction    │           │ anisometropia    │         │  amblyopia           │
└─────────────────┘           └──────────────────┘         └──────────────────────┘
        │                             ▲
        ▼                             │
┌─────────────────┐           ┌──────────────────┐
│ Fundus          │──────────▶│  Normal fundus   │
│ examination     │           └──────────────────┘
└─────────────────┘                   │
        │                             ▼
        ▼                   ┌──────────────────┐      5  ┌──────────────────────┐
┌─────────────────┐         │ VA remains reduced│────────▶│  Strabismic          │
│ Abnormal fundus │         │   with correction │         │  amblyopia           │
└─────────────────┘         └──────────────────┘         └──────────────────────┘
        │
        ▼
   1 ┌─────────────────┐
     │ Organic cause of│
     │ reduced VA      │
     └─────────────────┘
```

1.13   Decentered Corneal Light Reflex

(1) A decentered corneal light reflex in one or both eyes of a patient who is fixating on a point light source held directly in front of him or her may indicate that the visual axis of one eye is not aligned with the fixation target; when this occurs a manifest strabismus is present. Many tests for strabismus, for instance the Hirschberg and Krimsky tests, depend on the examiner's judgment of the position of the light reflection. However, there are other nonstrabismic causes for a decentered light reflex that must be considered for correct interpretation of this finding.

(2) On covering the fixating eye, the eye with the decentered reflex has made a corrective movement to take up fixation. Depending on the direction of this movement the patient has an esotropia, exotropia, right or left hypertropia or hypotropia.[56 p.38]

(3) The angle kappa is defined as the angle between the visual line (which connects the point of fixation with the nodal points and the fovea) and the pupillary axis (which is a line through the center of the pupil perpendicular to the cornea). A positive angle kappa (displacement toward the nose) of up at 5° is physiologic. A positive angle kappa may hide a small angle esotropia or cause pseudoexotropia, whereas a negative angle may simulate esotropia or hide exotropia.[56 p.32]

(4) Approximately 44% of patients with strabismic amblyopia have eccentric fixation, which may cause the light reflex in the amblyopic eye to become decentered.[59] For instance, in nasal peripheral eccentric fixation the light reflex is displaced temporally. In patients with parafoveolar or paramacular fixation, the displacement of the light reflex may be too minute to be detected by the examiner. In such cases the diagnosis of eccentric fixation can only be made with the Visuscope or an ophthalmoscope with a fixation target that can be projected on the fundus. The patient fixates this target while the sound eye is occluded. The examiner notes the position of the fixation target on the patient's fundus.[57 p.219]

(5) A large positive angle kappa results from temporal dragging of the macula in cases of retinopathy of prematurity (ectopic macula) when this eye is used for fixation. Such patients have pseudoexotropia. Visual acuity in such eyes is usually reduced but may remain normal or near normal despite the retinal distortion. A vertical angle kappa occurs infrequently and may be caused by scar formation (*toxocara canis* infection) with vertical dragging of the macula.

(6) Corectopia (decentered pupil) or coloboma of the iris may confuse the examiner regarding correct interpretation of the position of the light reflex.

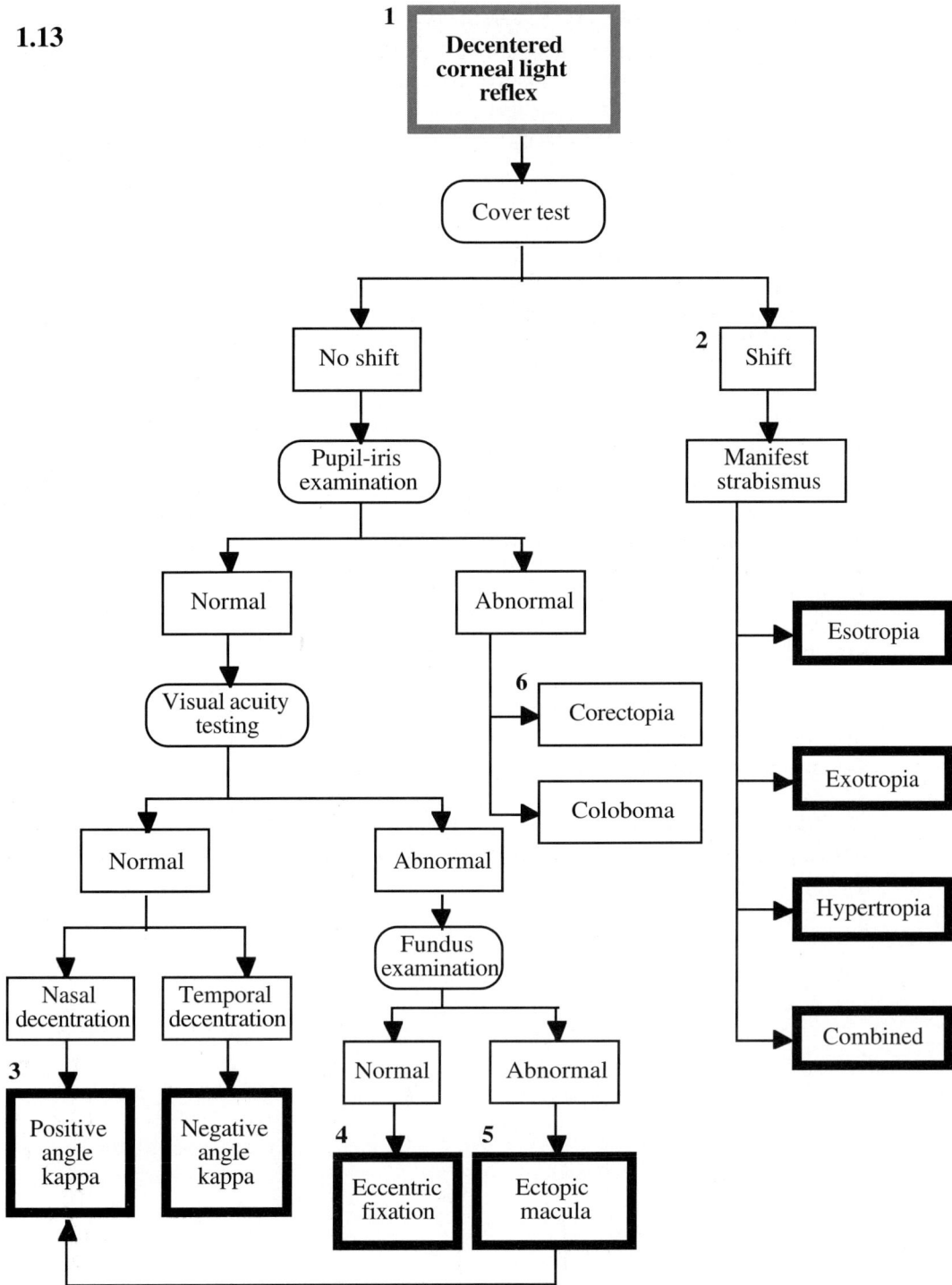

1.13

1

Decentered corneal light reflex

Cover test

No shift

2 Shift

Pupil-iris examination

Manifest strabismus

Normal

Abnormal

6 Corectopia

Coloboma

Esotropia

Exotropia

Hypertropia

Combined

Visual acuity testing

Normal

Abnormal

Nasal decentration

Temporal decentration

Fundus examination

Normal

Abnormal

3 Positive angle kappa

Negative angle kappa

4 Eccentric fixation

5 Ectopic macula

1.14   Strabismus: Generic Classification

(1) A generic classification of strabismus accommodates all the different clinical forms. For the beginner it is useful to approach an unknown ocular motility problem by answering the questions listed in Boxes 2 to 5. The boxes in the right portion of the flowchart list various entry points from which further leads can be obtained.

(2) The direction of a deviation should always be assessed in reference to the patient's head posture. For instance, in a V pattern strabismus the patient may have an exotropia when the chin is depressed and an esotropia with the chin elevated. Likewise, in Duane syndrome type III of the right eye, an exotropia may be present with the head turned to the right and an esotropia with a head turn to the left.

(3) Whether a strabismus is latent, intermittent, or manifest is determined with the cover test.[56 p.38] **(see 1.15 and 1.16).**

(4) To determine comitancy (similarity of angle of deviation in all positions of gaze), the angle of strabismus is measured in the diagnostic positions of gaze. In incomitant strabismus not only the magnitude of the angle may change in different gaze positions but the direction of the strabismus may also reverse. For instance, a patient with a right orbital floor fracture may have a right hypotropia in upward gaze and a right hypertropia in downward gaze.[23 p.516]

(5) Strong fixation preference for one eye (unilateral strabismus) may imply poor(er) visual acuity in the nonpreferred eye. Alternating fixation implies equal visual acuity in each eye.

(6) Whether limitation of a duction movement is caused by paralysis of an extraocular muscle or mechanical restriction requires careful evaluation and is further discussed at **1.30.**

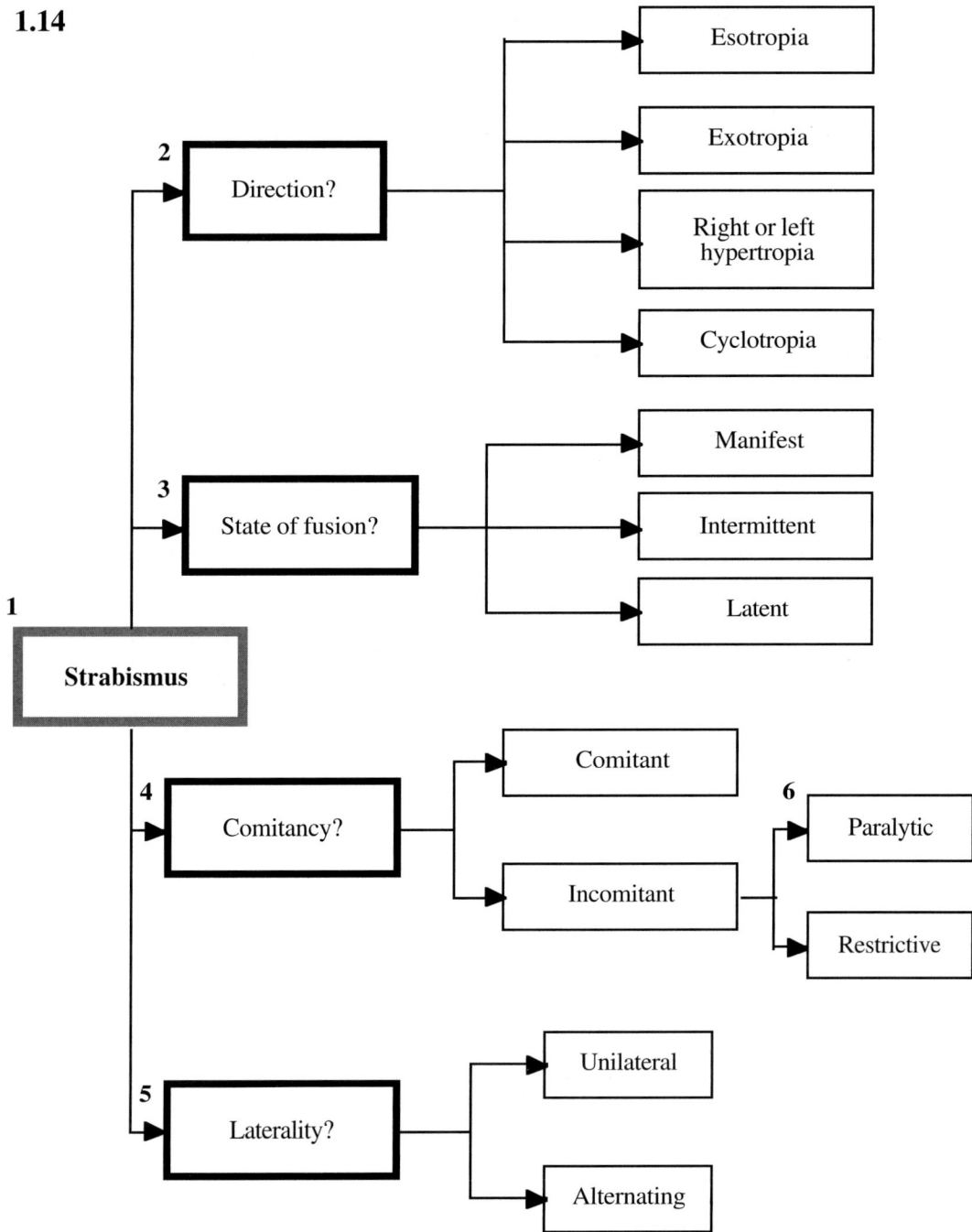

1.14

```
                                                    ┌─────────────────┐
                                                ┌──►│    Esotropia    │
                                                │   └─────────────────┘
                                                │   ┌─────────────────┐
                                                ├──►│    Exotropia    │
        ┌──────────────┐                        │   └─────────────────┘
   2    │              │                        │   ┌─────────────────┐
     ──►│  Direction?  │────────────────────────┼──►│  Right or left  │
        │              │                        │   │   hypertropia   │
        └──────────────┘                        │   └─────────────────┘
                                                │   ┌─────────────────┐
                                                └──►│   Cyclotropia   │
                                                    └─────────────────┘

                                                    ┌─────────────────┐
                                                ┌──►│    Manifest     │
        ┌──────────────┐                        │   └─────────────────┘
   3    │              │                        │   ┌─────────────────┐
     ──►│State of      │────────────────────────┼──►│  Intermittent   │
        │  fusion?     │                        │   └─────────────────┘
        └──────────────┘                        │   ┌─────────────────┐
                                                └──►│     Latent      │
                                                    └─────────────────┘
   1
   ┌──────────────┐
   │  Strabismus  │
   └──────────────┘
                                                    ┌─────────────────┐
                                                ┌──►│    Comitant     │
        ┌──────────────┐                        │   └─────────────────┘           6
   4    │              │                        │                          ┌──►┌──────────┐
     ──►│  Comitancy?  │────────────────────────┤   ┌─────────────────┐    │   │Paralytic │
        │              │                        └──►│   Incomitant    │────┤   └──────────┘
        └──────────────┘                            └─────────────────┘    │   ┌──────────┐
                                                                           └──►│Restrictive│
                                                                               └──────────┘

                                                    ┌─────────────────┐
                                                ┌──►│   Unilateral    │
        ┌──────────────┐                        │   └─────────────────┘
   5    │              │                        │   ┌─────────────────┐
     ──►│  Laterality? │────────────────────────┴──►│   Alternating   │
        │              │                            └─────────────────┘
        └──────────────┘
```

1.15   Is Latent Strabismus Present?

(1) The cover-uncover test detects ocular deviations that are controlled by the motor fusion mechanism that keeps the eyes aligned. Such latent deviations are absent when both eyes are open. By covering either eye, fusion is disrupted and one eye may turn in, out, up, or down. On removal of the cover, a corrective eye movement of the just uncovered eye occurs as a result of fusional vergence. The direction of this movement is noted by the examiner. Occasionally, the uncovered eye fails to make this corrective movement; in such cases, the latent deviation has become manifest (intermittent heterotropia). A negative cover test result, although it denotes motor fusion, does not justify the conclusion that normal sensory fusion is also present. In the presence of microtropia "with identity," the cover test result is negative but the 4 prism diopter base-out test reveals a foveal suppression scotoma in one eye that generally is also amblyopic **(see 2.11).**[27]

(2) A small degree of heterophoria occurs in most normal subjects and must be considered physiologic. For this reason, the condition of *orthophoria* must be considered as an ideal state of ocular alignment, rarely achieved even in the normal population. The term *orthotropia* is clinically more meaningful because it denotes an absence of a manifest deviation.[57 p.129]

(3) Many cases of hyperphoria, especially those associated with essential infantile esotropia, are eventually identified as dissociated vertical deviation **(see 2.16).**

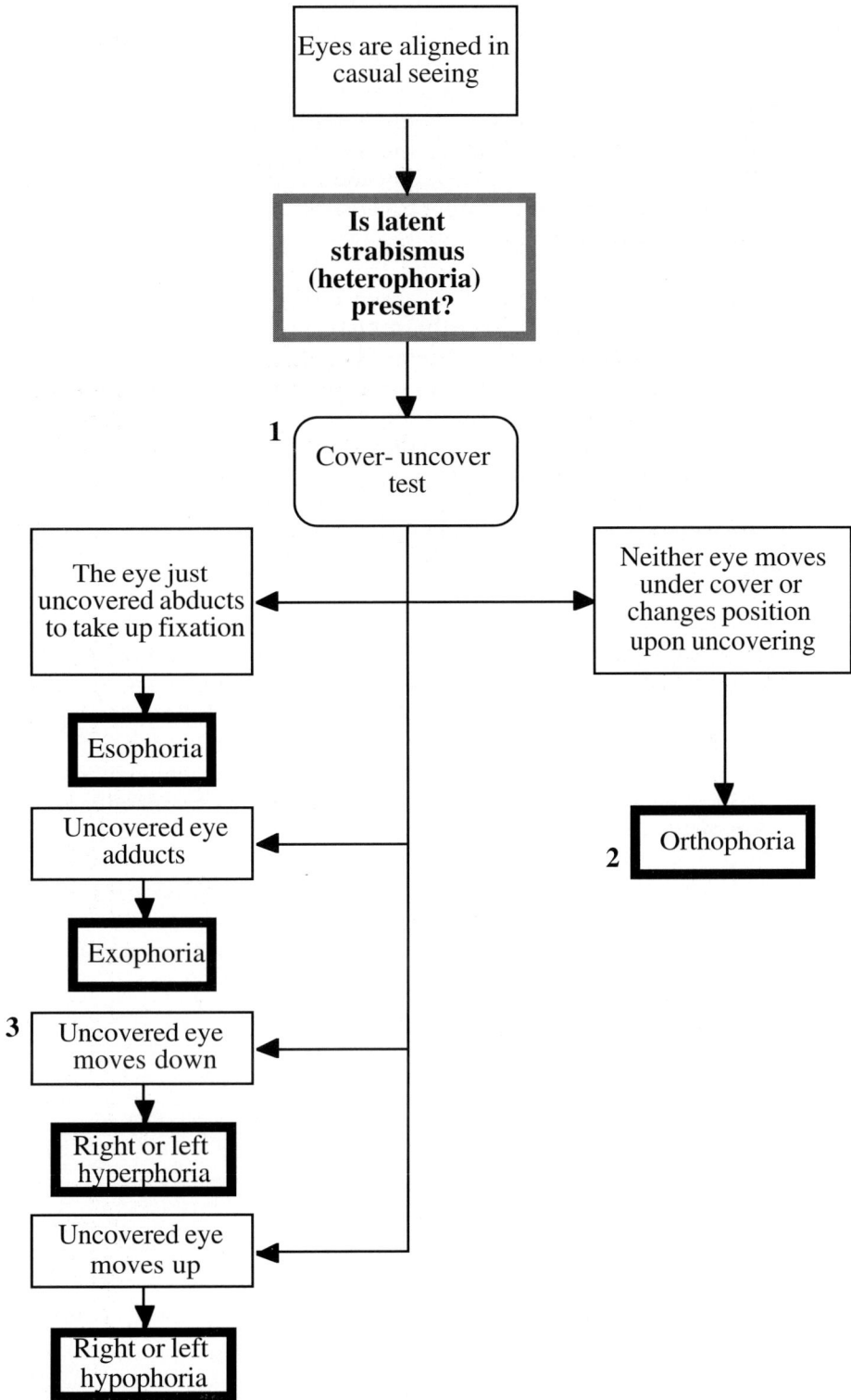

1.15

```
┌─────────────────────┐
│ Eyes are aligned in │
│    casual seeing    │
└─────────────────────┘
          │
          ▼
╔═════════════════════╗
║   **Is latent**     ║
║   **strabismus**    ║
║   **(heterophoria)**║
║   **present?**      ║
╚═════════════════════╝
          │
          ▼
   ╭─────────────────╮
 1 │  Cover- uncover │
   │      test       │
   ╰─────────────────╯
```

1 Cover- uncover test

The eye just uncovered abducts to take up fixation

Esophoria

Neither eye moves under cover or changes position upon uncovering

2 **Orthophoria**

Uncovered eye adducts

Exophoria

3 Uncovered eye moves down

Right or left hyperphoria

Uncovered eye moves up

Right or left hypophoria

1.16   **Is Manifest Strabismus Present?**

(1) The cover test is the most important qualitative test in the diagnosis of strabismus. It is simple, quick, and tells the examiner in a few seconds whether manifest strabismus is present and in which direction the nonfixating eye is turning. The patient must be able to maintain fixation on a visual object at 33 cm and 6 M fixation distance, which limits the use of this test to cooperative subjects. Deviations of 2^Δ or less may escape detection with this test. A fixation light is not recommended as a fixation target because accommodation is uncontrolled when the patient fixates on a light.

(2) Orthotropia is defined as absence of a manifest strabismus as determined with the cover test.[57 p.129] Orthotropia is present when both eyes are aligned at a particular viewing distance, under the influence of fusion, and with accommodation controlled. Orthotropia is confirmed by noting the absence of a refixation movement of either eye when the fellow eye is covered. Orthotropia is not synonymous with absence of an ocular motility problem because patients may be orthotropic at one fixation distance and heterotropic at another, or could have clinically significant degrees of heterophoria or a microtropia. Thus the cover test must always be used in conjunction with the cover-uncover test **(see 1.15)**.

(3) A negative cover test result does not automatically imply bifoveal fixation. A negative cover test result accompanied by reduced visual acuity in one eye strongly suggests the presence of microtropia **(see 2.11)** or of amblyopia with eccentric fixation **(see 2.01)**. A microtropia (esotropia or, less frequently, exotropia) may be present when the corrective movement of the deviating eye on covering the fixating eye is either absent or inconspicuously small.[27,36,57 p.309] Microtropia may occur as a desirable end stage of therapy of essential infantile esotropia,[60] be associated with anisometropic amblyopia or, less frequently, occur as a primary anomaly.

(4) A patient with amblyopia and eccentric fixation either has no corrective movement of the amblyopic eye when the sound eye is covered or this movement is so small that it may escape observation by the examiner.

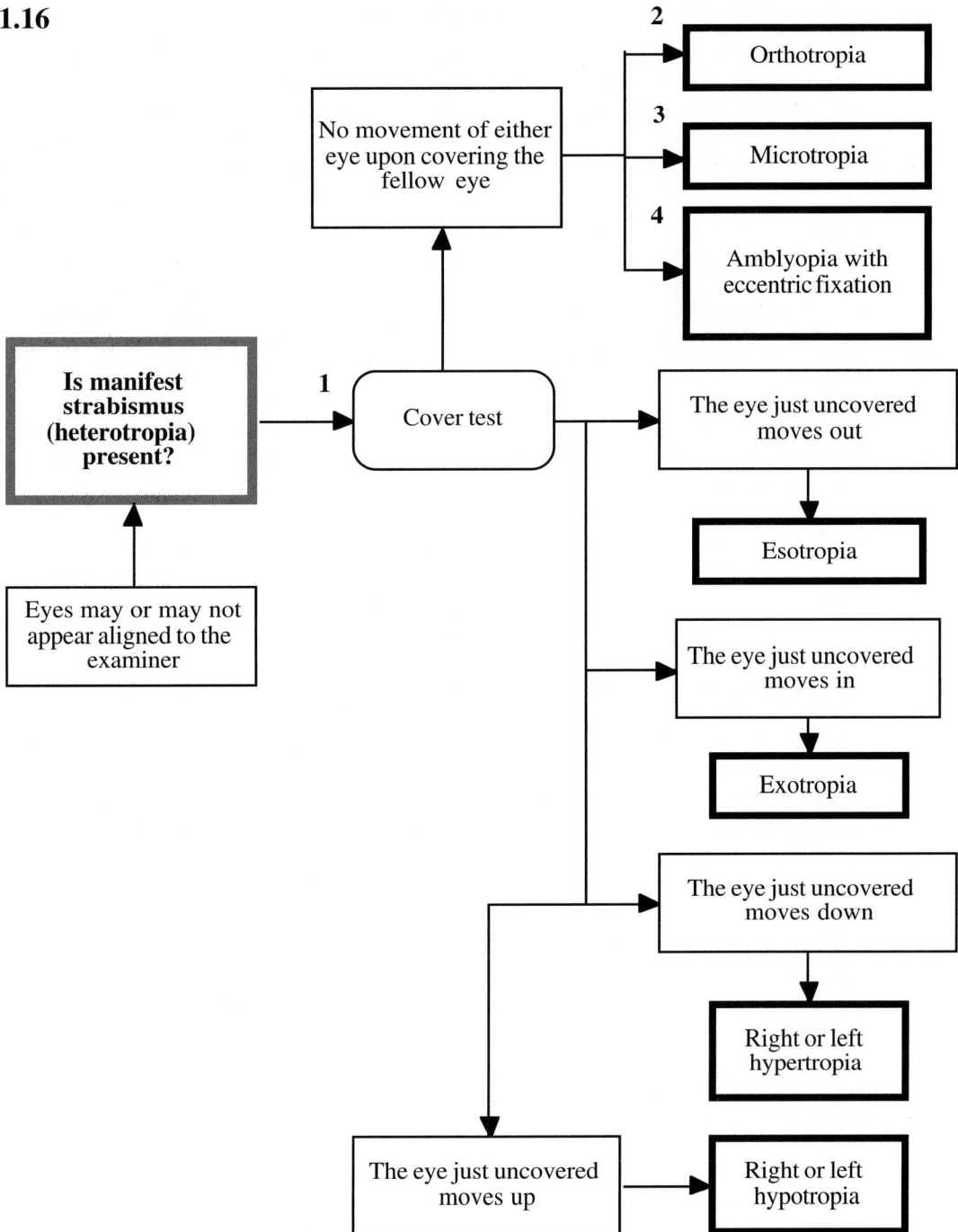

1.16

2 Orthotropia

No movement of either eye upon covering the fellow eye

3 Microtropia

4 Amblyopia with eccentric fixation

Is manifest strabismus (heterotropia) present?

1 Cover test

The eye just uncovered moves out

Esotropia

The eye just uncovered moves in

Exotropia

Eyes may or may not appear aligned to the examiner

The eye just uncovered moves down

Right or left hypertropia

The eye just uncovered moves up

Right or left hypotropia

1.17   Essential Infantile Esotropia: Etiology

*Essential infantile esotropia** is defined as a manifest esodeviation with an onset between birth and 6 months of age in an otherwise neurologically normal infant. It is frequently associated with rather typical clinical characteristics and is not eliminated by correction of hypermetropia.[57, p.293] This condition must be distinguished from other forms of esotropia with an onset at birth or shortly thereafter, such as the nystagmus compensation syndrome **(see 2.33)**, refractive accommodative esotropia **(see 2.07)**, Duane syndrome type I **(see 2.50)**, congenital sixth nerve palsy, and Möbius syndrome. The prefix "essential" emphasizes the obscure etiology of this condition. We favor a hypothesis according to which various strabismogenic forces impinge on a sensorially immature and therefore fragile visual system in the presence of a congenitally deficient or underdeveloped motor fusion reflex.[22; 23 p.391; 57 p.294]

(1) During the first 4 months of life the visual system is still immature. Ocular alignment is unstable and esodeviations and exodeviations occur frequently in a normal population.[1,39]

(2) Several known, and perhaps, some unknown strabismogenic forces impinge on the immature visual system to counteract ocular alignment in developing infants.

(3) When delayed maturation or a congenitally defective motor fusion mechanism interferes with a corrective fusional divergence response to nasal retinal disparity (esodeviation), induced by the esotropogenic factors listed under (2), esotropia ensues.

(4) Currently it is not clear what differences exist in terms of etiology between essential infantile esotropia with and without manifest latent nystagmus. In our experience, manifest latent nystagmus occurs in approximately 20% of children with essential infantile esotropia.

(5) Esotropia disrupts normal binocular vision. This in turn interferes with maturation of the OKN response. A nasotemporal pursuit defect that is present in all normal infants during the first few months of life persists in the patient with esotropia.[13]

(6) A normal fusional vergence response, on the other hand, maintains ocular alignment despite an immature sensory visual system and various strabismogenic factors.

(7) OKN responses become symmetric with maturation in the presence of normal binocular vision.

---

*The term "essential infantile esotropia" can be used interchangeably with "congenital esotropia." Experts are describing the same condition but choose one term or the other based on their interpretation of the etiology and the importance of the deviation *not* being connatal.

1.17

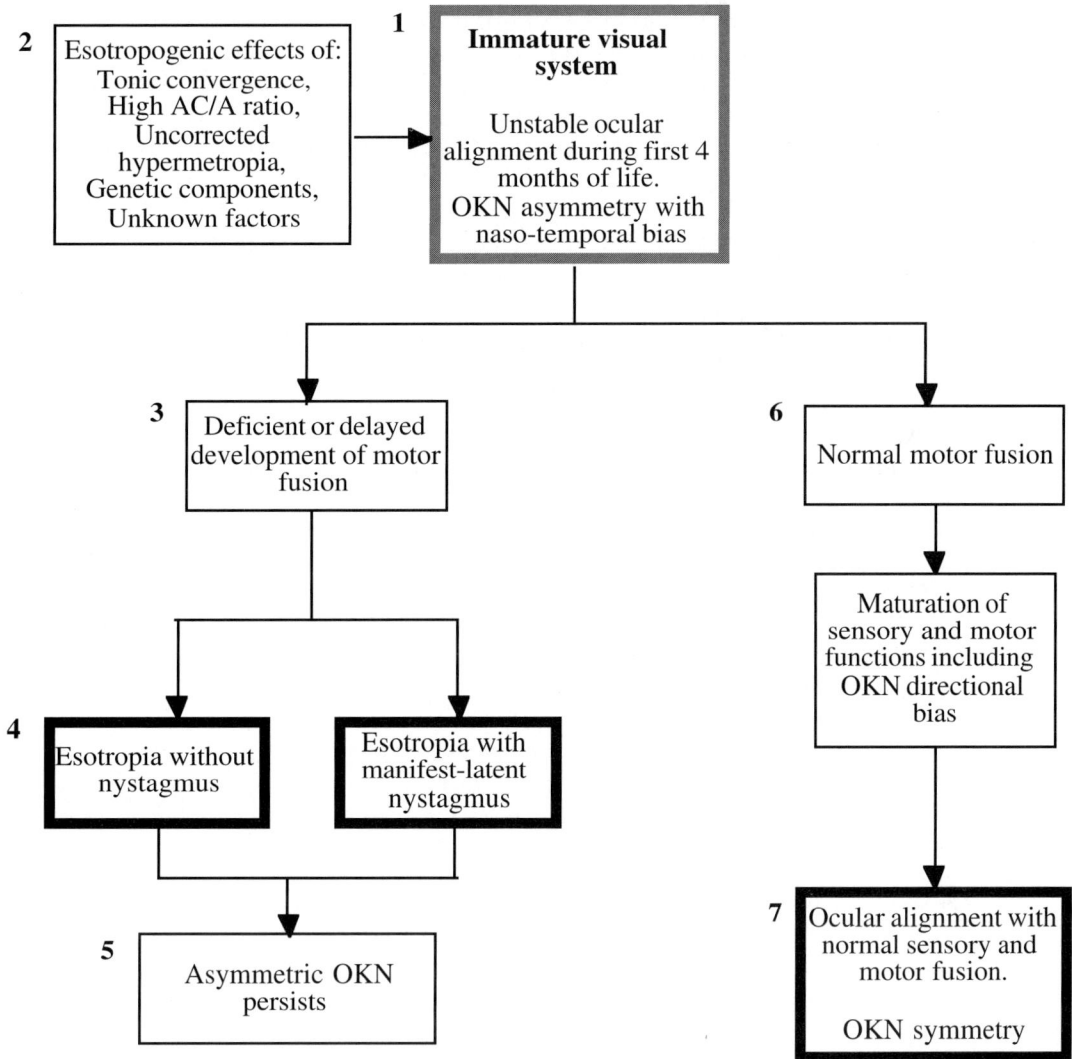

1.18   Esodeviation: Initial Decision Making

When examining a patient with esotropia several preliminary questions must be answered before the correct diagnosis can be made.

(1) Small differences in the angle of strabismus in different gaze positions are common and not inconsistent with the diagnosis of comitant strabismus. Essential infantile esotropia, refractive and nonrefractive accommodative esotropia, nonaccommodative convergence excess, and acute and cyclic esotropia are included in this group. In most instances gross incomitancy denotes a paralytic or restrictive type of strabismus.

(2) An esodeviation confirmed by a reliable observer before the age of 6 months narrows the diagnosis to only a few possibilities **(see 1.20).**

(3) Unlike exodeviations, which are frequently intermittent or latent, most esodeviations are manifest.

(4) An esodeviation is frequently greater at near than at distance fixation because of the effect of accommodative and proximal convergence **(see 2.07 and 2.08).**

(5) In all cases of esotropia the refractive error must be determined after complete cycloplegia. For management of refractive accommodative esotropia, **see 2.07.**

(6) In patients with an esotropia greater at near than at distance fixation, the effect of the AC/A ratio is determined with the gradient method[57 p.89] **(see 2.08).**

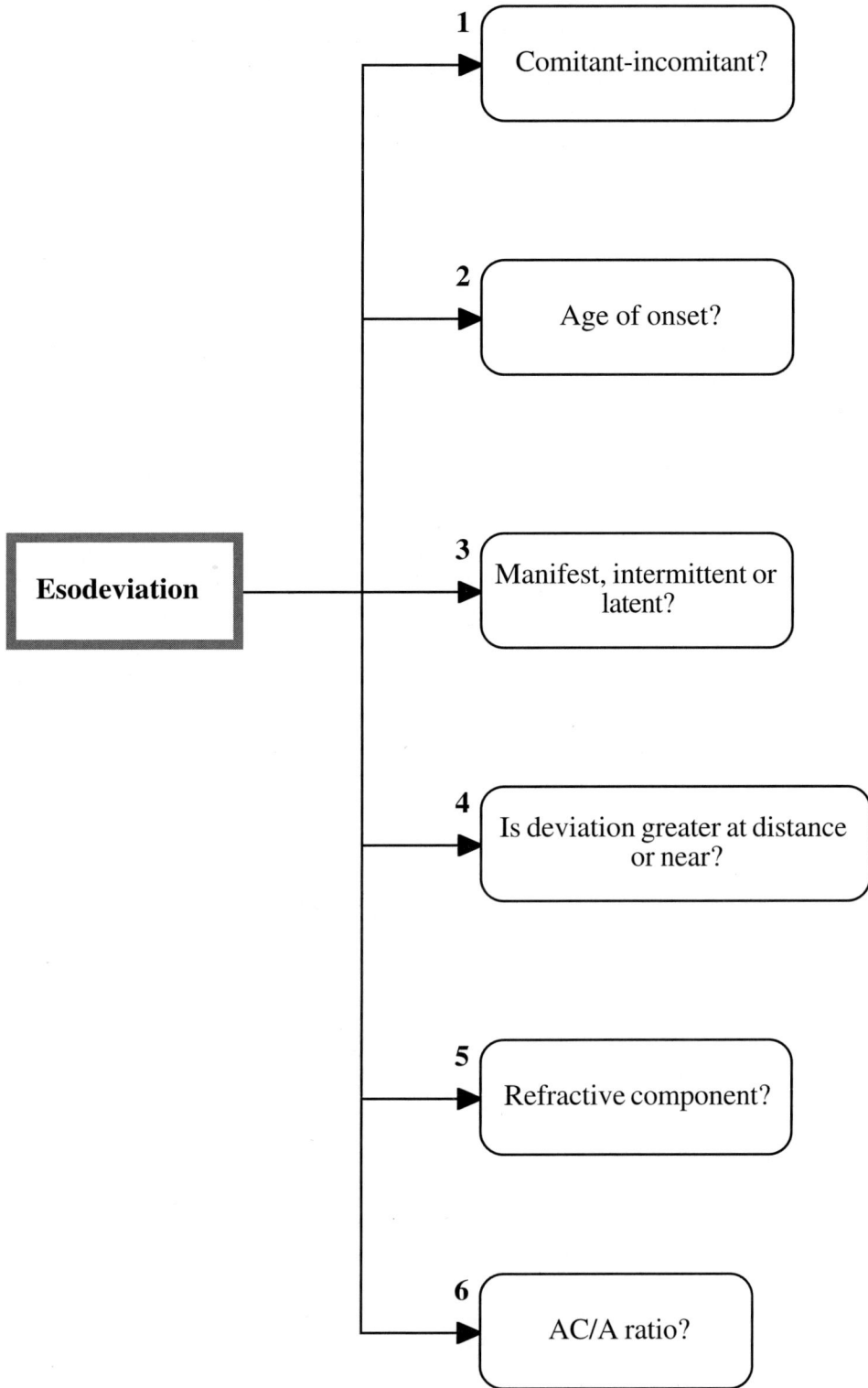

1.18

Esodeviation

1 Comitant-incomitant?

2 Age of onset?

3 Manifest, intermittent or latent?

4 Is deviation greater at distance or near?

5 Refractive component?

6 AC/A ratio?

1.19   Esotropia According to the State of Comitance

(1) The determination of whether an ocular deviation is comitant or incomitant should be made at the beginning of a motility analysis. For a preliminary overview, the patient is asked to maintain fixation on a muscle light, or in the case of a young child, a toy, presented to the patient in the diagnostic positions of gaze. The examiner notes whether ductions are full or whether there is lag of muscle action in any gaze position. This is followed by measurement of the ocular deviation with the prism and cover test at distance and near fixation in the primary position. These measurements are also done with the eyes in dextroversion and levoversion and in 30° elevation and depression, if a V or A pattern is suspected **(see 2.23 and 2.24).**

(2) Accommodative and nonaccommodative esotropia are rather loosely used terms that indicate only that excessive accommodative convergence, whether from uncorrected hypermetropia or from a high AC/A ratio, contributes to the etiology of an esodeviation.

(3) The forced duction test is of important diagnostic value in determining whether strabismus is of purely innervational or of mechanical-restrictive origin. Absence or weakness of abduction in the presence of an esodeviation with unrestricted passive ductions inculpates the ipsilateral abducens nerve. However, in paralyses of longer standing, the unopposed antagonist, the ipsilateral medial rectus muscle, may become tight and secondary contracture may develop. This causes the forced duction test result to become positive in the presence of a sixth nerve palsy *(dotted arrow).*

(4) A positive forced duction test result in the absence of a sixth nerve palsy indicates a mechanical obstacle other than secondary medial rectus muscle contracture that prevents the eye from being pulled into abduction. This is associated with a brisk saccade over a limited excursion **(see 1.30).**

(5) Refractive accommodative esotropia is defined as an esotropia that is caused by an uncorrected hypermetropic refractive error and that is fully corrected at near and distance fixation by prescription of the appropriate glasses or contact lenses.

(6) **See 1.17.**

(7) Nonaccommodative convergence excess is an increase of an esodeviation at near fixation of 15$^\Delta$ or more over the distance deviation in a patient with a normal AC/A ratio.[57] p.89 This increased near deviation is caused by excessive convergence from sources other than accommodation (tonic convergence?).

(8) Increased esotropia with accommodative effort at near when the refractive error is fully corrected occurs in patients with a high AC/A ratio.[57] p.89 **(see 1.21 and 2.07).**

(9) An esotropia is considered acquired when its onset occurs after the age of 6 months. Esotropia can result from a variety of causes.

(10) A residual esotropia that remains after correction of a full hypermetropic refractive error is referred to as partially accommodative.

(11) **See 2.33.**

(12) **See 2.10.**

(13) A rare but fascinating form of esotropia depends on a clock mechanism, usually regular and 48 hour: A 24-hour period of normal binocular vision is followed by 24 hours of manifest esotropia. Surgical treatment is based on the full amount of esotropia that occurs on the strabismic days and has been successful in restoring normal binocular functions.[21,57 p.414]

(14) Enlargement of the globe in high axial myopia may cause limitation of ocular motility.[12]

(15) **See 2.11.**

(16) Congenital fibrosis syndrome is characterized by limited elevation, chin-up position, and increasing esotropia on attempted up gaze. It is an autosomal dominant trait and is associated with ptosis.[23 p.518]

(17) **See 2.55.**

(18) **See 2.54.**

(19) **See 2.50.**

1.19

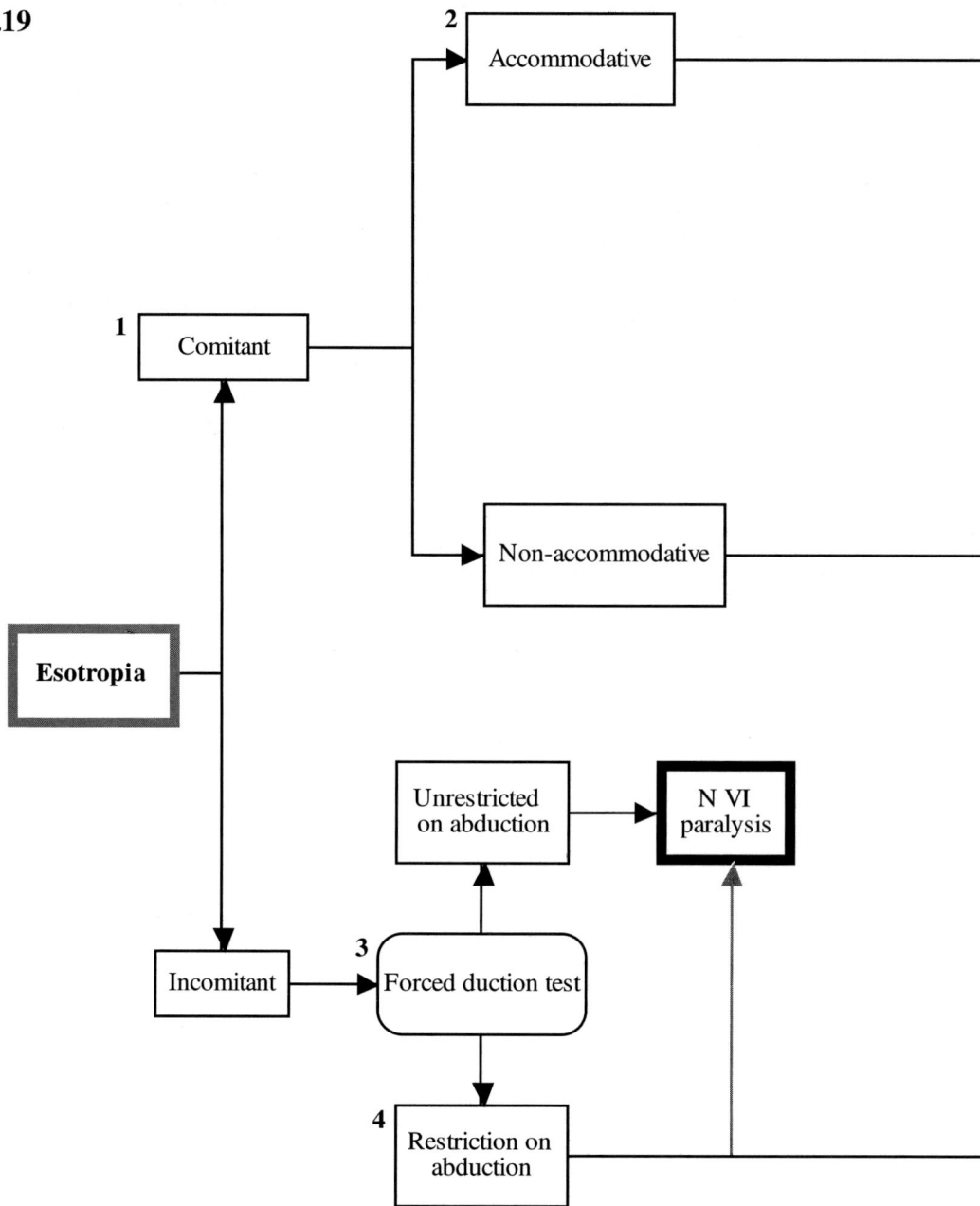

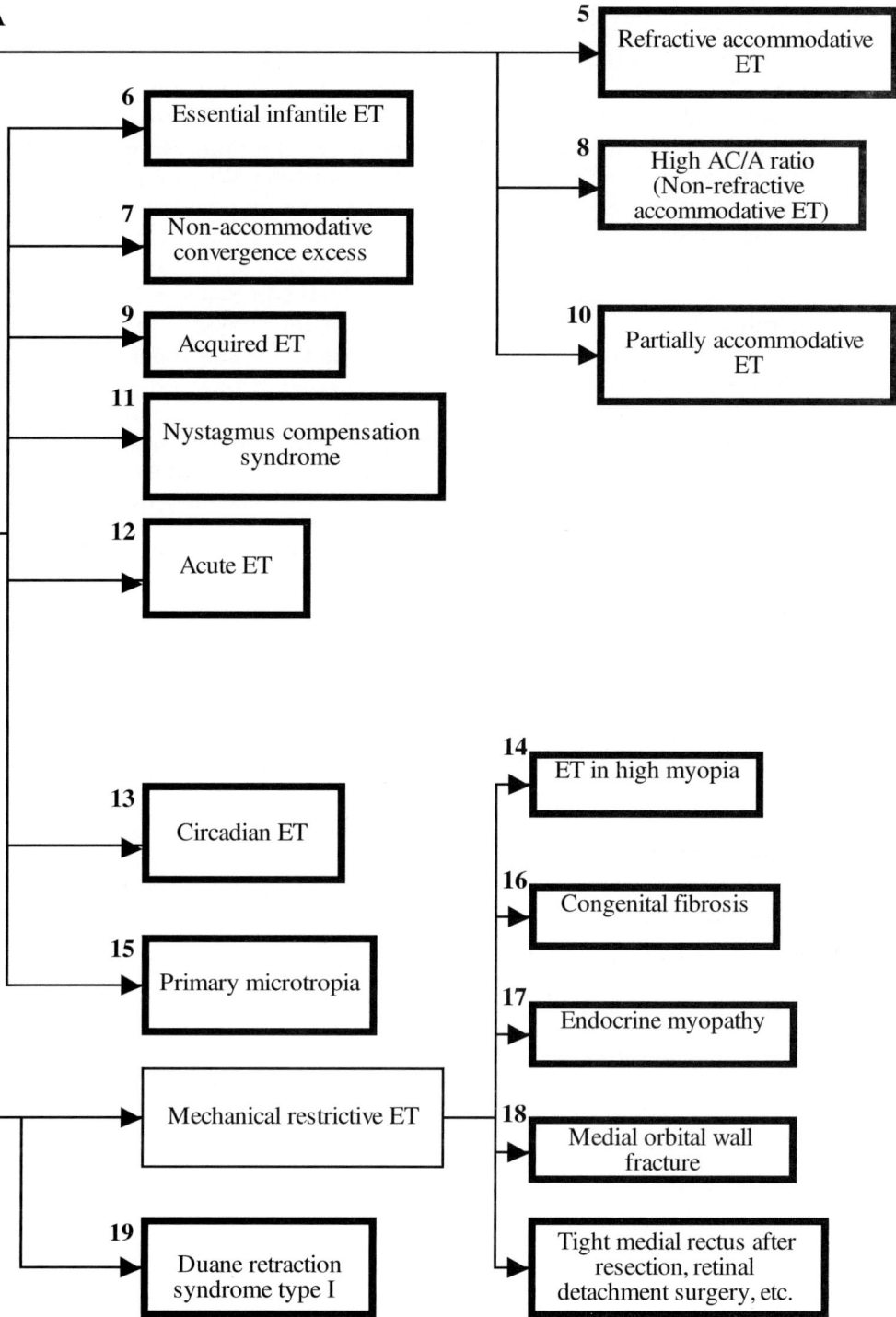

1.19 A

5 Refractive accommodative ET

6 Essential infantile ET

7 Non-accommodative convergence excess

8 High AC/A ratio (Non-refractive accommodative ET)

9 Acquired ET

10 Partially accommodative ET

11 Nystagmus compensation syndrome

12 Acute ET

13 Circadian ET

14 ET in high myopia

15 Primary microtropia

16 Congenital fibrosis

17 Endocrine myopathy

Mechanical restrictive ET

18 Medial orbital wall fracture

Tight medial rectus after resection, retinal detachment surgery, etc.

19 Duane retraction syndrome type I

1.20   Esotropia With Onset Before 6 Months of Age

(1) The question is often asked by primary care physicians and ophthalmologists alike: "When is an esodeviation in any infant significant and reason for referral?" Recent study of a large number of newborns has shown that in the first hours and days of life, two thirds of the neonates had intermittent exotropia.[1,39] None of these had a typical infantile (congenital) esotropia. When reexamined later, several patients had essential infantile esotropia. During the first 2 months of life the ocular alignment is unstable and biased toward exotropia. Between the second and fourth months of life, alignment becomes stable and stereopsis can be demonstrated with special tests. An esodeviation that persists after the fourth month of life in a neurologically normal infant without a significant hypermetropic refractive error is essential infantile esotropia and should be brought to the attention of a specialist.[23 p.391]

(2) Refractive accommodative esotropia usually occurs between the ages of 2 and 3 years. Occasionally, however, it occurs during the first 6 months of life and responds readily to prescription of the hypermetropic refractive error.[45]

(3) Nystagmus compensation (blockage) syndrome is an esotropia acquired in infancy; it is caused by a sustained convergence effort to decrease the intensity of manifest congenital nystagmus **(see 2.33).**

(4) An apparent limitation of abduction in an infant with esotropia is usually caused by crossed fixation or by manifest latent nystagmus with null point in adduction of the fixating eye. However, if this limitation persists after unilateral occlusion and with the doll's head maneuver, further study is indicated. Sixth nerve palsy in infants is often transient and without further sequelae.

(5) Bilateral abducens and facial paralysis is known as Möbius syndrome. Esotropia may be present, and atrophy of the distal part of the tongue is a characteristic feature.[23 p.519]

(6) **See 2.50.**

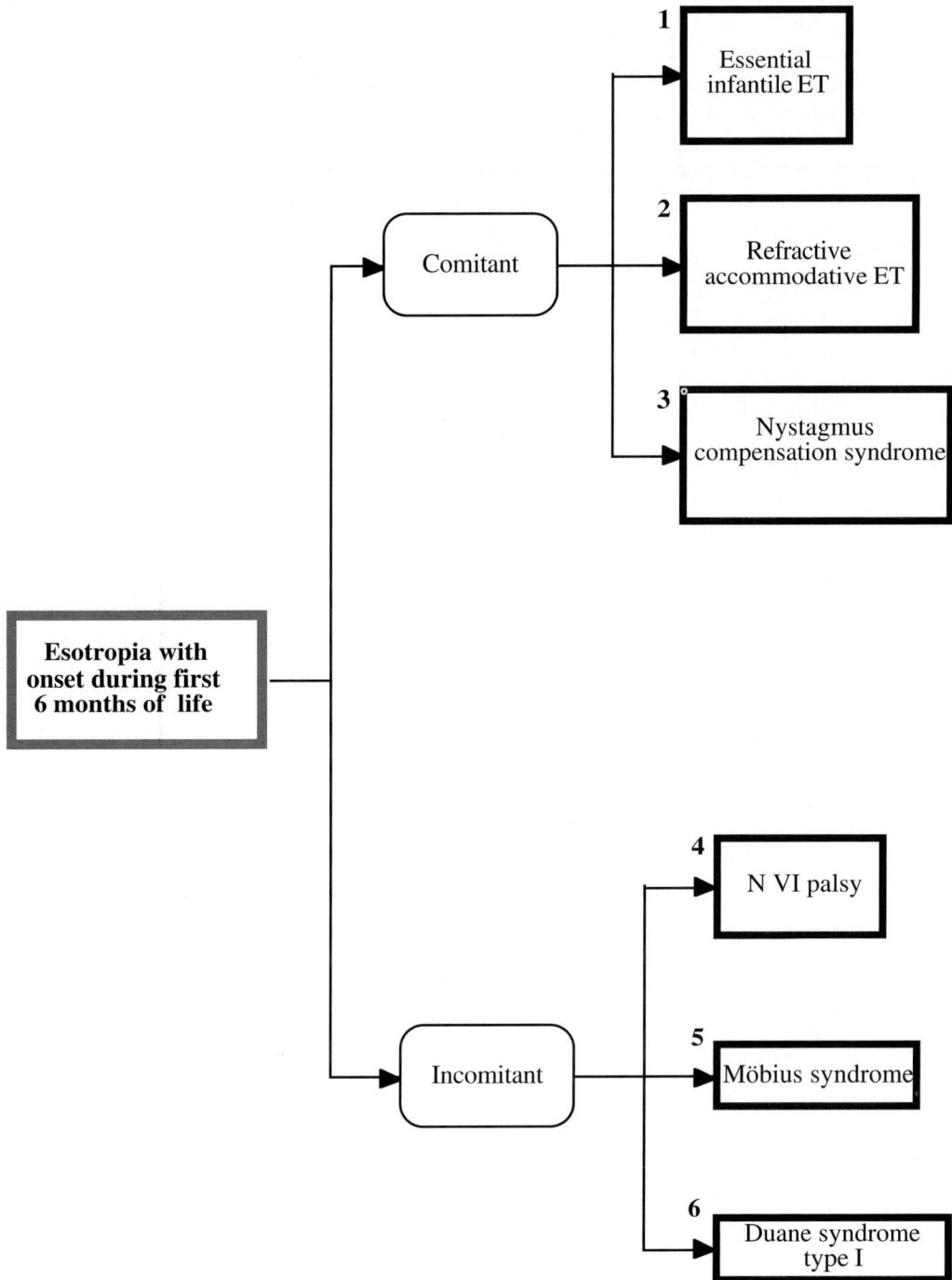

1.20

1 Essential infantile ET

2 Refractive accommodative ET

3 Nystagmus compensation syndrome

Comitant

Esotropia with onset during first 6 months of life

4 N VI palsy

5 Möbius syndrome

6 Duane syndrome type I

Incomitant

1.21   Esotropia According to Near/Distance Disparity

(1) Most forms of esotropia show a slight increase of the angle of strabismus at near fixation (33 cm) when this measurement is compared with the distance (6 M fixation distance) deviation. This is caused by a physiologic increase of convergence tonus at near fixation.

(2) *Any* esodeviation that is greater at distance than at near fixation should alert the examiner to search for neurologic causes. This finding is usually restricted to acquired esotropia and often occurs in paresis of the abducens nerve(s). In such cases, examination of ductions may show mild limitation of abduction in association with an increase of the deviation in lateroversion. Less frequently, divergence paralysis or paresis may be the cause. There is no limitation of abduction, and the angle of the esotropia is the same in primary position and lateral gaze.

(3) **See 2.08.**

(4) **See 2.08.**

(5) **See 2.45.**

(6) **See 2.47.**

1.21

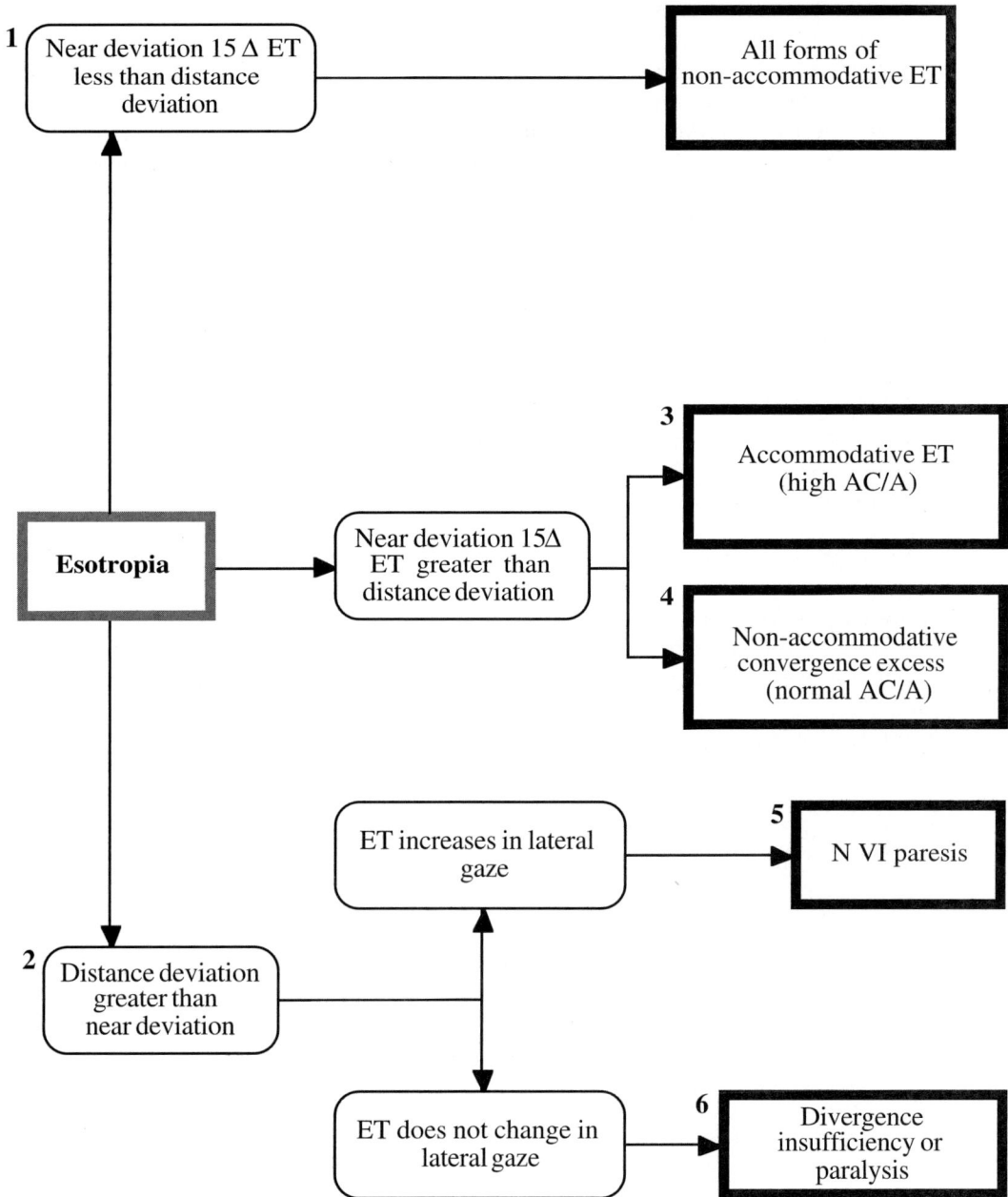

1.22   Exodeviations: Classification

(1) This classification pertains only to primary exodeviations and was introduced by Duane nearly 100 years ago.[15] In this classification exodeviations are distinguished according to differences between the near and distance deviation. A classification according to other criteria is also possible (e.g., considering the state of fusional control, primary versus secondary deviations). It should be emphasized that the terms "convergence insufficiency type" or "divergence excess type" do not imply a causative mechanism. In fact, there is no evidence that insufficiency of convergence or excess of divergence innervation causes exodeviations. However, as confusing as these terms may be, they have been widely used in clinical ophthalmology since their reintroduction by Burian and Miller.[9] For the treatment of exodeviations, **see 2.12.**

(2) Assuming the AC/A ratio[57 p.89] is normal, most exodeviations are 10^Δ to 15^Δ smaller at near fixation because of the influence of accommodative convergence. Thus only an increase of more than 15^Δ is considered clinically significant.

(3) As stated earlier (1), an exodeviation that is greater at near fixation (convergence insufficiency type) should not imply that the patient has a convergence insufficiency. In fact, functional convergence insufficiency **(see 2.48)** may occur in the presence of esophoria, orthophoria, or exophoria.

(4) Patching one eye for about 30 to 45 minutes[48] disrupts fusional and tonic convergence and may cause additional exodeviation at near fixation (simulated divergence excess). Even momentary binocular viewing after removal of the patch must be prevented because it may reinstate the powerful convergence mechanism by which a patient has learned to control the near deviation.[56 p.126]

(5) A true divergence excess type of exodeviation occurs less frequently than a simulated divergence excess type.[8]

(6) A simulated divergence excess type of exodeviation is merely a basic exodeviation with a powerful convergence mechanism that obscures the exodeviation at near fixation.

1.22

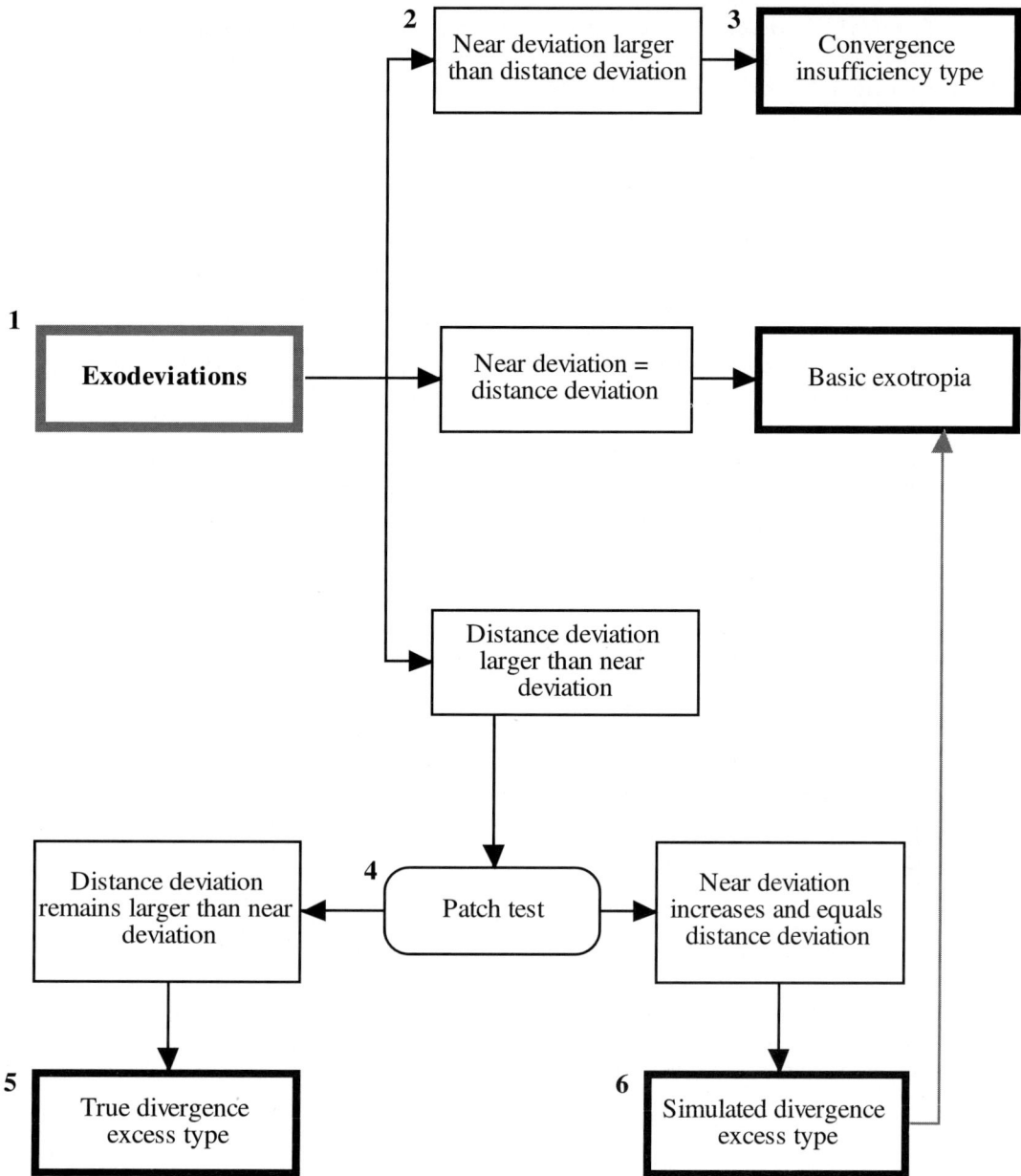

1.23 Exodeviations: Initial Decision Making

(1) The degree of fusional control determines whether a strabismus is manifest, intermittent, or latent. An exophoria may be controlled by fusion in the morning and become a manifest exotropia as the day progresses and the patient becomes fatigued. To determine how a patient copes with an exodeviation, repeated examinations at different times during the day are performed. Generally, intermittent deviations occur in patients with equal vision, full ductions, and a horizontally comitant deviation, although an **A** or **V** pattern may be present.

(2) With an intermittent exodeviation, it is necessary to determine during what percentage of time the eyes are exotropic. This is clinically more important than the angle of deviation. For instance, an exotropia of 50^Δ that is manifest only 5% of the time may not be a clinically significant deviation. Conversely, an intermittent exodeviation of only 20^Δ that is manifest 80% of the time is significant.[23 p.435]

(3) A difference between the angle of exodeviation at near and distance fixation may determine the type of surgery necessary to correct the strabismus **(see 2.12)**.

(4) A constant exotropia is clinically significant regardless of the angle of deviation or the cause. The larger the angle, the more likely the patient will benefit from surgical correction. However, when visual acuity is normal in both eyes, peripheral vision is reduced by aligning the eyes. The patient's awareness of the reduction in peripheral field always disappears.

(5) A patient with comitant constant exotropia may have equal vision or decreased vision in one eye. In fact, the exotropia may have been caused by the poor vision (sensory exotropia). When vision is decreased in one eye, surgery is ordinarily limited to this eye.[23 p.508]

(6) Incomitant constant exotropia may be associated with equal vision or decreased vision in one eye.

(7) Mechanical restriction of adduction may be the result of injury, prior eye muscle surgery (tight lateral rectus), surgery for retinal detachment, or congenital causes, such as Duane syndrome types II or III **(see 2.51 and 2.52)**.

(8) Exotropia with paresis of the medial rectus, usually from third nerve palsy, may be associated with ptosis and a hypotropia of the paretic eye. Restriction of adduction may be caused by contracture of the lateral rectus muscle **(see 2.36)**.

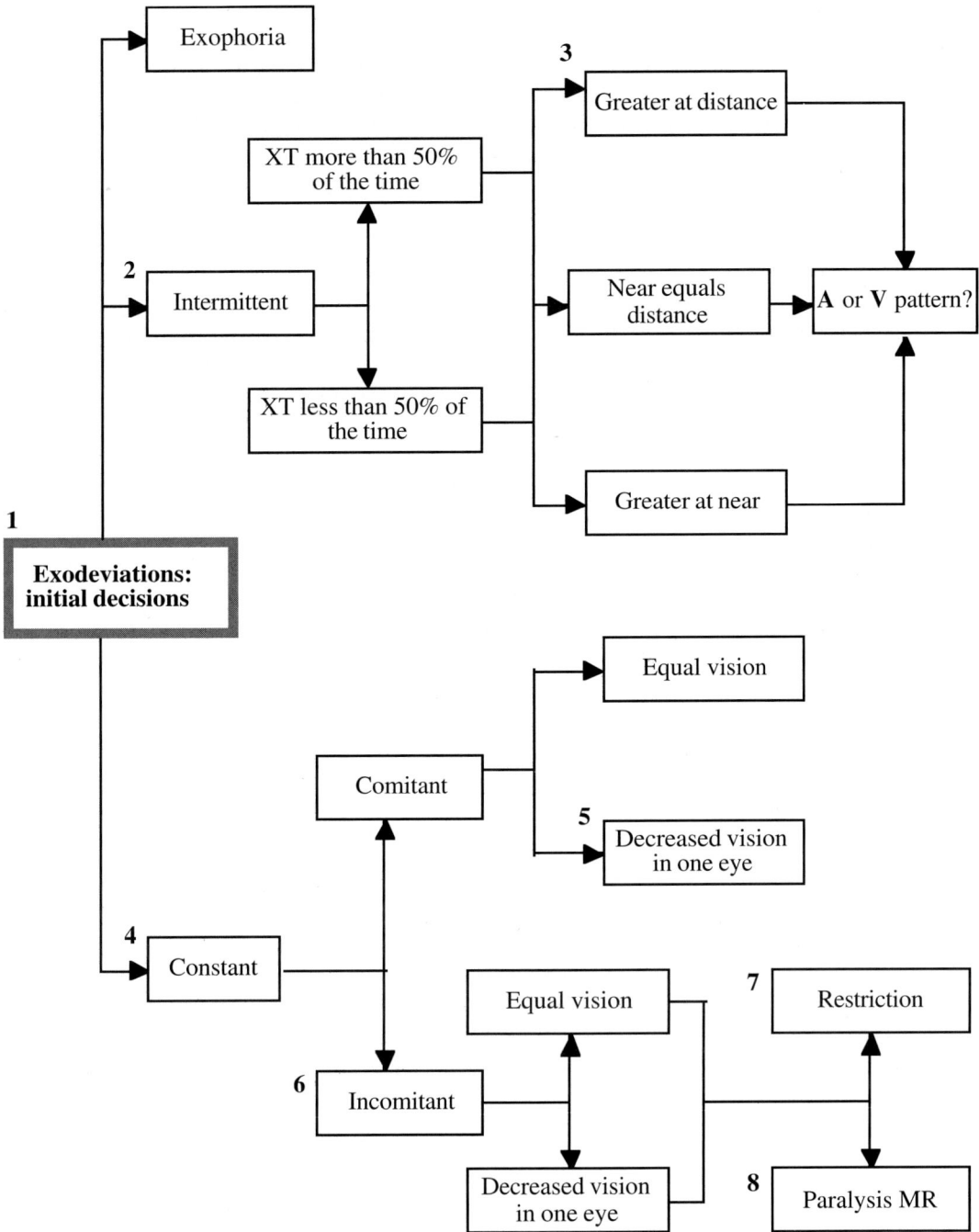

1.23

Exophoria

3
Greater at distance

XT more than 50%
of the time

2
Intermittent

Near equals
distance

A or **V** pattern?

XT less than 50% of
the time

Greater at near

1
Exodeviations:
initial decisions

Equal vision

Comitant

5
Decreased vision
in one eye

4
Constant

7
Restriction

Equal vision

6
Incomitant

Decreased vision
in one eye

8
Paralysis MR

1.24 Cyclovertical Deviations: Classification

(1) Cyclovertical deviations include vertical strabismus, isolated cyclotropia, and a combination of both.

(2) Vertical diplopia, sometimes accompanied by image tilting (cyclotropia) may be present, and compensatory anomalous head postures are frequent. The most common cause of symptomatic cyclotropia is a traumatic fourth nerve paralysis, especially when the palsy is bilateral. A careful history should be taken at the beginning of the examination and may often provide important clues as to the nature of the condition **(see 2.41 and 2.42).**

(3) Measurements of the deviation in the diagnostic positions of gaze establish which of the vertical rectus or oblique muscles are overacting or underacting and establish whether the strabismus is incomitant **(see 2.14, 2.15, and 2.21).**

(4) The forced duction test determines whether the strabismus is caused by innervational factors (paralysis or paresis) or restrictive factors **(see 1.30).**

(5) In muscle paralysis of recent onset the forced duction test result is negative.

(6) Dissociated vertical deviations (DVD) differ in several aspects from true hyperdeviations **(see 2.16)** and may coexist with hypertropia and A or V patterns.

(7) Comitant hyperdeviations are rare. It is unusual to find a patient with a significant hyperdeviation of the same magnitude in all gaze positions. In many instances such patients may have at one time had a paretic cyclovertical deviation that became comitant over time. In others, the hypertropia may have been caused by inadvertent raising or lowering of the muscle insertions during a previous operation for horizontal strabismus.

(8) Paralytic strabismus, although incomitant in its initial stage, may become increasingly comitant with the passage of time.

(9) **(See 2.30).** An acquired comitant vertical deviation is called skew deviation. It usually occurs in an older individual and is caused by a brainstem microvascular insult. The condition may be self-limiting. If not, it may be treated at least temporarily with vertical prism. The deviation is usually of small amplitude, being less than 10 prism diopters. Persistent skew deviation may be treated with recession of one or more vertical rectus muscles.[23] p.520

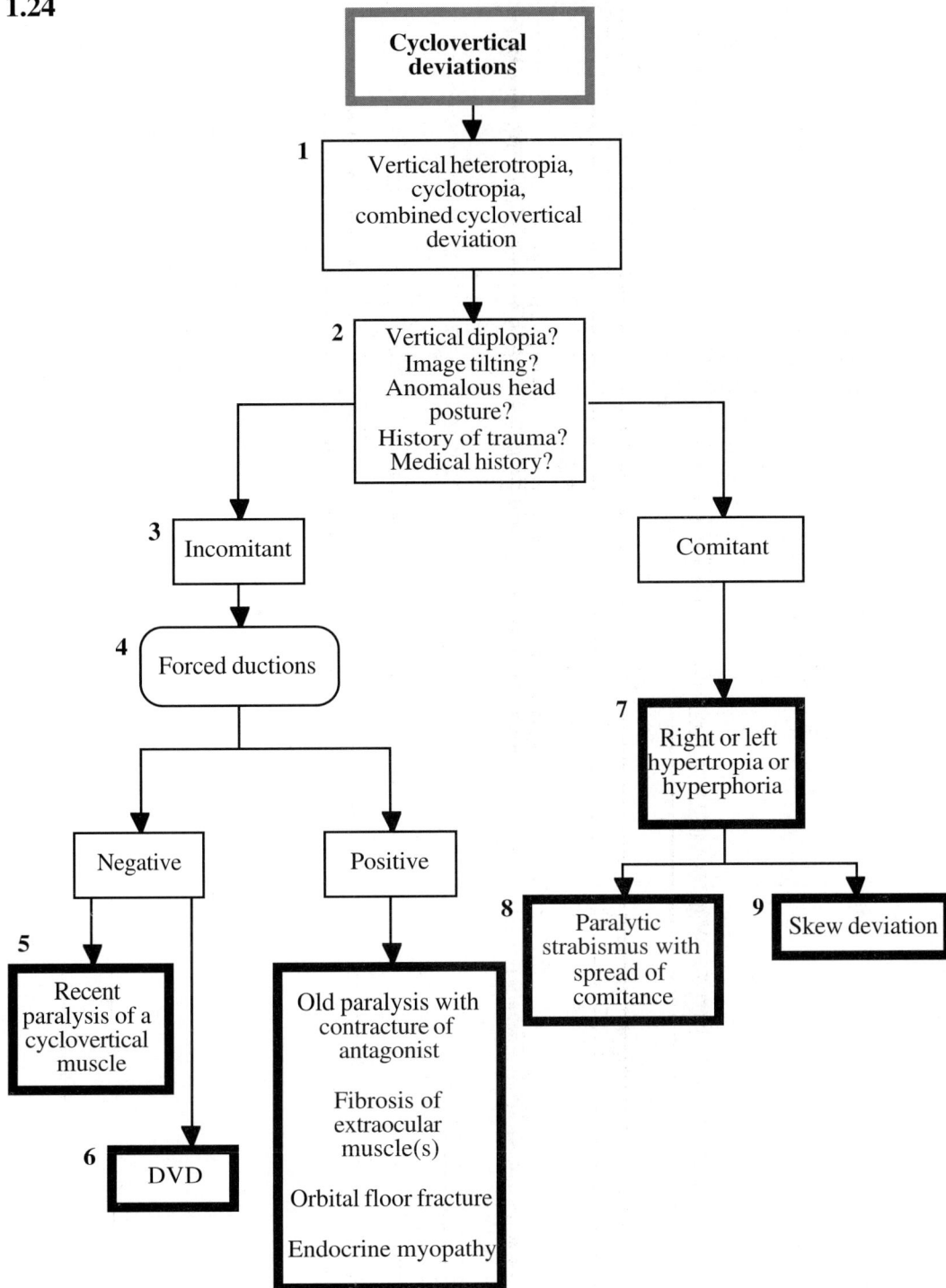

1.24

```
            ┌─────────────────────┐
            │   Cyclovertical     │
            │    deviations       │
            └─────────────────────┘
                      │
                      ▼
         ┌─────────────────────────┐
    1    │  Vertical heterotropia, │
         │      cyclotropia,       │
         │  combined cyclovertical │
         │       deviation         │
         └─────────────────────────┘
                      │
                      ▼
         ┌─────────────────────────┐
    2    │   Vertical diplopia?    │
         │     Image tilting?      │
         │   Anomalous head        │
         │        posture?         │
         │   History of trauma?    │
         │    Medical history?     │
         └─────────────────────────┘
```

3   Incomitant

4   Forced ductions

Negative   Positive

5   Recent paralysis of a cyclovertical muscle

6   DVD

Old paralysis with contracture of antagonist

Fibrosis of extraocular muscle(s)

Orbital floor fracture

Endocrine myopathy

Comitant

7   Right or left hypertropia or hyperphoria

8   Paralytic strabismus with spread of comitance

9   Skew deviation

1.25   **Anomalous Head Posture**

An anomalous head posture becomes readily apparent during the initial part of the examination. In children it is best observed under casual conditions (e.g., while directing attention to the parents while the history is obtained). The parents or the patient may be unaware of an anomalous head posture. In most instances of incomitant strabismus, the head is rotated to avoid diplopia. For this reason, an anomalous position is often referred to as a "compensatory" head posture. Less frequently and when fusion becomes impossible or is difficult to maintain, the head is rotated such that the separation between the double images is maximized (paradoxic head posture).[70] An ocular head tilt or head turn unrelated to incomitant strabismus occurs with nystagmus and a null point in certain gaze positions. Another ocular cause, unrelated to an ocular motility problem, is an uncorrected refractive error. When obtaining the history it is important to ascertain whether the anomalous posture is constant, if its direction is always the same, and whether it occurs at all or only at certain fixation distances. An anomalous head posture should always raise concern because it may cause neck strain; if left untreated, secondary scoliosis, contracture of the neck muscles,[57 p.371] and facial asymmetry[74] may occur.

(1) **See 1.26.**

(2) **See 1.27.**

(3) **See 1.28 and 1.29.**

(4) **See 1.26, 1.27, 1.28, and 1.29.**

1.25

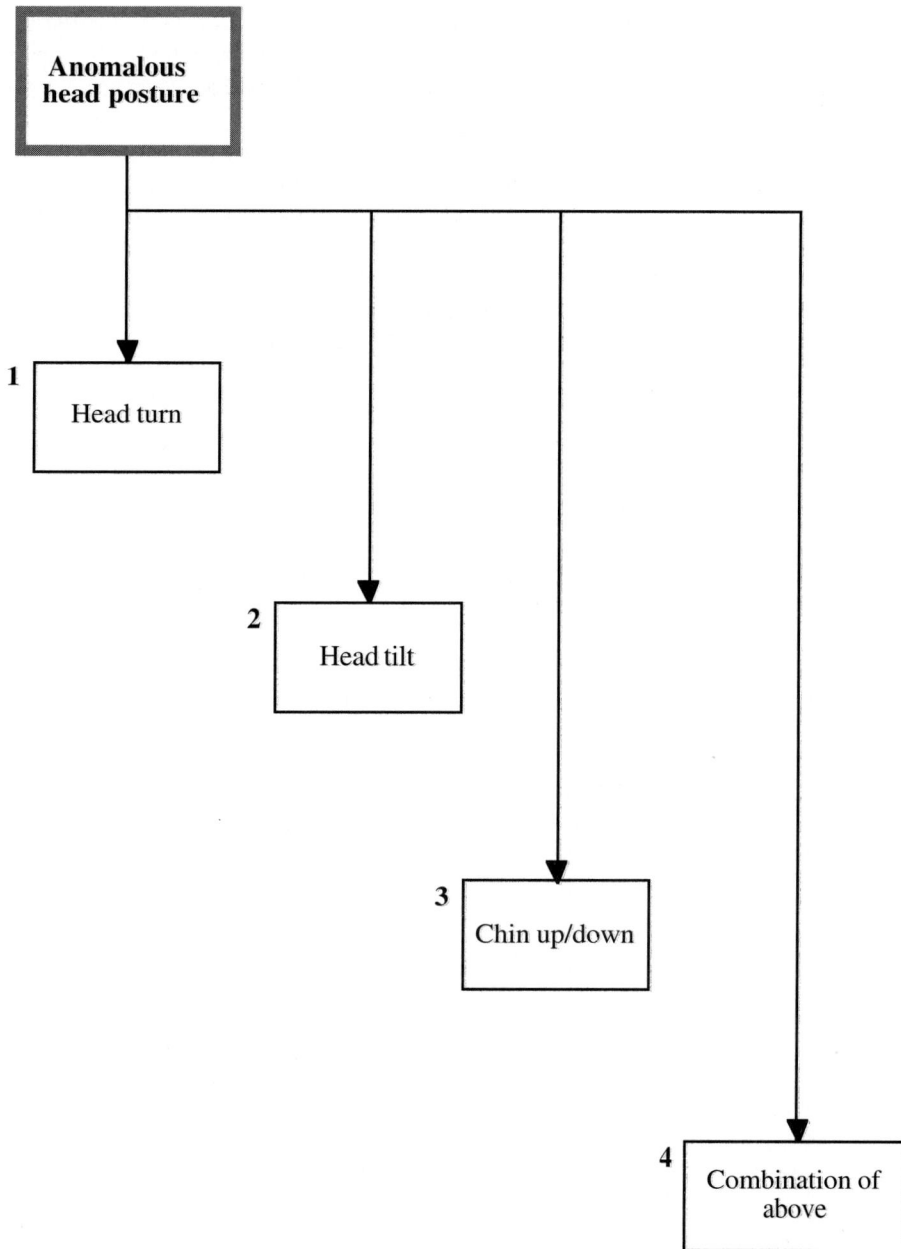

1.26   Head Turn

A patient turns his or her head (face) to one side and looks to the opposite side for two reasons: (1) He or she is unable to look to one side and therefore looks to the other side, or (2) he or she chooses to look to one side because it is more comfortable, improves visual acuity, or avoids diplopia. While most head turns are caused by strabismus or nystagmus, an uncorrected refractive error or a unilateral hearing defect may also have to be considered as causes.

(1) The patient turns his or her face to use an eye position in which the nystagmus is least pronounced (null point, neutral zone). In that position visual acuity is optimal but decreases when the head is passively straightened. In casual seeing the eyes (head) may be straight, but when looking at smaller objects or during visual attention (e.g., during visual acuity testing or while watching TV), the face turn is accentuated. Periodic alternating nystagmus causes an alternating face turn **(see 2.33 and 2.34)**.[23 p.542]

(2) Patients with essential infantile esotropia and manifest latent nystagmus frequently prefer to hold their dominant eye in a position of extreme adduction. The reason for this is that the nystagmus is generally dampened in this gaze position. A head turn in the direction of the fixating eye consequently develops.[23 p.421; 69]

(3) Dissociated vertical or horizontal deviations may be associated with a head turn **(see 2.16)**.

(4) In other cases the nose may be used to "occlude" the adducted eye to avoid double vision. The head is turned toward the side of the adducted eye.

(5) When an eye cannot adduct or abduct, the patient usually fixates in a gaze position opposite to that of the restricted duction. This allows the eye with restricted abduction or adduction some horizontal range of movement. For instance, when abduction is limited the preferred gaze position is one of adduction. The head turn is usually used to avoid diplopia.

(6) In some cases of unilateral third nerve palsy, the patient fixates with the paralyzed eye and the fellow eye may be amblyopic. In such cases, the head is turned toward the nonparalyzed side **(see 2.36)**.

(7) In cases of Duane syndrome type II with exotropia, the face is turned away from the involved eye, a response opposite to the more common Duane syndrome type I with esotropia and a head turn toward the side of the involved eye **(see 2.50, 2.51, and 2.52)**. A head turn may be seen in any of the classes of Duane syndrome.

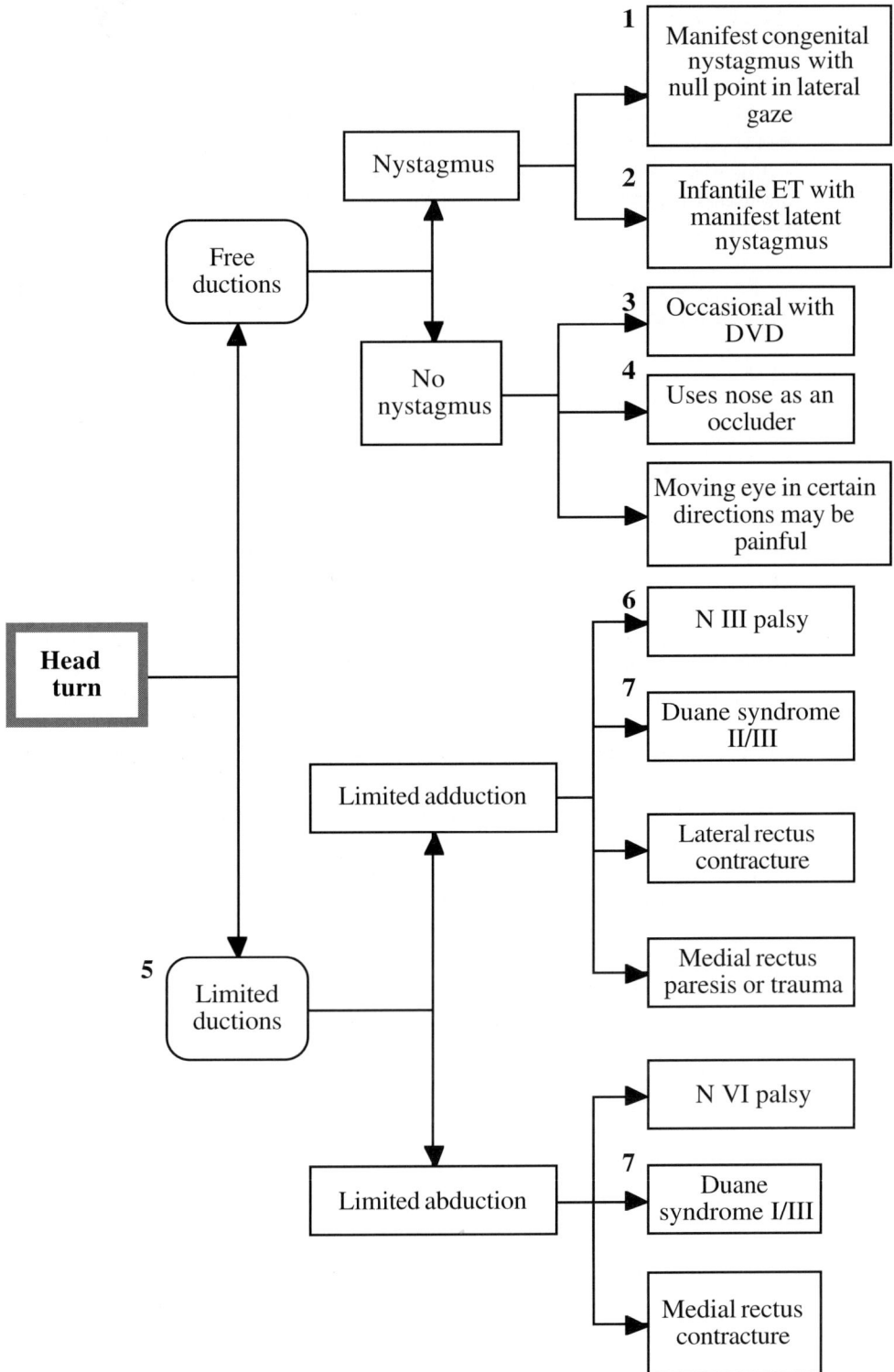

1.26

```
                                                    1  Manifest congenital
                                                       nystagmus with
                                                       null point in lateral
                                                       gaze

                            Nystagmus
                                                    2  Infantile ET with
                                                       manifest latent
                                                       nystagmus

         Free
         ductions                                   3  Occasional with
                                                       DVD

                            No                      4  Uses nose as an
                            nystagmus                  occluder

                                                       Moving eye in certain
                                                       directions may be
                                                       painful


                                                    6  N III palsy


                                                    7  Duane syndrome
                                                       II/III

                            Limited adduction
                                                       Lateral rectus
                                                       contracture

  Head
  turn
                                                       Medial rectus
                                                       paresis or trauma


      5    Limited
           ductions                                    N VI palsy


                                                    7  Duane
                            Limited abduction          syndrome I/III


                                                       Medial rectus
                                                       contracture
```

1.27   Head Tilt to Either Shoulder

(1) A patch is placed over the right and then the left eye while the patient is observed for changes in the head posture. Patients with nonocular head tilt do not respond to the patch test. The patient is encouraged to sit up straight during this observation. The patient's attention is directed toward a distant fixation target. It is important that he or she be unaware of the purpose of the test and remain relaxed during observation. In children it is advisable to ask the child to walk to the end of the room and back.

(2) The head tilt compensates for the tilt of the visual environment. It disappears on patching of the eye with cyclotropia.

(3) A compensatory head posture with the chin elevated and pointing toward the opposite shoulder permits fusion in Brown syndrome.[23 p.408; 57 p.404]

(4) The head tilt, often in combination with a face turn, avoids diplopia in cyclovertical strabismus. Infrequently, the head is tilted to cause maximal separation of the double images when fusion cannot be maintained.[70] The direction of the head tilt is of no diagnostic significance. Patching one eye eliminates diplopia and the head straightens.

(5) Congenital nystagmus with null point in tertiary gaze may cause a head tilt to either shoulder. The patient has optimal visual acuity with the head tilted. The nystagmus may be of minimal amplitude and escape detection.[67]

(6) A long-standing ocular head tilt may cause tightness of the neck muscles, deformities of the cervical spine,[57 p.371] and facial asymmetry.[74] These sequelae of ocular head tilt may maintain an abnormal head posture even after the ocular cause has been removed.

(7) Fibrosis of the sternocleidomastoid muscle may be caused by intramuscular hemorrhage during birth. Unlike ocular head tilt, congenital torticollis may be present as early as 6 months after birth. The tightness of the muscle is palpable and prevents passive tilting of the head toward the noninvolved side.

(8) This unusual cause of a severe head tilt[55] should be considered during the differential diagnosis.

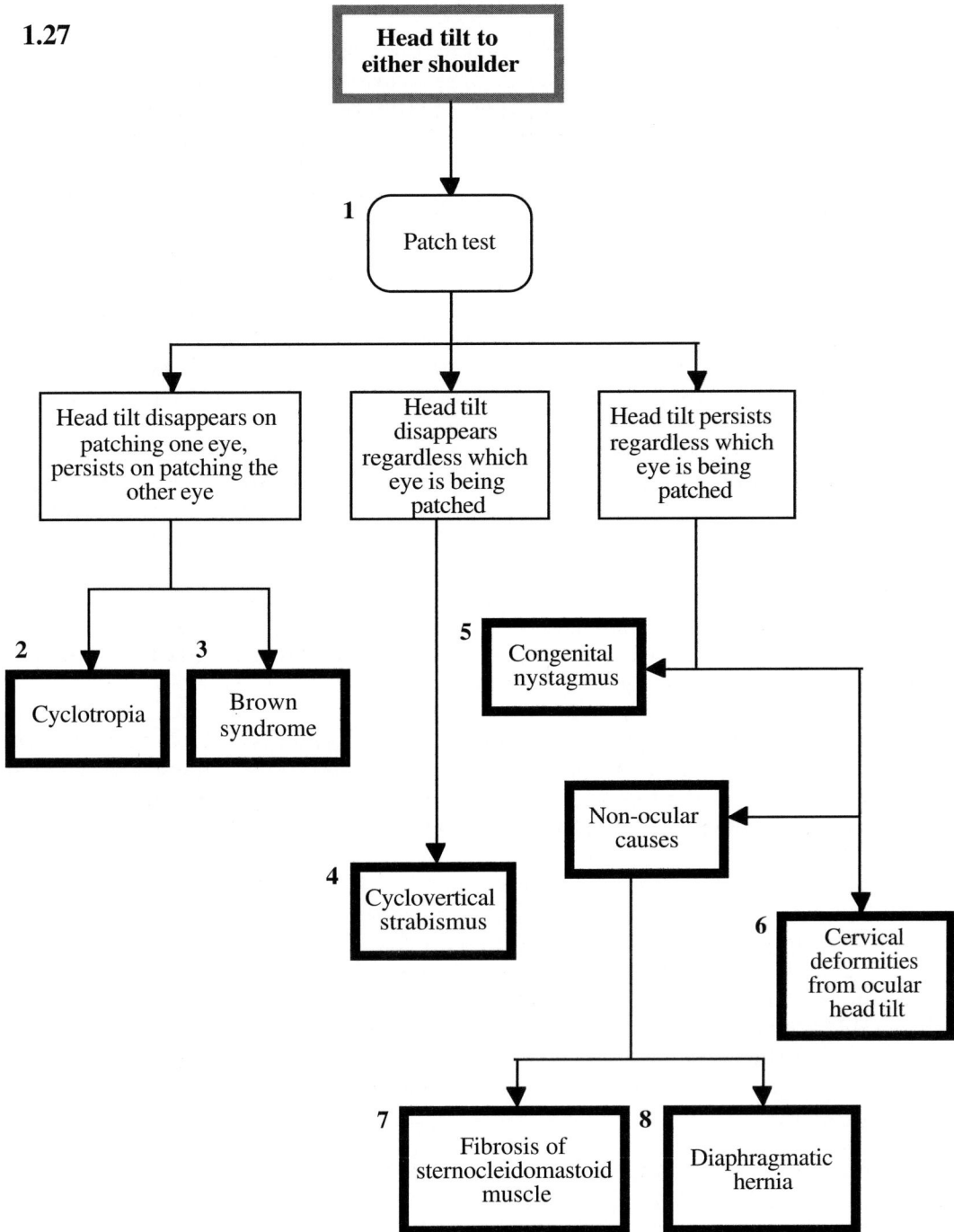

1.27

```
Head tilt to
either shoulder
```

1 → Patch test

Head tilt disappears on patching one eye, persists on patching the other eye

Head tilt disappears regardless which eye is being patched

Head tilt persists regardless which eye is being patched

2 Cyclotropia

3 Brown syndrome

5 Congenital nystagmus

4 Cyclovertical strabismus

Non-ocular causes

6 Cervical deformities from ocular head tilt

7 Fibrosis of sternocleidomastoid muscle

8 Diaphragmatic hernia

1.28   **Chin Elevation**

(1) A patient may assume a chin-up anomalous head posture because comfortable binocular vision or improved visual acuity can be obtained when both eyes are in a position of depression. The primary position of the eyes is avoided because double vision or decreased visual acuity may be present in that position.

(2) The first diagnostic step should determine whether both eyes elevate normally. If they do, vertical strabismus from innervational or mechanical restrictive causes can be excluded.

(3) When the cover test **(see 1.16)** shows a heterotropia in upward gaze and no shift on covering either eye in downward gaze, horizontal strabismus with incomitance in vertical gaze (**A** or **V** pattern) is present. Some patients may note double vision when the head is passively straightened but not when the chin is elevated.

(4) The prism cover test is performed with the fixation target in 30° elevation and depression to diagnose an **A** or **V** pattern strabismus[23 p.535; 57 p.358] **(see 2.22 and 2.23).**

(5) Manifest nystagmus is usually diagnosed by direct observation. Occasionally, the nystagmus amplitude may be so small that it escapes casual clinical examination and can only be diagnosed with magnification by ophthalmoscopy or biomicroscopy (micronystagmus) **(see 2.33).**

(6) Congenital or acquired nystagmus may have a null point with the eyes in depression. In that case, the patient elevates the chin to gain better vision. This improvement may be too subtle to measure on the acuity chart but sufficiently important for the patient to maintain an uncomfortable head posture.[23 p.541]

(7) **See 2.33.**

(8) Forced ductions must be performed when examination of ductions and versions shows limitation of elevation of the eye(s). In most instances such limitations indicate mechanical restriction of elevation from a number of causes listed below. In cooperative subjects the test is performed in the office after local anesthesia is obtained with topical 4% lidocaine hydrochloride. It is important to instruct the patient to look up while determining whether there is a restriction to elevation.

(9) Restriction of elevation from endocrine myopathy of the inferior rectus muscle is usually asymmetric. However, in most instances both eyes are involved, and surgery on both muscles may be required **(see 2.55).**[23 p.489; 57 p.410]

(10) **See 2.54.**

(11) **See 2.29.**

(12) **See 2.53.**

(13) **See 2.37 and 2.40.**

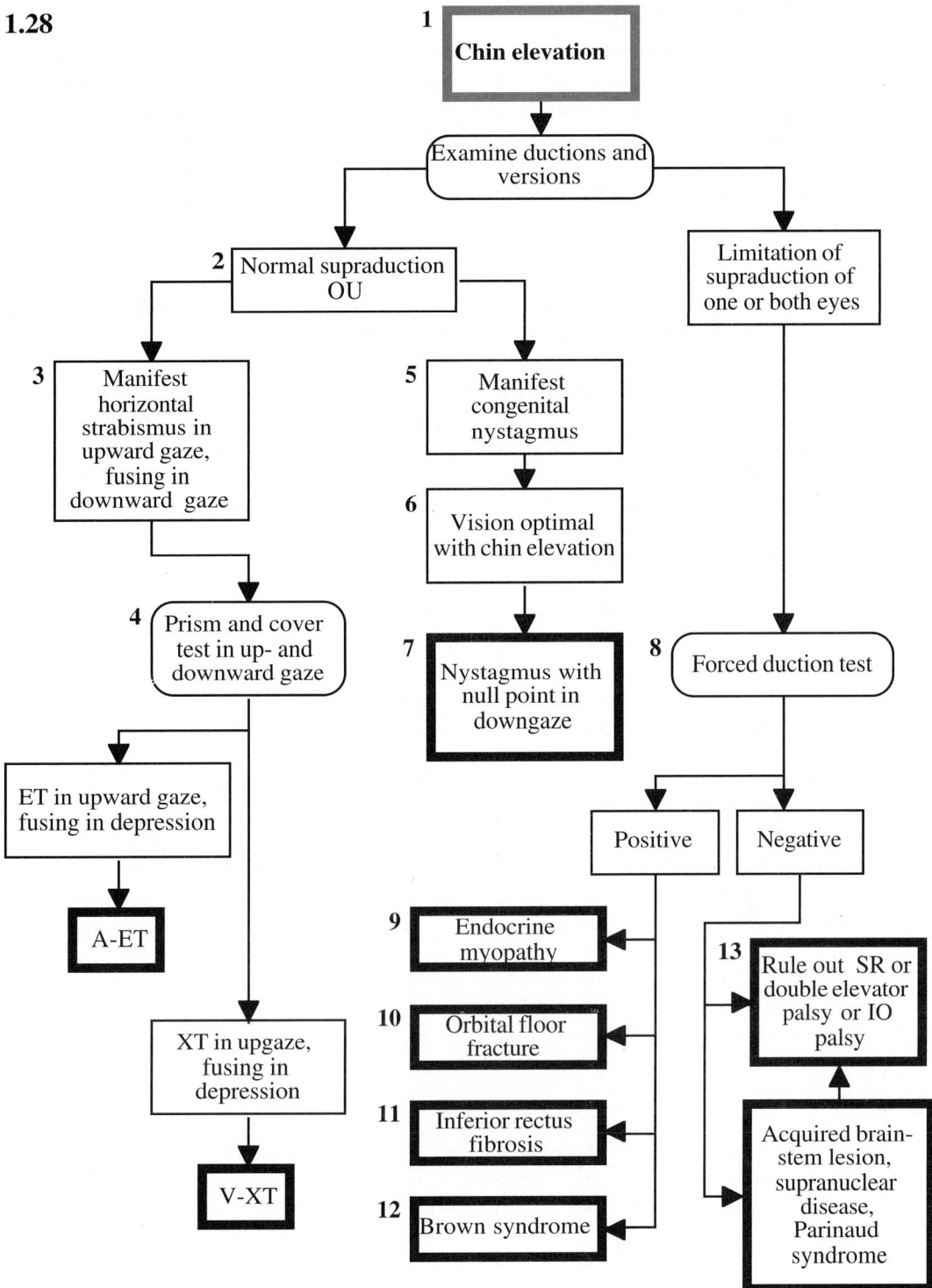

1.28

1 **Chin elevation**

Examine ductions and versions

2 Normal supraduction OU

Limitation of supraduction of one or both eyes

3 Manifest horizontal strabismus in upward gaze, fusing in downward gaze

5 Manifest congenital nystagmus

6 Vision optimal with chin elevation

7 Nystagmus with null point in downgaze

4 Prism and cover test in up- and downward gaze

8 Forced duction test

ET in upward gaze, fusing in depression

A-ET

Positive

Negative

XT in upgaze, fusing in depression

V-XT

9 Endocrine myopathy

13 Rule out SR or double elevator palsy or IO palsy

10 Orbital floor fracture

11 Inferior rectus fibrosis

Acquired brain-stem lesion, supranuclear disease, Parinaud syndrome

12 Brown syndrome

1.29   **Chin Depression**

(1) A chin depression helps the patient to avoid the downward gaze position and to obtain comfortable binocular vision or improved visual acuity in upward gaze. With the eyes lowered, the patient may experience double vision or visual discomfort from sustained efforts to maintain fusion in the presence of a muscle imbalance (muscular asthenopia). Chin depression causes neck strain much as chin elevation does and for this reason requires treatment.

(2) At the beginning of an examination it must be determined whether the eyes are capable of depressing synchronously or whether there is restricted depression in one eye. Such limitation is usually of innervational origin and is less likely to be caused by mechanical restriction **(see 1.09 and 1.10).**

(3) In some patients visual acuity improves when the chin is depressed and decreases when the eyes are in primary position or downward gaze. This is caused by a manifest congenital nystagmus which, as a rule, is visible on examination of the eyes and has its neutral point when the eyes are elevated. In some instances the amplitude of the nystagmus may be so small that it escapes gross observation by the examiner. Magnification with the slit lamp or ophthalmoscopy while the patient fixates a visual target built into the optical system of an ophthalmoscope helps to detect the nystagmus in such cases. Acquired upbeating nystagmus can also have a null point with better vision in upgaze, which causes chin depression **(see 1.35).**

(4) **See 2.24.** Other causes of chin depression are bilateral abducens **(see 2.45)** and trochlear nerve pareses and paralyses **(see 2.41 and 2.42).**

(5) **See 2.23.**

(6) Paralysis of the inferior rectus muscle **(see 2.38)** may cause rapid contracture of the ipsilateral superior rectus muscle. The resulting diplopia forces the patient to depress the chin and avoid the hypertropia of the paralyzed eye in primary position and downward gaze.

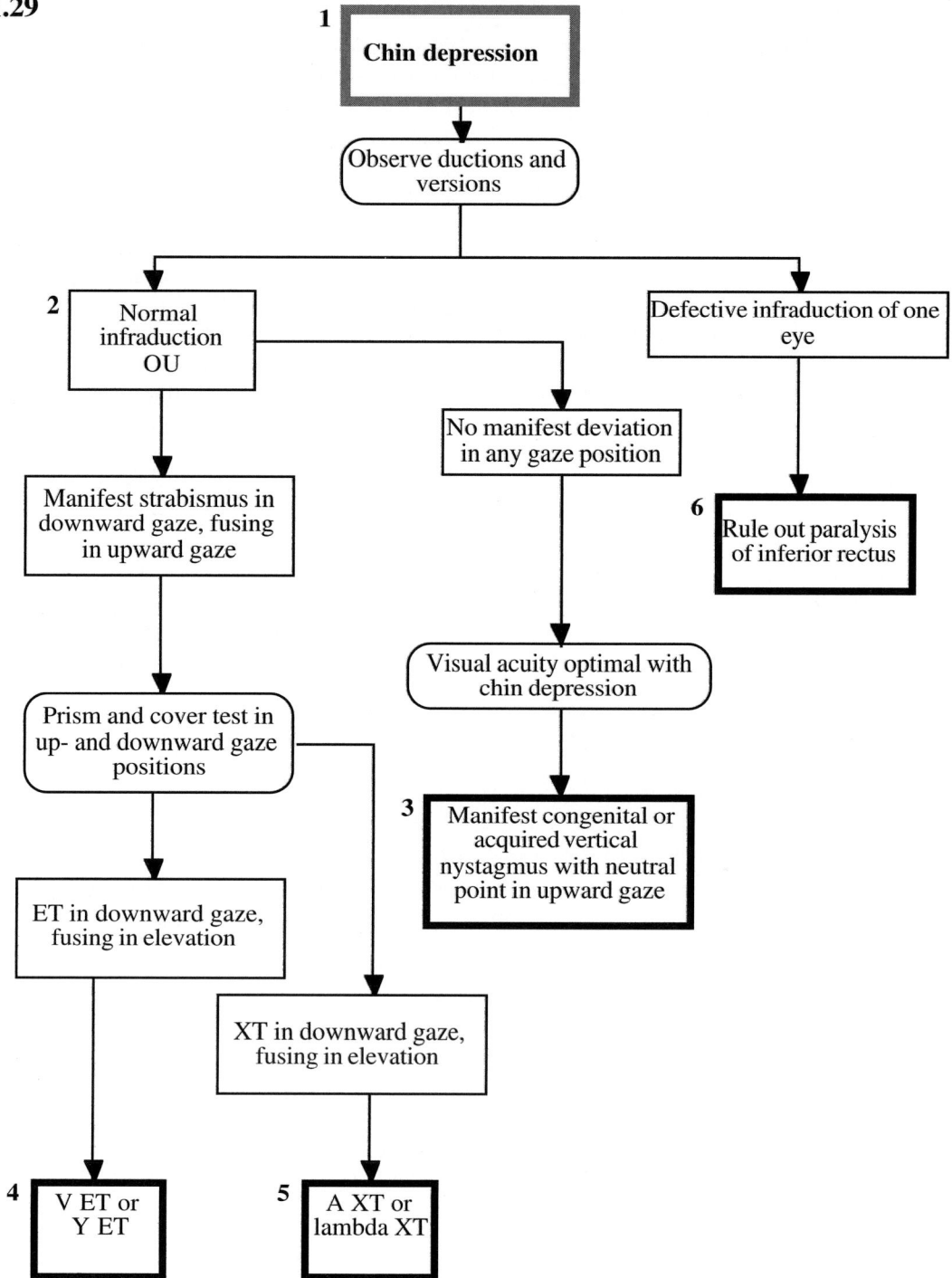

1.29

1 Chin depression

Observe ductions and versions

2 Normal infraction OU

No manifest deviation in any gaze position

Defective infraction of one eye

Manifest strabismus in downward gaze, fusing in upward gaze

6 Rule out paralysis of inferior rectus

Prism and cover test in up- and downward gaze positions

Visual acuity optimal with chin depression

3 Manifest congenital or acquired vertical nystagmus with neutral point in upward gaze

ET in downward gaze, fusing in elevation

XT in downward gaze, fusing in elevation

4 V ET or Y ET

5 A XT or lambda XT

1.30   **Innervational Versus Restrictive Strabismus**

(1) When an eye fails to fully execute a duction, the question arises whether this limitation of ocular motility is caused by a paresis or paralysis, a mechanical restriction, or a combination of the two.

(2) Provided the patient is cooperative, forced ductions are performed in the office after anesthetizing the conjunctiva with several drops of proparacaine hydrochloride, tetracaine, or 4% lidocaine. The conjunctiva is then grasped with a forceps close to the limbus, and the examiner tries to complete the limited duction while the patient looks into the direction of the apparently underacting muscle. Care has to be taken not to press the eye into the orbit during this test because this may simulate free forced ductions when, in fact, restrictions are present. If passive ductions are free, a paresis or paralysis is assumed to be present. If the ductions are restricted, a mechanical obstacle to ocular motility is present.

(3) The generated muscle force is estimated in the manner described in our texts.[23 p.257;57 p.375] Saccadic velocity is observed or measured and recorded when the necessary equipment is available.

(4) Whenever possible, a distinction should be made between paresis (incomplete paralysis) and paralysis of an extraocular muscle or muscle group.

(5) In patients with restricted forced ductions, generated muscle force may be positive within a limited scope of eye movement. In this case, the intraocular pressure (IOP) increases when the eye attempts to look in the field of limited movement.[23 p.269] This is an indirect measure of generated force. In addition, in this limited area of movement, the saccade may be brisk rather than floating. When intraocular pressure increases in the presence of a limited duction or if a brisk saccade is seen in the limited duction, restriction of motility with intact innervation can be inferred. In such cases, release of the restriction may suffice in realigning the eyes.

(6) If there is no generated muscle force in the presence of restriction, surgical removal of the restriction in addition to muscle transposition procedures may be indicated to restore ocular alignment in primary position.[23 p.291]

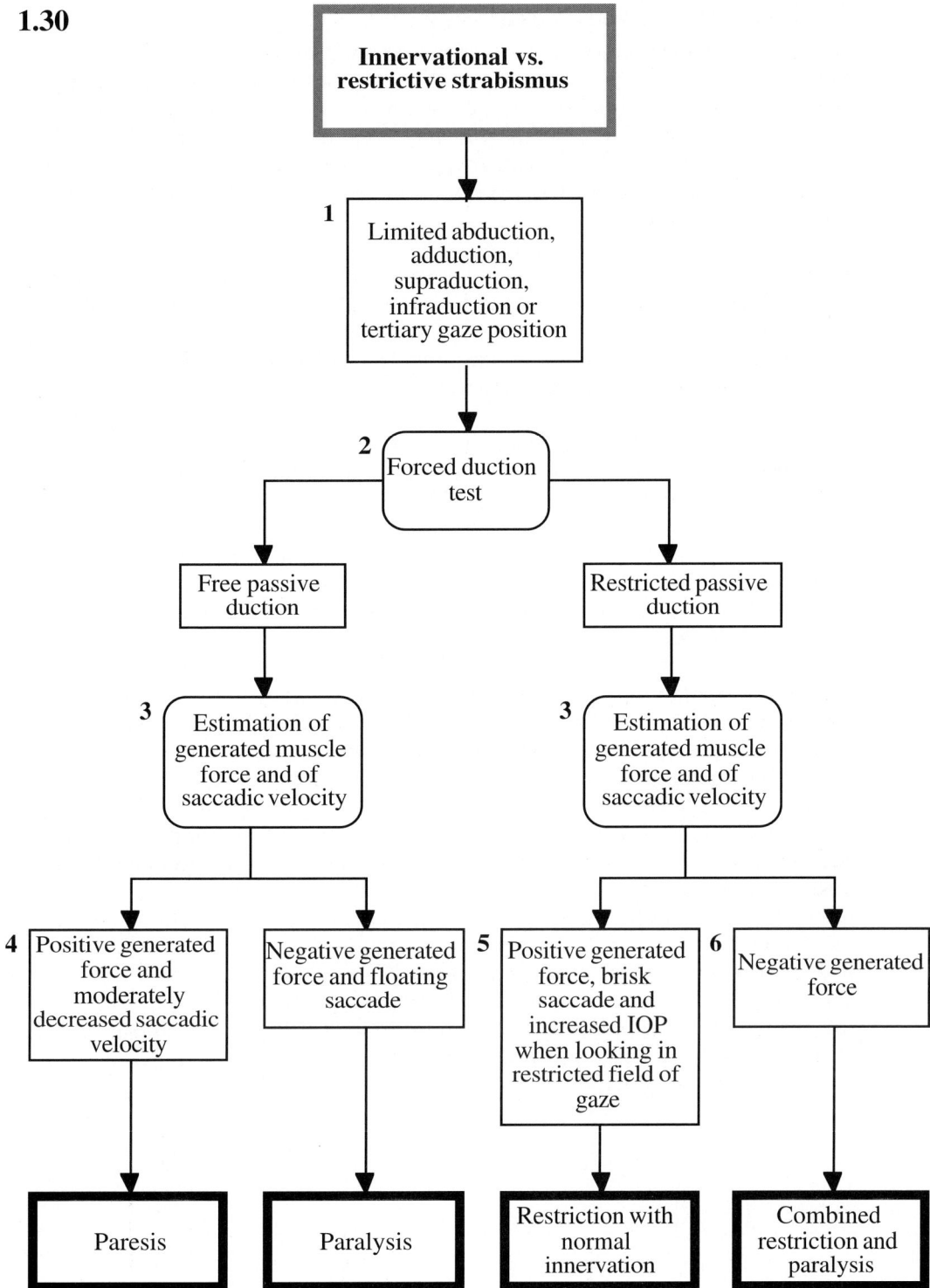

1.30

```
┌─────────────────────────┐
│   Innervational vs.     │
│  restrictive strabismus │
└─────────────────────────┘
             │
             ▼
```

1 Limited abduction, adduction, supraduction, infraduction or tertiary gaze position

2 Forced duction test

Free passive duction

Restricted passive duction

3 Estimation of generated muscle force and of saccadic velocity

3 Estimation of generated muscle force and of saccadic velocity

4 Positive generated force and moderately decreased saccadic velocity

Negative generated force and floating saccade

5 Positive generated force, brisk saccade and increased IOP when looking in restricted field of gaze

6 Negative generated force

Paresis

Paralysis

Restriction with normal innervation

Combined restriction and paralysis

1.31   Old Versus Recent Paralysis

The decision whether a paralysis is of recent onset or has been present for a long time or even since birth is of paramount importance in deciding the extent of the medical workup for a patient, as well as for medicolegal reasons in some cases. Some of the features listed in the table may assist the examiner in making this decision in cases without a clear history of antecedent trauma or other pertinent medical events, or when the patient is intentionally misleading the examiner when compensation is involved.

(1) Diplopia is the most prominent complaint of patients with extraocular muscle paralysis of recent onset. In infants and small children who are less likely to complain, voluntary closure of one eye may be a sign that double vision is present. In cases of paralyses of long duration, the patient will have learned to avoid diplopia by assuming a compensatory head posture.

(2) Complaints about image tilt occur almost exclusively in patients with a recent onset of trochlear paralysis, especially bilateral paralysis, and have not been observed by us in cases with congenital onset.[19]

(3) The patient, relatives, and other close associates may be unaware that a patient has an anomalous head posture. Old photographs, preferably frontal views (driver's license or passport pictures, graduation or wedding photographs), are of inestimable value in dating the onset of an anomalous head posture.

(4) Facial asymmetry is a common feature in patients who have had a head tilt since infancy and is not limited to congenital torticollis of nonocular causes. The face toward the side of the head tilt is hypoplastic (the face on the side of the paralysis is fuller).

(5) Because of secondary changes in the antagonist or the yoke of a paralyzed muscle, incomitant strabismus may eventually become increasingly comitant. As a rule, this spread of comitance signals a condition that has been present for a long time. This should not distract from the fact that spread of comitance may occasionally develop in a matter of a few weeks, and in some patients a paralysis may be present for many years and yet remain highly incomitant.

(6) Testing for past-pointing is infrequently used today to diagnose paralytic strabismus. Occasionally, this test may be useful to distinguish a paralysis of recent onset from an older one.[57 p.372]

TABLE 1-31 *Old Versus Recent Paralysis*		
	Old or congenital	**Recent**
Diplopia **(1)**	Only in paretic gaze position	Prominent complaint
Image tilt **(2)**	Absent	Diagnostic
Old photos **(3)**	May show anomalous head posture	Normal head posture
Facial asymmetry **(4)**	Common with fourth nerve palsy	Absent
Forced ductions	May show contracture	Negative
Amblyopia	May be present	Normal vision in each eye
Comitance **(5)**	Spread of comitance	Incomitant
Past-pointing **(6)**	Absent	Common

1.32   Asthenopia

(1) The patient with asthenopia may complain about eye strain, blurred vision, intermittent double vision, headaches, or pain in and around the eyes. Such complaints are usually related to near work or prolonged periods of reading or studying although they may also occur after driving and other tedious visual tasks. Typically, asthenopia develops during or after work and symptoms are not present on awakening in the morning. The two principal causes of asthenopia are sustained efforts to maintain fusion in the presence of an oculomotor imbalance (muscular asthenopia) or an uncorrected refractive error or accommodative insufficiency (refractive asthenopia).

(2) To distinguish between muscular and refractive asthenopia, we instruct the patient to wear a patch over either eye for several days during near work or studying. If asthenopia persists during monocular vision, it clearly is not of muscular origin.

(3) Improvement of symptoms after wearing the patch implies that asthenopia is caused by sustained efforts to maintain binocular vision against the obstacle of an oculomotor imbalance. Of the numerous types of latent or intermittent strabismus that may cause such imbalance, only the most frequently encountered conditions are listed here and are discussed in greater detail elsewhere **(see 1.15, 1.16, 1.22, and 2.12).**

(4) Accommodative insufficiency may occur without obvious cause in healthy young individuals as an isolated anomaly[11] or in association with convergence insufficiency.[64] The first condition may require reading adds and the second a combination of bifocals and base-in prisms for near vision.

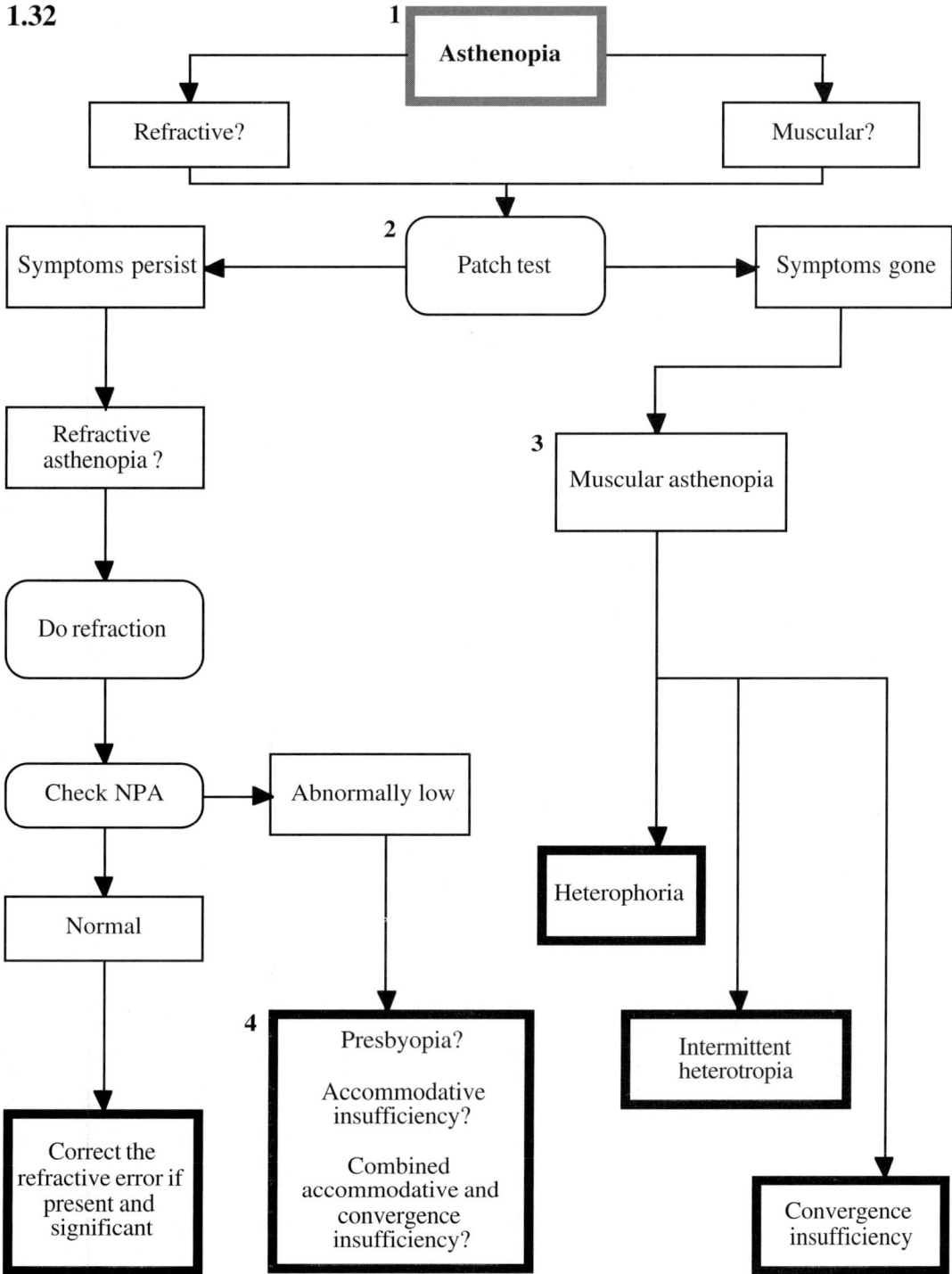

1.32

1 Asthenopia

Refractive? Muscular?

2 Patch test

Symptoms persist Symptoms gone

Refractive asthenopia ?

3 Muscular asthenopia

Do refraction

Check NPA Abnormally low

Normal

Heterophoria

Correct the refractive error if present and significant

4 Presbyopia?

Accommodative insufficiency?

Combined accommodative and convergence insufficiency?

Intermittent heterotropia

Convergence insufficiency

1.33 Diplopia

(1) Before a complete ocular motility evaluation, the examiner should first determine whether the patient really sees double or has blurred vision, overlay of images or sees a halo. This information is obtained by a careful history and may be supplemented by asking the patient to draw a picture of what he or she sees.

(2) Unless the cause of double vision is obvious by the presence of a gross strabismus, either eye is briefly covered while the patient is asked whether double vision persists under monocular conditions.

(3) Most people ignore physiologic diplopia. However, occasionally a patient becomes aware of it and may seek medical advice. This phenomenon is readily explained to the patient.[57 p.18]

(4) Monocular diplopia that persists when the patient looks through a pinhole occurs infrequently and only transiently from sensory causes during the treatment of amblyopia,[57 p.358] in the presence of subretinal neovascular membranes,[6] after traumatic brain injury, or after a cerebrovascular accident. In such cases, the patient frequently sees multiple images of the same fixation object (polyopia).[57 p.201]

(5) Monocular diplopia from optical causes disappears when the patient looks through a pinhole; this type of diplopia is far more frequent than sensory monocular diplopia. In most instances, slit lamp examination of the lens shows incipient cataract with zones of increased optical density in the anterior and posterior subcapsular or nuclear layers. This condition also occurs occasionally in pseudophakia with otherwise excellent vision.

(6) A red filter is held before the fixating eye while the patient views a fixation light at the end of the examination lane. The patient is asked to indicate the position of the red light in relation to the fixation light. The diplopia field can then be mapped.

(7) Traumatic fusion deficiency, also called central disruption of motor fusion, is caused by brain concussion and consists of a defect of motor fusion.[57 p.143] The patient alternates between crossed and uncrossed diplopia. Motor fusion can be achieved for a fleeting moment but cannot be maintained although sensory fusion may be intact.

(8) Crossed diplopia in esotropes and uncrossed diplopia in exotropes may occur transiently after strabismus surgery and is caused by persistence of anomalous retinal correspondence.[57 p.258] In such cases the postoperative position of the eyes no longer corresponds to the preoperatively established angle of anomaly. The red-filter test is indispensable to distinguish paradoxic diplopia from postoperative diplopia caused by surgical overcorrection in a patient who reports double vision after muscle surgery.

(9) In certain cases of long-standing strabismus without adequate suppression and without the capacity for motor or sensory fusion, the two foveas actually repel each other, producing constant or at least frequent diplopia.[57 p.137]

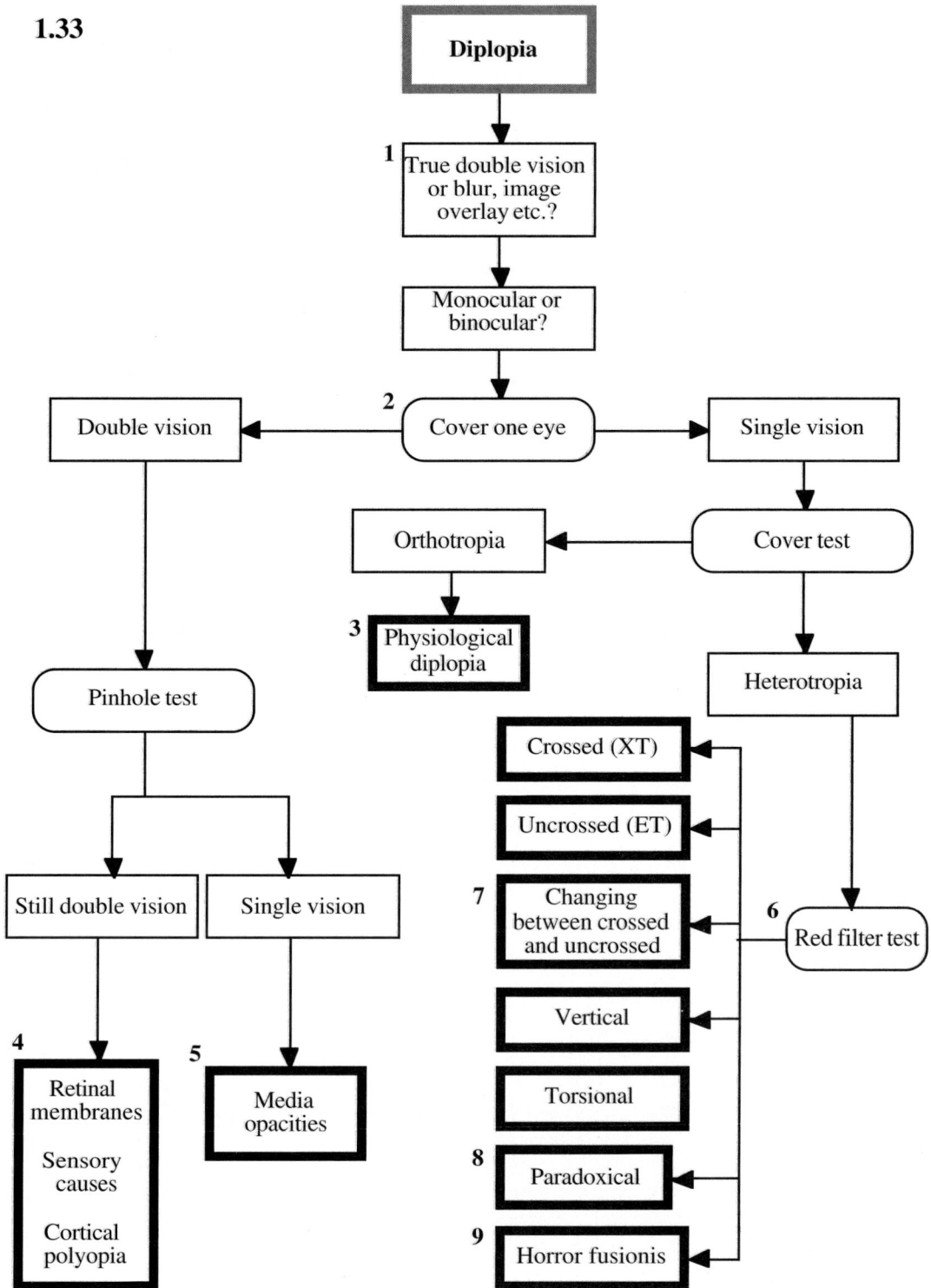

1.33

```
                    ┌─────────────────┐
                    │    Diplopia     │
                    └────────┬────────┘
                             │
                             ▼
              1  ┌────────────────────┐
                 │ True double vision │
                 │ or blur, image     │
                 │ overlay etc.?      │
                 └─────────┬──────────┘
                           │
                           ▼
                 ┌────────────────┐
                 │  Monocular or  │
                 │   binocular?   │
                 └───────┬────────┘
                         │
                         ▼
```

2 Cover one eye

Double vision ◄─── Cover one eye ───► Single vision

Orthotropia ◄─── Cover test

Double vision → Pinhole test

3 Physiological diplopia

Single vision → Cover test → Heterotropia → Red filter test

Pinhole test → Still double vision / Single vision

Crossed (XT)

Uncrossed (ET)

7 Changing between crossed and uncrossed

6 Red filter test

Vertical

Torsional

4 Retinal membranes

Sensory causes

Cortical polyopia

5 Media opacities

8 Paradoxical

9 Horror fusionis

1.34   Congenital Nystagmus: Clinical Characteristics

(1) So-called congenital nystagmus is rarely present at birth but develops within the first 2 to 4 months of life. Congenital nystagmus occurs in two basic forms: "jerk," with a slow drift away from fixation and a rapid corrective saccade, and "pendular," in which to-and-fro movements of the eyes are essentially of the same speed. The amplitude and frequency of both jerk and pendular nystagmus can vary.

(2) Latent nystagmus occurs in its pure form when one eye is covered. More common is a nystagmus that occurs with both eyes open but intensifies when one eye is covered (manifest-latent nystagmus). Both forms are commonly associated with infantile esotropia but may also occur with other types of strabismus or without any strabismus. The waveform of latent nystagmus differs from the waveform of manifest nystagmus inasmuch as it has a *decelerating* velocity slow phase.[69]

(3) Manifest jerky congenital nystagmus is presumably caused by a defect in the brainstem. It is only infrequently associated with infantile esotropia, in which it may cause nystagmus compensation syndrome **(see 2.33).**

(4) Pendular nystagmus may occur in patients with normal eyes. In such cases, a neurologic workup should be considered. The workup should start with an electroretinogram, which may uncover ophthalmoscopically undetectable retinal disease. Pure pendular nystagmus is rare; more frequent is pendular nystagmus that becomes jerky in peripheral gaze positions.

(5) When the eyes are abnormal, such as in macular hypoplasia, aniridia, albinism, or Leber's amaurosis, the pendular nystagmus is caused by reduced visual input. This has been called "sensory" nystagmus.

(6) **See 2.33.**

1.34

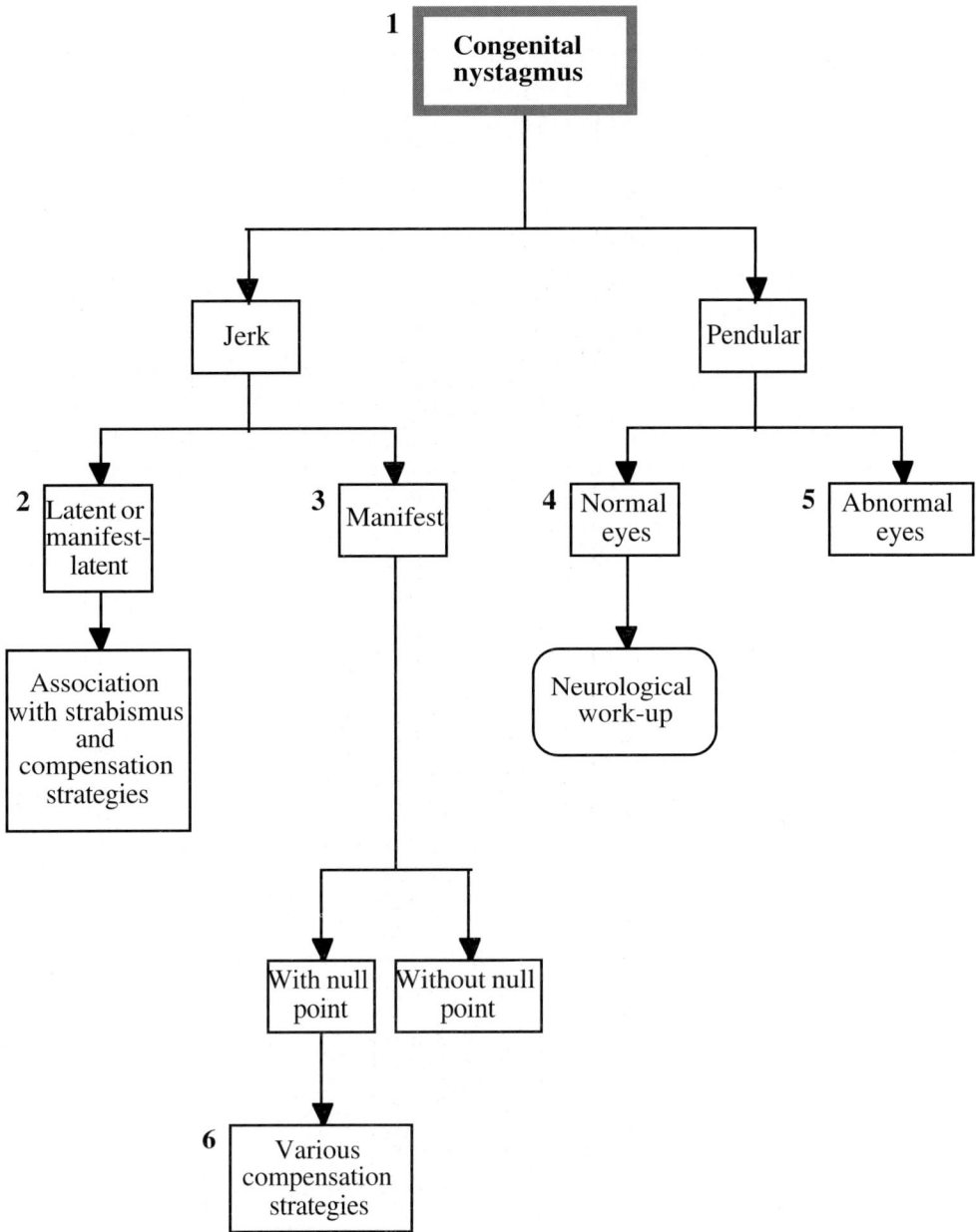

1 **Congenital nystagmus**

Jerk

Pendular

2 Latent or manifest-latent

3 Manifest

4 Normal eyes

5 Abnormal eyes

Association with strabismus and compensation strategies

Neurological work-up

With null point

Without null point

6 Various compensation strategies

1.35   Acquired Nystagmus in Childhood

(1) Acquired nystagmus in childhood may be a sign of serious neurologic problems and should alert the clinician to several possibilities.

(2) Vertical nystagmus acquired in childhood may occur with or without retraction during the upbeat. It suggests the possibility of a chiasmal lesion and, therefore, neuroimaging, preferably by magnetic resonance imaging, is indicated. Downbeat nystagmus is equally serious and suggests the possibility of posterior fossa or brainstem lesion. As with upbeat nystagmus, downbeat nystagmus indicates that neuroimaging is needed.

(3) Ocular flutter or opsoclonus occurs in patients with neuroblastoma. Chaotic horizontal, vertical, and rotary large amplitude eye movements may occur in a so-called central nervous system crisis from a variety of causes, including fever or seizure disorders. Nystagmus or nystagmoid (nonrhythmic) eye movements can occur from a variety of brainstem lesions that may be vascular, traumatic, demyelinating, or pressure induced. A special category of acquired nystagmus in childhood is spasmus nutans, which is a unilateral, usually horizontal nystagmus with head nodding and torticollis. Recent studies have indicated the importance of neuroimaging in such patients.[23 p.362]

1.35

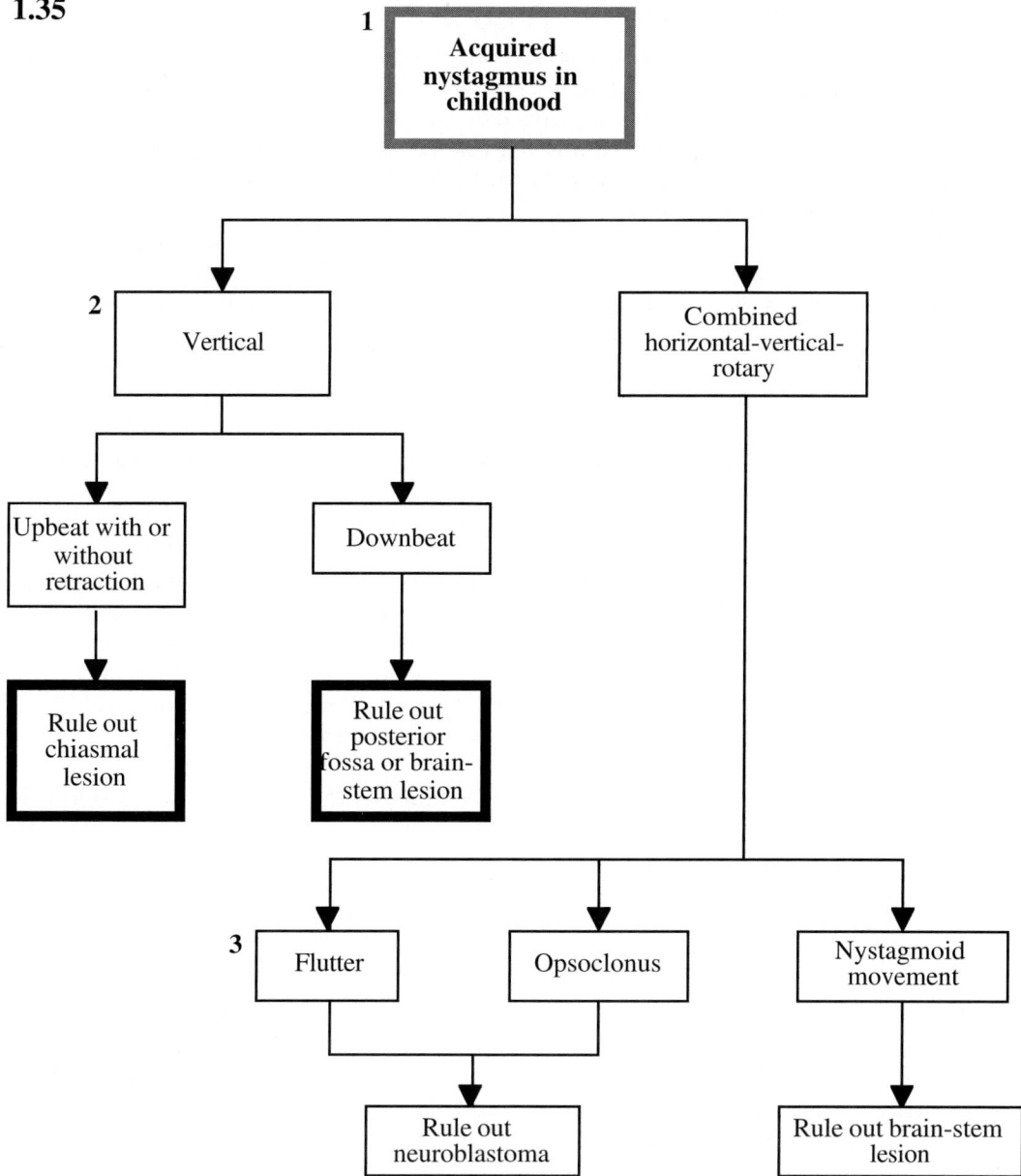

1.36   **Evaluation of Fusional Vergence**

The alignment of the eyes is maintained by motor fusion. This reflex is driven by retinal image disparity. In the normal state retinal image disparity produces diplopia. Motor fusion then triggers a vergence response to align the images of the object of regard on the two foveas. Visual objects brought closer to the observer produce temporal disparity and elicit convergence. Divergence is triggered when visual objects move farther away and produce nasal disparity. Similarly, vertical vergence (sursumvergence and deorsumvergence) and cyclovergence correct for vertical and torsional retinal image disparities. For clinical purposes, testing of fusional vergences is performed to assess the power and stability of motor fusion and the patient's capacity to compensate for underlying heterophorias.

(1) The amplitudes of fusional vergences are tested by artificially inducing retinal image disparity. Methods to measure the amplitude vary according to the preferences of different examiners.

(2) A prism bar with gradually increasing horizontal or vertical prisms is moved before one eye while the patient fixates on a muscle light at 33 cm and 6 M fixation distance. When the patient experiences double vision, the **breakpoint** of fusion has been reached. The prism power is then reduced until the double images can be fused again to determine the **recovery point.** Fusional divergence is always measured first.[57 p.191] The fusional amplitude depends on the amount of fusable material in the field of view of the person examined.

(3) The use of a rotary prism has the advantage of increasing or decreasing prismatic power more smoothly than with prism bars.

(4) Two disadvantages of use of the haploscope are that the fusible material is decreased and that proximal convergence may play a role.

(5) For averages of horizontal and vertical fusional amplitudes in normal subjects, see reference 57. [p.193]

(6) Cyclofusion occurs predominantly on a sensory basis. The amplitudes of cyclofusion are infrequently measured and no standard testing procedure exists. Such measurements, although of theoretic interest, are clinically of lesser value.

1.36

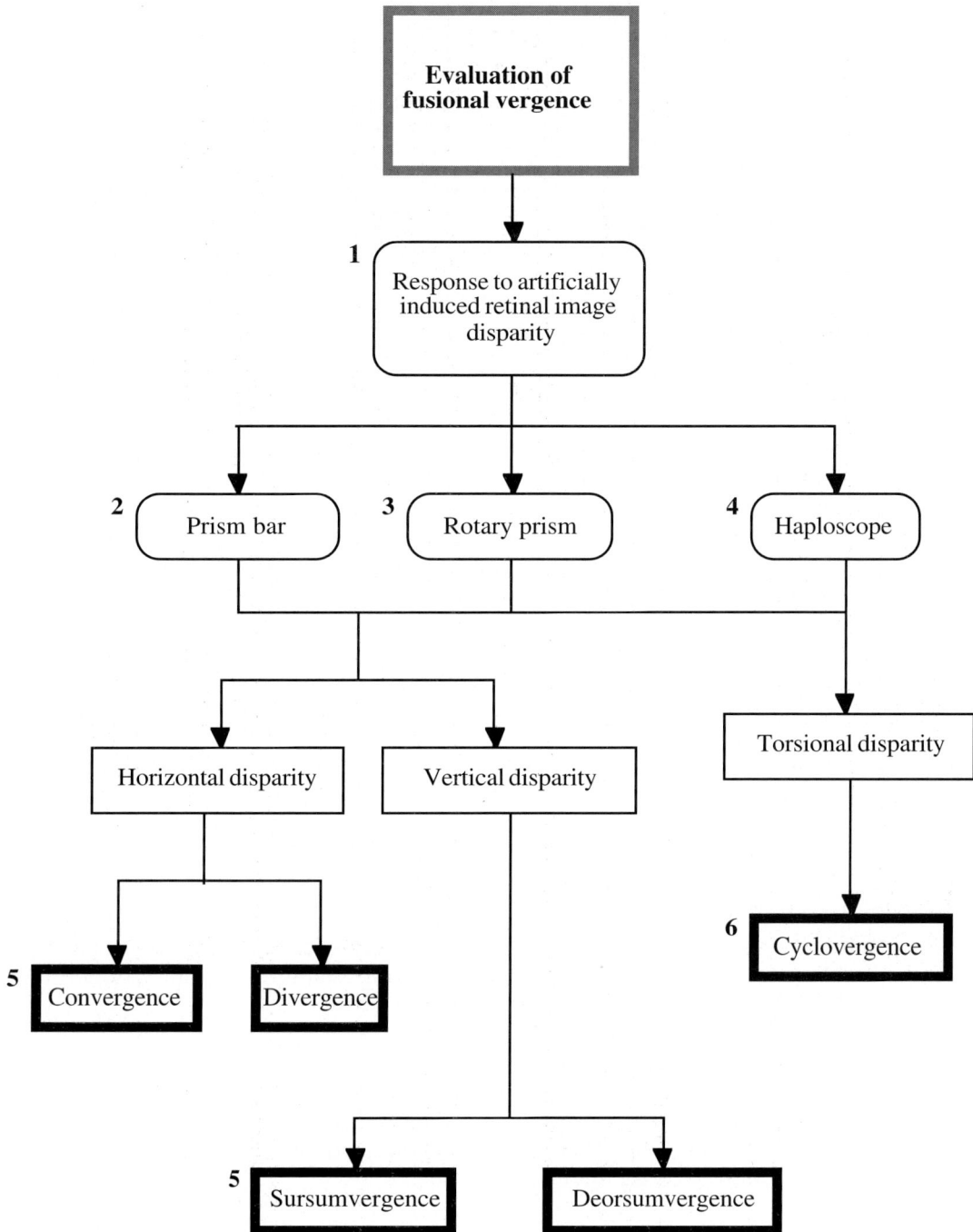

1.37   Evaluation of the Sensory State

(1) The sensory state is evaluated while the patient performs certain visual tasks with both eyes open.

(2) **See 1.33.**

(3) Visual confusion occurs when the patient notes the overlap of two different images at the same point in visual space.[57 p.201] Visual confusion is not often reported spontaneously but may be a most distressing symptom in strabismus of recent onset. It is caused by subjective localization of different foveal images in a common visual direction during the initial phase of strabismus, before suppression develops or the patient has learned to ignore the second image.[57 p.207]

(4) Some patients with manifest strabismus deny seeing double because they are ignoring the image seen by the deviating eye. Further questioning by the examiner may reveal that the patient actually does see double. In others a light red filter held before one eye quickly makes the patient aware of the second image.

(5) The Worth 4-dot and the Bagolini tests should be performed at near and distance fixation.[56 pp.70,90]

(6) A "normal" response (4 dots on the Worth or a cross on the Bagolini test) may indicate fusion or, in the presence of a manifest strabismus, abnormal binocular vision on the basis of anomalous retinal correspondence.

(7) The diagnosis of motor and sensory fusion is not sufficient to establish the presence of normal binocular vision. This is present only when fusion is accompanied by normal stereopsis.

(8) When the patient sees either 3 or 2 dots instead of 4 dots on the Worth test or one instead of two lines on the Bagolini test, suppression is present. Five lights on the 4-dot test or two stripes with the Bagolini lenses with the intersection below or above the midpoint, indicates diplopia.[57 p.251]

(9) The afterimage and Bagolini striated lenses are used most commonly in clinical practice to assess the state of retinal correspondence. At times the patient may give different responses on both tests. This is important information to determine the depth of the sensorial adaptation in strabismus.[57 p.254]

(10) Amblyopia **(see 2.01)** and anomalous retinal correspondence may coexist in a patient who habitually prefers one eye for fixation. In that case, visual acuity may be reduced in the nonfixating eye and the tests for anomalous retinal correspondence may be positive. In alternating strabismus, amblyopia is absent but anomalous retinal correspondence may exist.

(11) **See 2.01.**

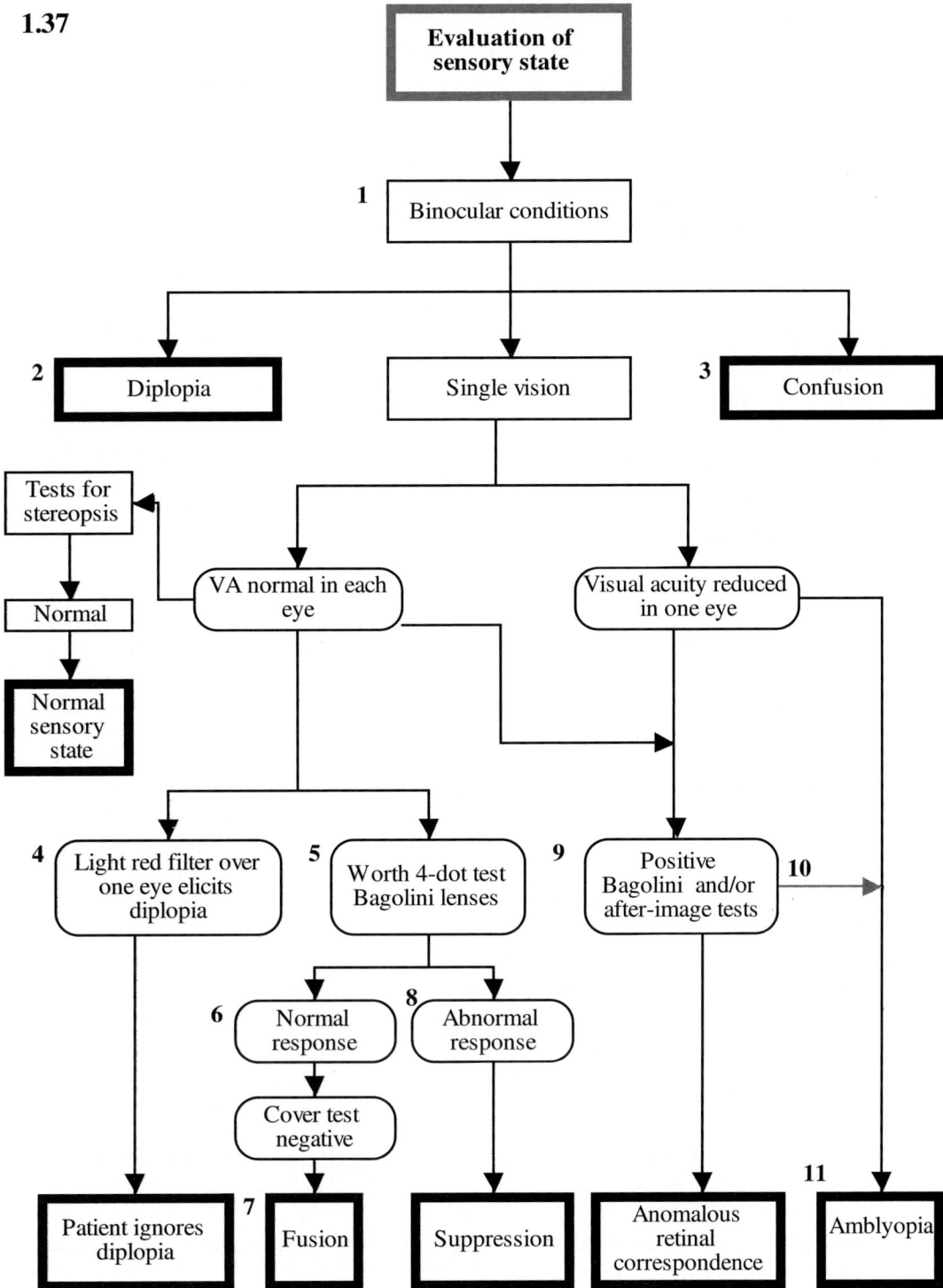

1.37

Evaluation of sensory state

1 Binocular conditions

2 Diplopia   Single vision   3 Confusion

Tests for stereopsis

Normal

Normal sensory state

VA normal in each eye   Visual acuity reduced in one eye

4 Light red filter over one eye elicits diplopia   5 Worth 4-dot test Bagolini lenses   9 Positive Bagolini and/or after-image tests   10

6 Normal response   8 Abnormal response

Cover test negative

Patient ignores diplopia   7 Fusion   Suppression   Anomalous retinal correspondence   11 Amblyopia

1.38   Ptosis in the Patient With Strabismus

(1) Ptosis is frequently found in the patient with strabismus. The ptosis may be true ptosis or a pseudoptosis. The ptosis may be related or unrelated to the cause of the strabismus.

(2) Ptosis is a common, almost constant, accompaniment of ocular myasthenia. The ptosis may be unilateral or bilateral but is always variable. Observing improvement of ptosis during the Tensilon test is an important diagnostic feature in ocular myasthenia. Changes in motility after administration of Tensilon are much less reliable predictors of a diagnosis of myasthenia.[23 p.525]

(3) Obtaining a positive family history for ptosis is an important part of the evaluation because ptosis from a variety of causes related to the levator itself or to the levator plus the extraocular muscles is common.

(4) Congenital fibrosis syndrome is transmitted as an autosomal dominant gene. It is characterized by bilateral blepharoptosis and deficient elevation with restricted elevation on forced ductions. Such patients characteristically keep the chin up and look downward.[23 p.518; 57 p.409]

(5) Patients with chronic progressive external ophthalmoplegia (CPEO) may be ocularly normal early in life, but ptosis and an inability to move the eyes in any direction gradually develop during the course of years. The main clinical symptoms are manifested during the teen years. This condition can be associated with heart block in the Kearns-Sayre syndrome. Patients with CPEO should always have an EKG to detect heart block.[23 p.524]

(6) When ptosis disappears while the patient fixates with the ptotic eye, pseudoptosis must be suspected. A common cause is an incomplete paralysis (paresis) of the superior rectus muscle, which causes hypotropia with pseudoptosis of the involved eye. A less common cause is a superior oblique muscle paralysis of the contralateral eye and habitual fixation preference with the paralyzed eye. When such a patient fixates in the field of action of the paralyzed superior oblique muscle, its yoke muscle, the contralateral inferior rectus, receives excess innervation according to Hering's law. According to Sherrington's law, the antagonist of the yoke muscle, the superior rectus, together with the levator palpebrae, receives less than normal innervation and hypotropia accompanied by ptosis develops. This has been called "inhibitional palsy of the contralateral antagonist".[57 p.367]

(7) Patients with third nerve palsy and double elevator palsy may have persistent ptosis when the nonptotic fixing eye is occluded.

(8) After extensive resection of the superior rectus muscle, ptosis may occur because the levator palpebrae is pulled forward.[23 p.318]

1.38

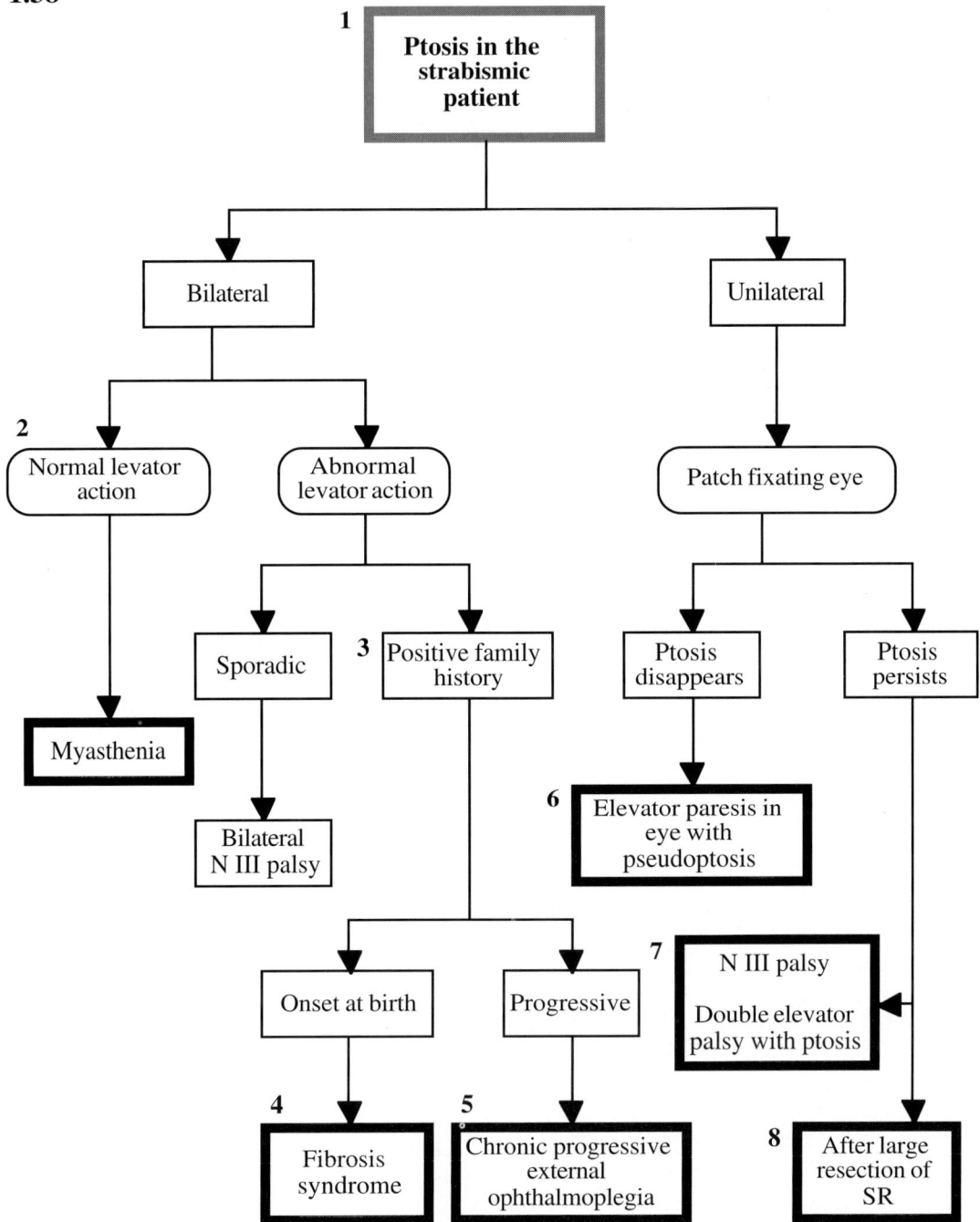

Flowchart: Ptosis in the strabismic patient

1 **Ptosis in the strabismic patient**

Bilateral

Unilateral

2 Normal levator action

Abnormal levator action

Patch fixating eye

Myasthenia

Sporadic

3 Positive family history

Ptosis disappears

Ptosis persists

Bilateral N III palsy

6 Elevator paresis in eye with pseudoptosis

Onset at birth

Progressive

7 N III palsy

Double elevator palsy with ptosis

4 Fibrosis syndrome

5 Chronic progressive external ophthalmoplegia

8 After large resection of SR

2

Diagnostic and Treatment Decisions

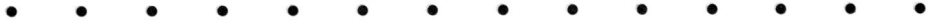

• • • • • • • • • • • • • • • •

2.01 Amblyopia: Diagnosis and Classification

(1) Amblyopia is defined as a unilateral or bilateral decrease of visual acuity for which no organic cause can be detected on physical examination of the eye and which in appropriate cases is reversible by therapeutic measures.[57] p.208 This algorithm is based on the assumption that visual acuity has been found to be decreased **(see 1.06)** and cannot be improved by corrective lenses.

(2) A negative cover test result rules out a manifest heterotropia. At this point in the examination, the examiner must establish that there is no history of previous strabismus that may have improved spontaneously or with glasses or after surgery. If this history is positive, strabismic amblyopia must be suspected **(see 2.02).**

(3) A refraction establishes whether anisometropic amblyopia is present. A fundus examination rules out organic causes for the decrease in visual acuity. A functional (i.e., reversible) amblyopia may be superimposed on a lesion of the optic disc or the macula (relative amblyopia). The fixation behavior must be checked in all cases of suspected unilateral amblyopia. This test is performed with a modified ophthalmoscope that contains a fixation target that is projected on the fundus and is seen by both the examiner and the patient.[57] p.220 The 4^Δ base-out prism test is positive in anisometropic amblyopia.[56] p.72

(4) The exact refractive difference between the eyes that causes amblyopia is unknown. However, most clinicians agree that a spherical equivalent of more than 1.5 diopters between the eyes may be amblyopiogenic.

(5) In the absence of a positive cover test result, a history of strabismus or of anisometropia, the examiner should question the patient or the parents carefully for a history of unilateral occlusion during infancy and early childhood. Causes for unilateral visual deprivation include a unilateral ptosis, cataract, orbital cellulitis with swelling of the lids, and prolonged wearing of an occlusive patch.

(6) In the absence of a positive cover test result, of anisometropia, a history of strabismus or of visual deprivation, an idiopathic amblyopia (i.e., an amblyopia without known cause) may be present.[58]

(7) Anisometropia is fairly common in a strabismic population. It is not always possible to ascertain whether the amblyopia in such patients is caused by the strabismus, the anisometropia, or a combination of both. Strabismus may also occur as a result of decreased vision in one eye, for instance, a macular retinoblastoma. A careful examination of the fundus is therefore indicated in all cases of

amblyopia associated with strabismus. The fixation behavior is recorded as foveolar, parafoveolar, parafoveal, or peripheral.[57 p.219]

(8) Uncorrected high bilateral hypermetropia of an equal degree may cause bilateral visual deprivation amblyopia. The patient makes no effort to accommodate and grows up with chronically blurred retinal images (bilateral visual deprivation). A manifest congenital nystagmus may have a similar effect on the development of normal visual acuity.

(9) When there is no detectable cause for bilaterally reduced visual acuity, special tests are indicated to rule out rare diseases such as cone deficiency disorder.

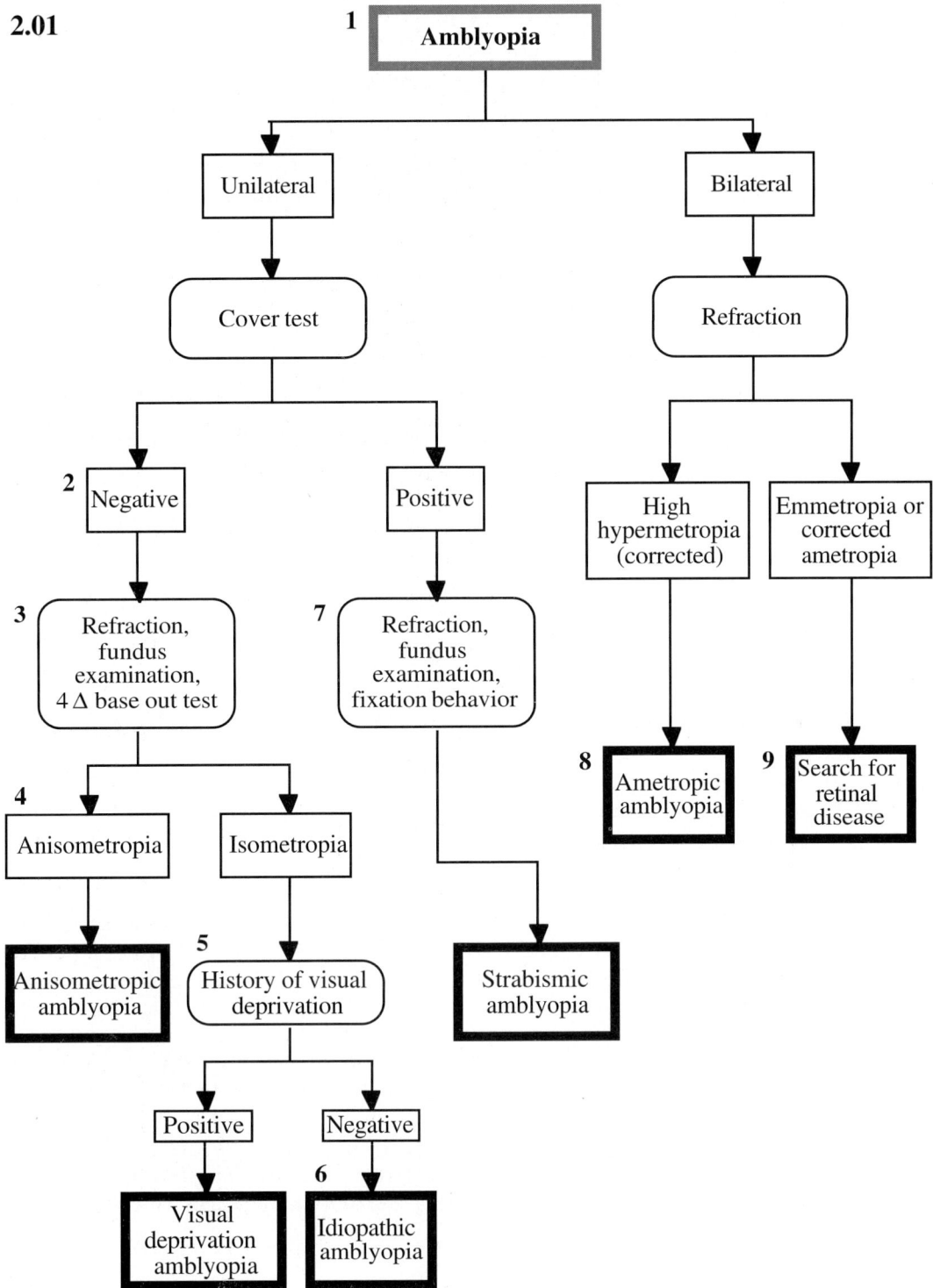

2.01

1 **Amblyopia**

Unilateral

Bilateral

Cover test

Refraction

2 Negative

Positive

High hypermetropia (corrected)

Emmetropia or corrected ametropia

3 Refraction, fundus examination, 4 Δ base out test

7 Refraction, fundus examination, fixation behavior

8 Ametropic amblyopia

9 Search for retinal disease

4 Anisometropia

Isometropia

Anisometropic amblyopia

5 History of visual deprivation

Strabismic amblyopia

Positive

Negative

6

Visual deprivation amblyopia

Idiopathic amblyopia

2.02   **Strabismic Amblyopia: Treatment**

(1) The goal of amblyopia treatment is to normalize visual acuity of the amblyopic eye or, when this is not possible, to improve it to its optimal level. Once this has been accomplished, visual acuity must be maintained at that level.

(2) Before occlusion treatment for amblyopia, a significant refractive error of the amblyopic eye should be corrected to create optimal functional conditions for that eye.

(3) We prefer to use an adhesive patch attached to the skin and occluding the sound eye regardless of the fixation behavior of the amblyopic eye.

(4) Children younger than 6 or 7 years of age are susceptible to visual deprivation, and amblyopia may develop in the occluded eye. This risk is higher during the first 2 years of life and decreases with increasing age. To prevent visual deprivation amblyopia, occlusion of the sound eye is combined with alternate occlusion of the amblyopic eye. The rhythm of this alternation must be modified according to the sensitivity to the treatment. The suggestions given in this algorithm are only general guidelines and may be modified according to each patient's individual sensitivity to occlusion treatment.[57 p.471]

(5) Older children tolerate constant patching of the sound eye for 4- to 6-week periods. Visual deprivation amblyopia, if it occurs, is rapidly reversible by brief periods of patching the amblyopic eye.

(6) Once visual acuity has been equalized, the goal of treatment has been reached.

(7) In children who cannot tolerate a patch (skin sensitivity, severe behavioral problems) penalization may be considered.[57 p.471] It is not as effective as occlusion treatment and should not be considered as a primary form of therapy.

(8) Total penalization blurs the sound eye at near and distance fixation. This can be accomplished by removing the spectacle lens from the sound eye of a patient with hypermetropia (distance penalization) and atropinization of that eye (near penalization).

(9) Partial penalization consists of blurring the sound eye optically at near or distance fixation; this has been less successful in our experience.[57 p.471]

(10) Alternating penalization is successful in preventing recurrence of amblyopia. Two pair of spectacles are prescribed, one overcorrecting the right eye and the other overcorrecting the left eye with +3.00 diopter spherical lenses.

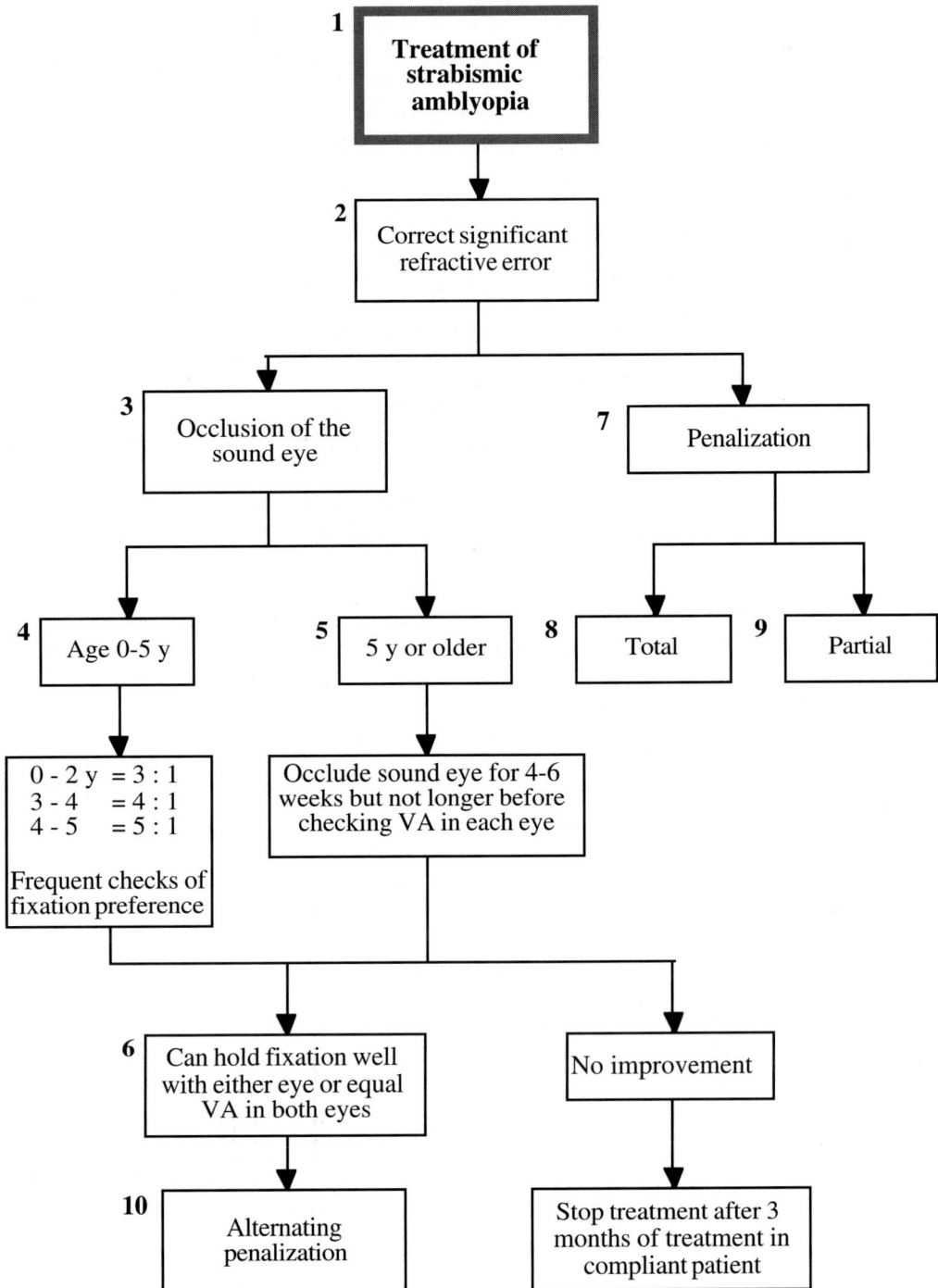

2.02

```
                              ┌─────────────────┐
                          1   │   Treatment of  │
                              │   strabismic    │
                              │    amblyopia    │
                              └────────┬────────┘
                                       │
                                       ▼
                          2   ┌─────────────────┐
                              │ Correct significant │
                              │ refractive error │
                              └────────┬────────┘
```

1 Treatment of strabismic amblyopia

2 Correct significant refractive error

3 Occlusion of the sound eye

7 Penalization

4 Age 0-5 y

5 5 y or older

8 Total

9 Partial

0 - 2 y = 3 : 1
3 - 4 = 4 : 1
4 - 5 = 5 : 1

Frequent checks of fixation preference

Occlude sound eye for 4-6 weeks but not longer before checking VA in each eye

6 Can hold fixation well with either eye or equal VA in both eyes

No improvement

10 Alternating penalization

Stop treatment after 3 months of treatment in compliant patient

2.03   Anisometropic Amblyopia: Treatment

(1) In patients with amblyopia who have never had optical correction, a trial with spectacle correction alone should be made before occlusion is considered or a contact lens is fitted. It is surprising how frequently visual acuity improves with no further therapy.

(2) If visual acuity continues to improve without occlusion, no additional treatment except correction of the refractive error is indicated. When no further improvement occurs, and provided visual acuity is not equal, occlusion of the sound eye is added to the therapy.

(3) If no improvement has occurred after spectacle correction for 6 weeks the sound eye is patched. The same precautions that were mentioned at **2.02** to prevent visual deprivation amblyopia of the sound eye apply during occlusion treatment of anisometropic amblyopia.

(4) As in cases of strabismic amblyopia, the goal of treatment of anisometropic amblyopia is to equalize visual acuity in both eyes and, when this is not possible, to optimize visual acuity of the amblyopic eye. Once treatment is discontinued, efforts should be made to maintain visual acuity in the formerly amblyopic eye by optical penalization.[57 p.471]

(5) Glasses or a contact lens are prescribed according to a patient's individual needs or tolerance. Successfully treated anisometropic amblyopia can result in equal vision and normal sensory fusion in some cases, especially with low degrees of anisometropia.

2.03

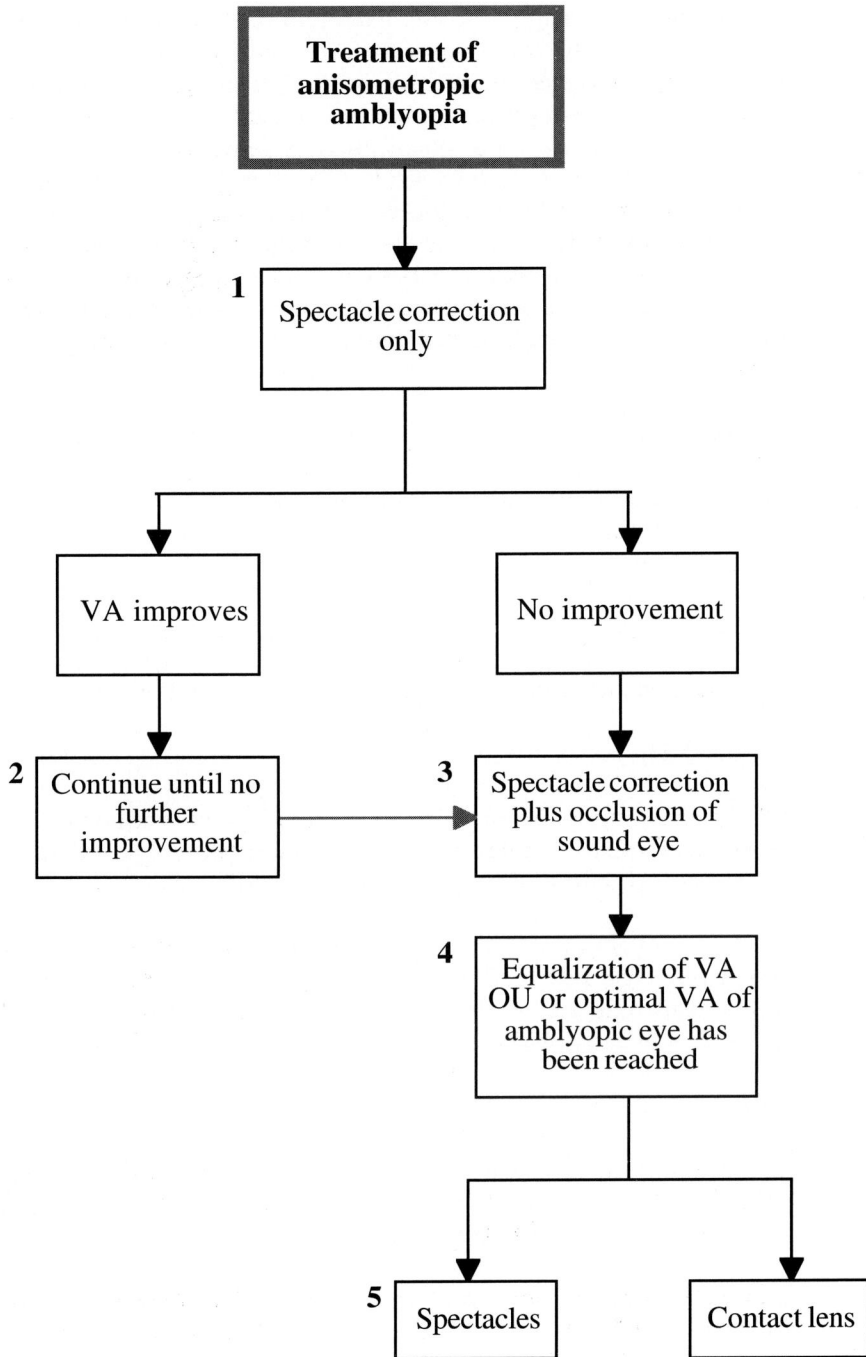

2.04 Essential Infantile Esotropia: Diagnostic Evaluation

(1) The infant with esotropia is usually brought for initial treatment by the parents while the child is held in the mother's arms. The complete evaluation of such an infant for the presence of essential infantile esotropia can be completed in a short time with little discomfort to the infant.[23 p.394]

(2) Before progressing with the examination, it is important to obtain a history **(see 1.02)** from the family and to record this history in the chart. The infant's birth weight and the family history for strabismus should always be recorded. The timing of onset of the deviation is essential. Most infants with essential infantile esotropia are reported by their parents to have had crossed eyes since birth or shortly after. Parents tend to fixate on the times that the child's eyes are crossed rather than the interludes of straight eyes. Technically, essential infantile esotropia can be diagnosed by age 4 months. Convention has established that an esotropia confirmed by a reliable observer by 6 months of age is considered to have been present sufficiently early to qualify for the diagnosis of infantile esotropia. An esodeviation that begins after 6 months may be an acquired esotropia.

(3) **See 1.03.**

(4) Gross motor evaluation usually reveals general developmental delay or cerebral palsy in an infant so affected. However, in the very young child, this may be overlooked at the initial examination.

(5) **See 1.25.**

(6) Spasmus nutans may require neurologic evaluation.[23 p.362]

(7) **See 2.33.**

(8) Determining whether an infant prefers fixation with one eye or the other can be challenging. Most infants object to having either eye occluded. The cover test in an infant should be done in a nonthreatening way.

(9) Motor evaluation is usually carried out binocularly by evaluating versions **(see 1.10).** This may be done by rotating the baby to elicit the oculocephalic or doll's head reflex. It is virtually impossible to evaluate ductions in infants because they usually object strongly to having one eye covered.

(10) **See 1.07.**

(11) The testing of sensory functions in infants is limited because of lack of reliable subjective responses. However, the presence of sensory anomalies can often be inferred from other findings during the examination.

(12) Retinoscopy is done in all infants with esotropia. A hypermetropia of +3.00 diopters or greater indicates the need to rule out a refractive accommodative component.

(13) Examination of the fundus and the media is essential in an infant with esotropia to rule out pathologic conditions such as cataract, coloboma, optic nerve hypoplasia, or atrophy and retinal tumors.

2.04

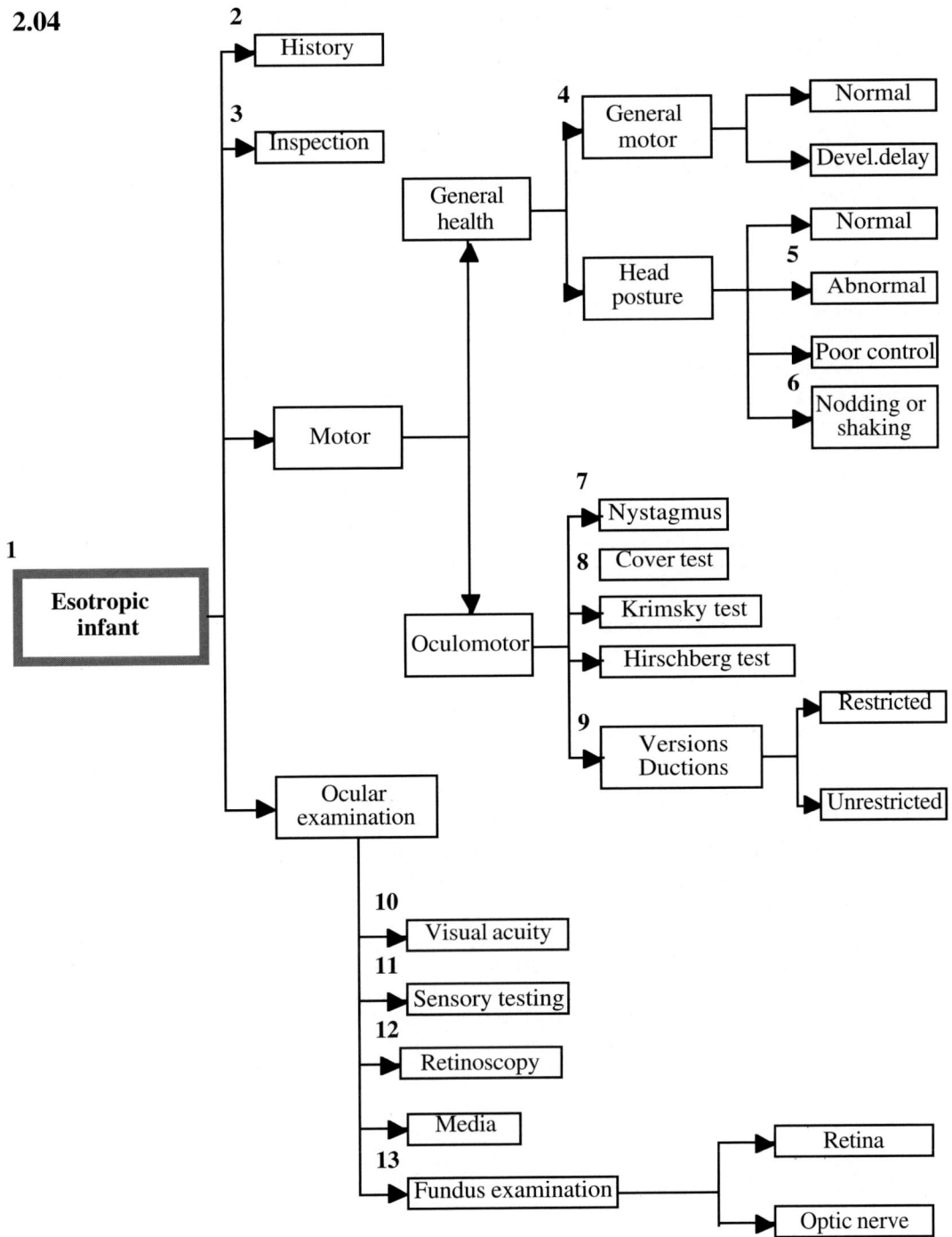

- **1** Esotropic infant
  - **2** History
  - **3** Inspection
  - Motor
    - General health
      - **4** General motor
        - Normal
        - Devel.delay
      - Head posture
        - Normal
        - **5** Abnormal
        - Poor control
        - **6** Nodding or shaking
    - Oculomotor
      - **7** Nystagmus
      - **8** Cover test
      - Krimsky test
      - Hirschberg test
      - **9** Versions Ductions
        - Restricted
        - Unrestricted
  - Ocular examination
    - **10** Visual acuity
    - **11** Sensory testing
    - **12** Retinoscopy
    - Media
    - **13** Fundus examination
      - Retina
      - Optic nerve

2.05 Essential Infantile Esotropia: Treatment

(1) A cycloplegic refraction and fundus examination must be performed at the end of the initial examination; the results determine the course of therapy. In uncooperative children this examination may have to be performed with the child under general anesthesia. Under no circumstances should therapy be initiated without knowledge of the refractive error and without having visualized the fundus.

(2) A mild hypermetropia of up to +3.00 diopters spherical is physiologic in infants and young children, and its optical correction usually has no significant effect on the esotropia. However, we routinely prescribe glasses, at least for a period of time, for hypermetropia in excess of that amount. Refractive accommodative esotropia, although usually seen between the first and second year of life, may occasionally occur in infants and respond well to optical correction.[23 p.553]

(3) Once the decision is made to correct the hypermetropia in a patient with esotropia, the full refractive error should be prescribed and is usually well accepted by the patient. In case of poor acceptance, atropinization of both eyes for 3 days is often helpful in getting the patient to tolerate the glasses.

(4) Spontaneous alternation signals the absence of amblyopia.

(5) **See 2.02.**

(6) The type of surgery for essential infantile esotropia depends on the fixation preference. With alternating fixation or in the absence of strong fixation preference, we prefer a recession of both medial rectus muscles. In case of strong fixation preference, we recess the medial rectus and resect the lateral rectus muscle of the nonfixating eye. The amount depends on the age of the child and the size of the deviation. For details see references 23 [p.418] and 57. [p.304]

(7) Botulinum injections into the medial rectus muscles have been recommended by some authors,[51] but this method of treatment has not been established as an acceptable alternative to surgical treatment of essential infantile esotropia.

2.05

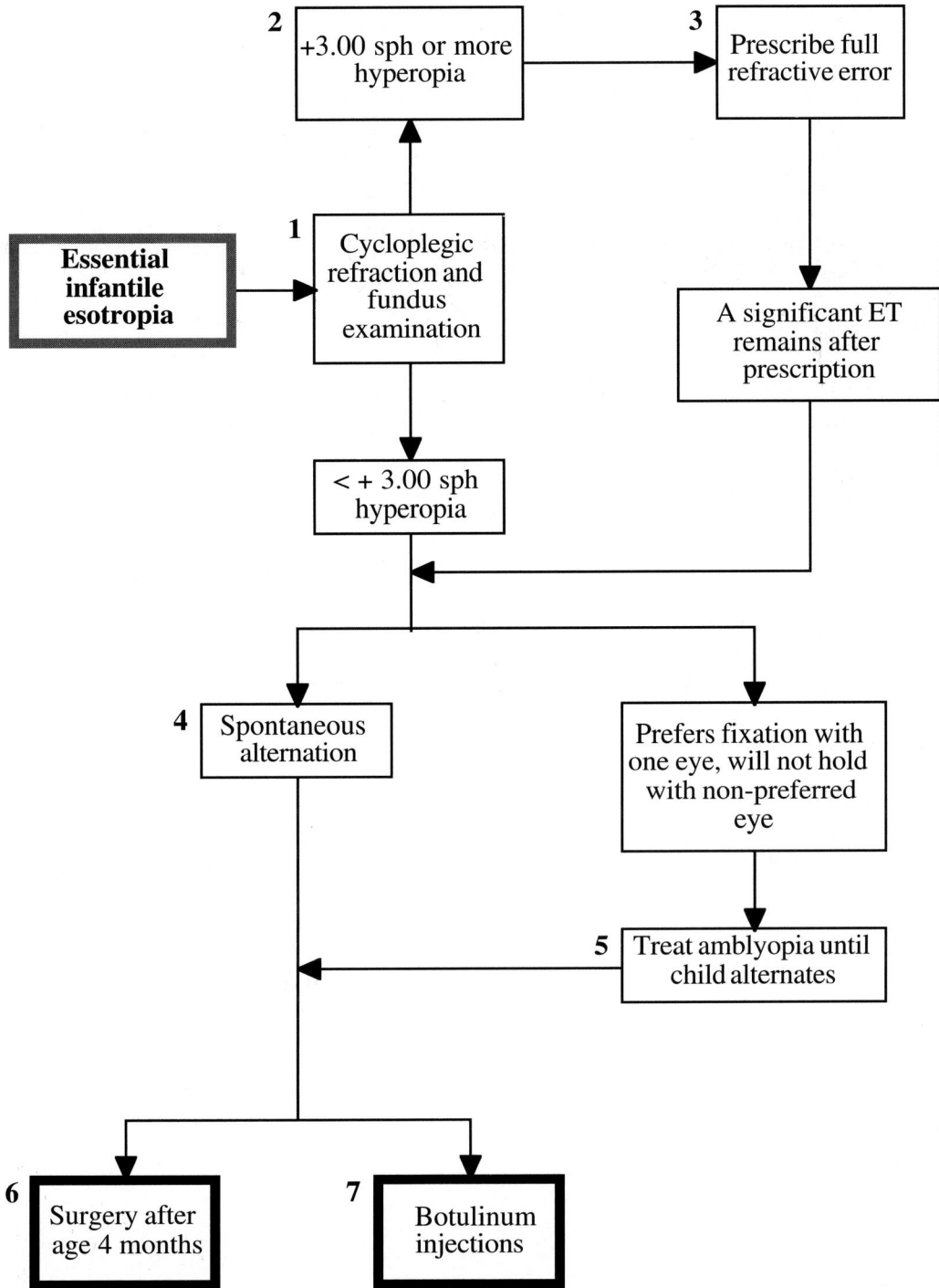

2.06   Acquired Esotropia

(1) Any esotropia that is not present at birth or which occurs during the first 6 months of life (essential infantile esotropia) is called acquired esotropia.

(2) Acute esotropia; **see 2.10.**

(3) Injury to or disinsertion of the lateral rectus muscle occurs infrequently. However, this extraocular muscle is more exposed to traumatic events than the others; we have seen disinserted lateral rectus muscles after a dog bite and other orbital trauma. More frequent is a lateral rectus muscle that becomes partially disinserted or is "lost" during surgery.[23 p.324] In the first case, abduction may only be slightly limited; in the second, the limitation is usually severe.

(4) The medial rectus muscle may become involved in endocrine orbitopathy **(see 2.55)** and cause restriction of abduction.

(5) After a sixth nerve palsy of extended duration, secondary contracture of the medial rectus muscle causes restriction of abduction **(see 2.45).** Forced duction testing confirms this diagnosis and estimation of the generated muscle force establishes whether residual lateral rectus function is present.[23 p.262; 57 p.375]

(6) This complication of strabismus surgery is accompanied by excessive adduction and a positive traction test result.

(7) Enlargement of a myopic globe may cause limitation of ductions.[12]

(8) A severe unilateral reduction of visual acuity in one eye during infancy may cause with equal frequency either esotropia or exotropia of that eye. In older children or adults an exotropia is more likely to occur.[52]

(9) **See 1.21.**

(10) **See 1.19.**

(11) **See 1.21 and 2.07.**

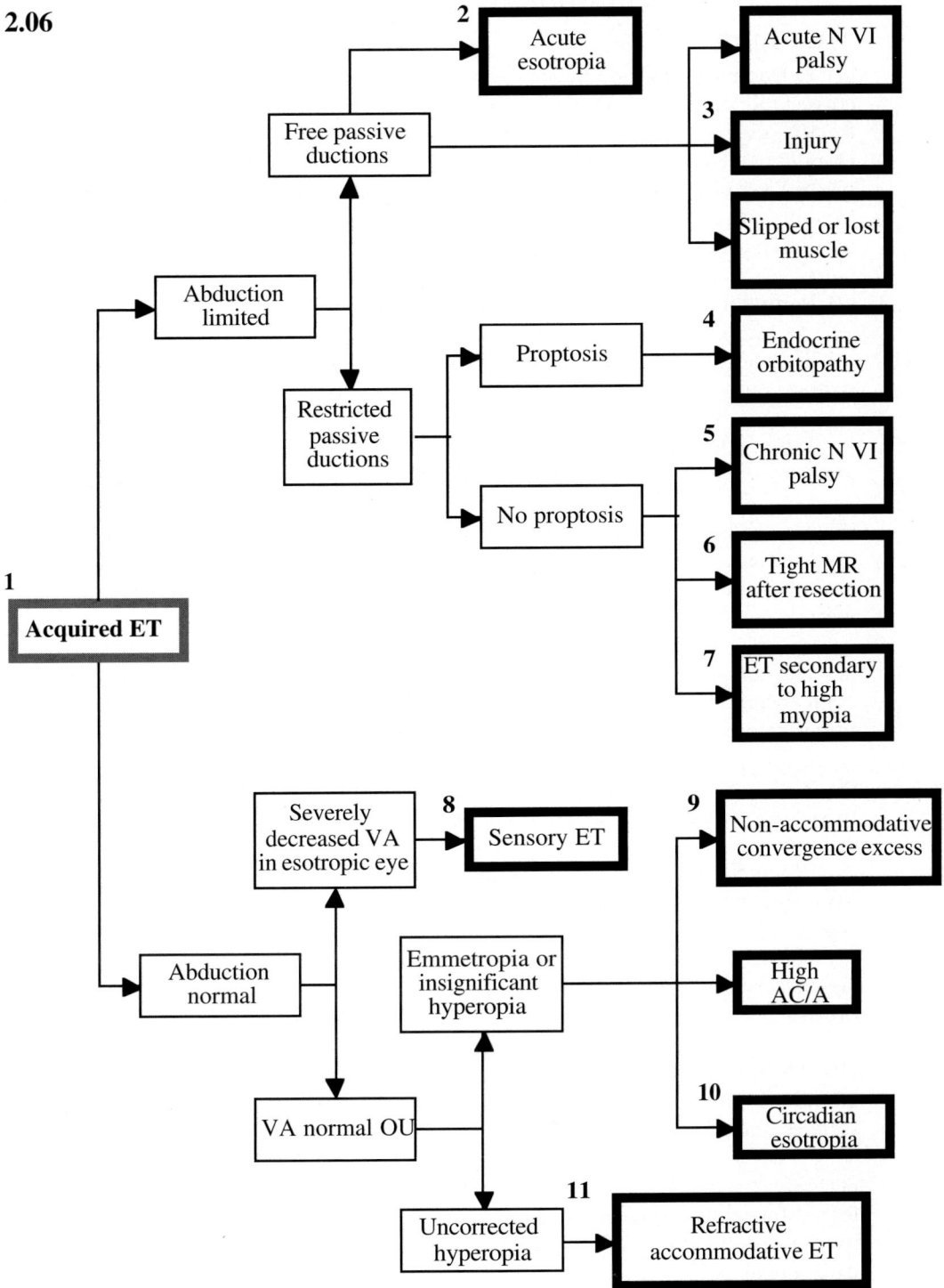

2.06

1
Acquired ET

Abduction limited

Free passive ductions

2 Acute esotropia

Acute N VI palsy

3 Injury

Slipped or lost muscle

Restricted passive ductions

Proptosis

4 Endocrine orbitopathy

No proptosis

5 Chronic N VI palsy

6 Tight MR after resection

7 ET secondary to high myopia

Abduction normal

Severely decreased VA in esotropic eye

8 Sensory ET

9 Non-accommodative convergence excess

Emmetropia or insignificant hyperopia

High AC/A

VA normal OU

10 Circadian esotropia

Uncorrected hyperopia

11 Refractive accommodative ET

2.07   Refractive Accommodative Esotropia: Etiology and Treatment

(1) Refractive accommodative esotropia is defined as an esotropia that is fully correctable at all fixation distances by optical correction of the hypermetropic refractive error. The mechanism of this form of strabismus has been known since Donders (1884) discovered the relationship between accommodation and convergence.[57 p.85] However, not all uncorrected hypermetropes become esotropic. Factors other than accommodation are important in the etiology of refractive accommodative esotropia and are included in this algorithm.

(2) Retinal image blur triggers accommodation to focus the image.

(3) This accommodative effort elicits accommodative convergence at distance fixation and at near fixation.

(4) When fusional divergence is sufficient to overcome this excessive convergence innervation, fusion is preserved but an esophoria is now present.

(5) No correction is required if the hypermetropia is mild or moderate, the patient remains asymptomatic, and fusion is stable. However, regular return visits are advisable if the esophoria becomes intermittent or if symptoms develop, in which case the refractive error should be corrected with glasses.

(6) The convergence innervation induced by accommodative effort is reduced or even absent in patients with a low or flat AC/A ratio. In such cases, the esodeviation is minimal or even absent, although the hypermetropia remains uncorrected.

(7) Such patients may have orthotropia despite a large uncorrected hypermetropic refractive error.[63] These patients are at risk for ametropic amblyopia.

(8) When fusional divergence is insufficient to overcome the excessive convergence innervation, constant esotropia develops.

(9) The AC/A ratio must be normal (or greater than normal) to produce excessive accommodative convergence from uncorrected hypermetropia and thus esotropia.

(10) Optical correction of the refractive error is required to treat refractive accommodative esotropia. Surgery is contraindicated in patients whose esotropia is fully corrected in this manner.

(11) Some patients with uncorrected hypermetropia prefer blurred but single vision rather than the constant effort required to focus the retinal images by accommodation and the resulting diplopia. Bilateral ametropic amblyopia and a reduced near point of accommodation may be the consequence of this scenario.[63]

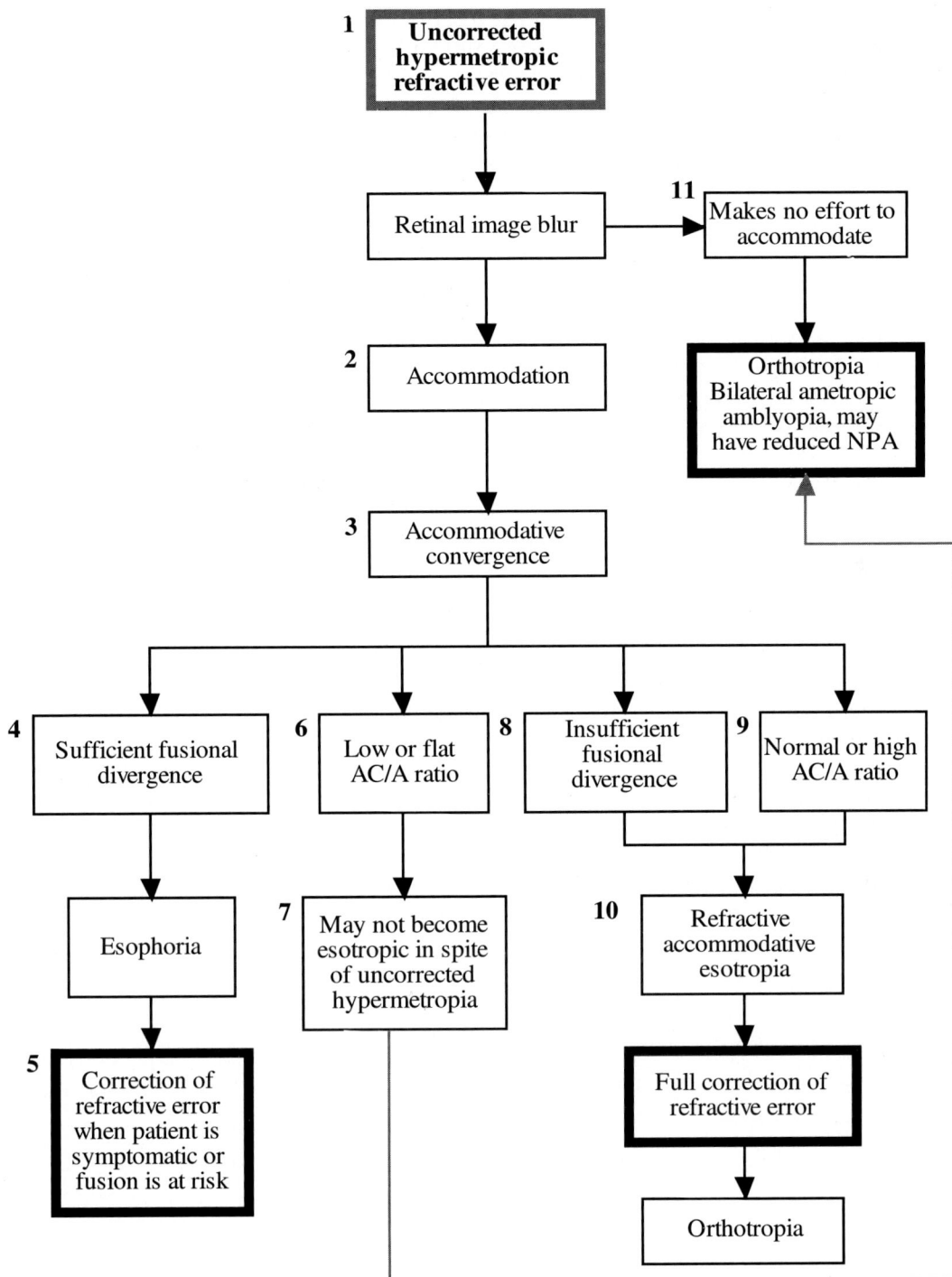

2.07

1 Uncorrected hypermetropic refractive error

↓

Retinal image blur → **11** Makes no effort to accommodate

↓ ↓

2 Accommodation

Orthotropia Bilateral ametropic amblyopia, may have reduced NPA

↓

3 Accommodative convergence

↓

4 Sufficient fusional divergence | **6** Low or flat AC/A ratio | **8** Insufficient fusional divergence | **9** Normal or high AC/A ratio

↓

Esophoria

↓

5 Correction of refractive error when patient is symptomatic or fusion is at risk

7 May not become esotropic in spite of uncorrected hypermetropia

10 Refractive accommodative esotropia

↓

Full correction of refractive error

↓

Orthotropia

2.08 Convergence Excess Type Esotropia

(1) There are different causes for esotropia with a near/distance disparity. It is not justified to conclude from the finding of an increased esodeviation at near fixation that a patient has a high AC/A ratio because other factors may be involved.[57 p.306] To determine the role of accommodation in causing the increased near deviation, the AC/A ratio is measured according to a simplification of the gradient method described below.[57 p.89]

(2) Plus 3.00 diopter lenses are added to the patient's prescription, and the deviation is measured while the patient fixates on an accommodative target at 33 cm distance. A decrease of the esodeviation of less than 15^Δ under these circumstances indicates a low AC/A ratio.

(3) Factors other than accommodative convergence must contribute to the increased near deviation. Among these, tonic and proximal convergence, or both, may contribute to nonaccommodative convergence excess.[57 p.141]

(4) Surgery consists of a recession of both medial rectus muscles with or without posterior fixation of these muscles. This approach has little effect on the esodeviation at distance fixation. The effect on the near deviation is variable; we have frequently observed a recurrence of the nonaccommodative convergence excess after an initial satisfactory response to surgery.[23 p.423; 57 p.306]

(5) Bifocals may be considered for a patient with orthotropia or who has a minimal angle of esotropia at distance fixation and an esotropia at near, that can be converted into an asymptomatic esophoria or orthotropia by means of additional plus lenses. The power of the bifocal lens needs to be titrated carefully; only the minimal lens power to achieve the treatment goal should be prescribed.[57 p.458]

(6) Two thirds of patients initially responsive to bifocals eventually require surgery.[68] Surgical intervention is indicated when a manifest deviation persists at near fixation despite maximal bifocal prescription. We use recession of both medial rectus muscles, supplemented by posterior fixations if the angle at near is variable.

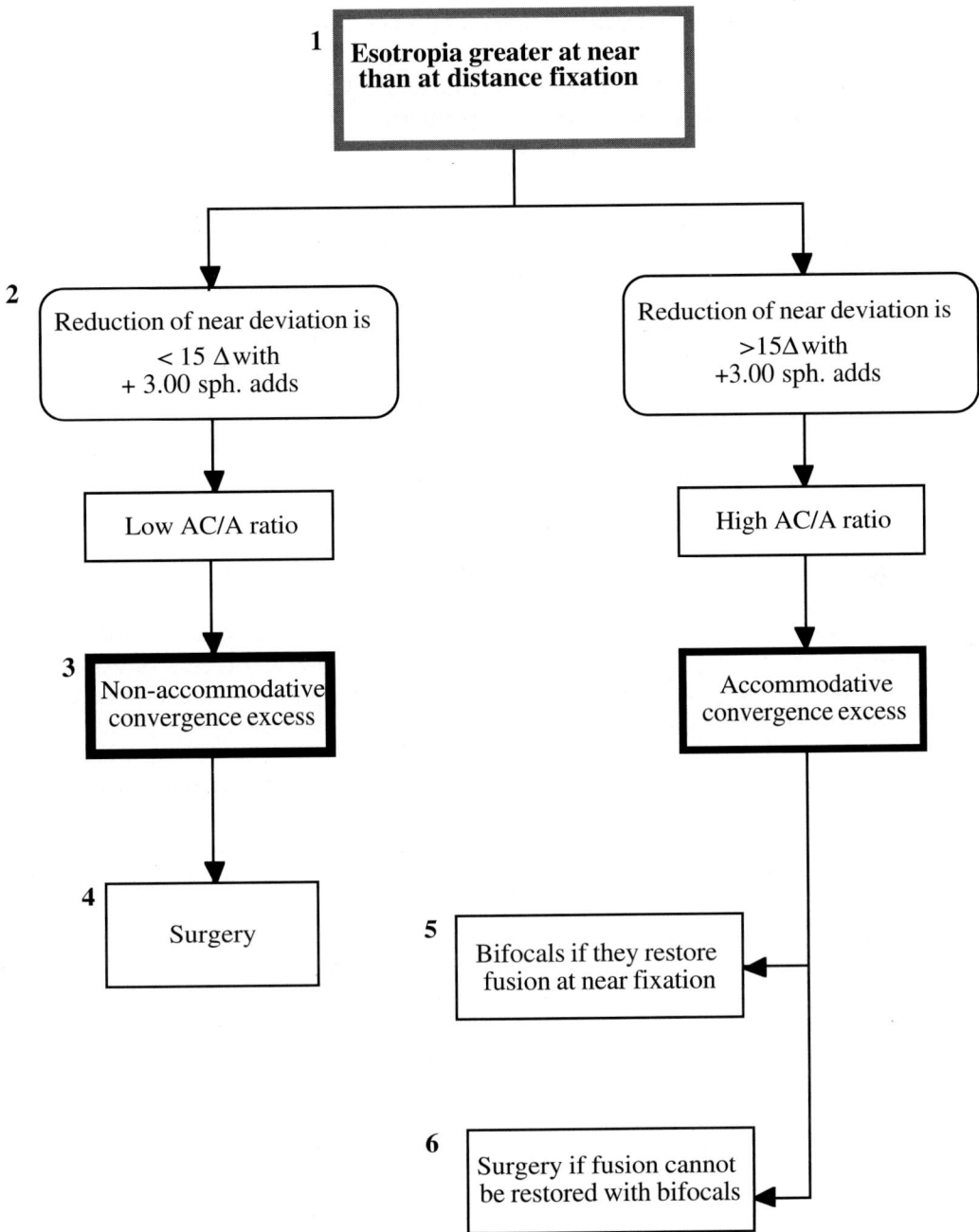

2.08

1 **Esotropia greater at near than at distance fixation**

2 Reduction of near deviation is
< 15 Δ with
+ 3.00 sph. adds

Reduction of near deviation is
>15Δ with
+3.00 sph. adds

Low AC/A ratio

High AC/A ratio

3 Non-accommodative
convergence excess

Accommodative
convergence excess

4 Surgery

5 Bifocals if they restore
fusion at near fixation

6 Surgery if fusion cannot
be restored with bifocals

2.09 Consecutive Esotropia

(1) An esodeviation is called consecutive when it occurs after surgery for exotropia or when an exotropia changes spontaneously into esotropia.

(2) When passive ductions are free in a patient with limited abduction, the lateral rectus muscle is not functioning properly.

(3) Postoperative lateral rectus underaction in the presence of normal passive ductions is caused by excessive recession of the lateral rectus muscle. This muscle must be brought forward to its original insertion with or without resection to restore normal abduction.[23 p.448]

(4) If no lateral rectus is found, a full tendon transfer shifting the superior and inferior rectus muscles to the insertion site of the lateral rectus is indicated.

(5) When passive ductions are restricted, the first requirement is to free the restriction. Restriction is usually caused by excessive resection of the medial rectus muscle and/or extensive scarring of the nasal conjunctiva.

(6) Recessing the medial rectus muscle and/or the nasal conjunctiva may be sufficient to release the restriction.[23 p.284]

(7) In larger consecutive esodeviations a resection or advancement of the lateral rectus muscle, or both is indicated in addition to medial rectus recession. If the esodeviation is greater at near and lateral rectus function is normal, bimedial rectus recession may be required.

(8) An esotropia occurs commonly after surgery for intermittent exotropia. If this consecutive deviation is relatively small (less than 10$^\Delta$) and if abduction is full or nearly full, it should not be treated. A slight overcorrection has been correlated with the most stable long term postoperative alignment of intermittent exotropia.

(9) An overcorrection larger than 10$^\Delta$ should be monitored and if treated it should be done so at first conservatively including some or all of the following: full plus correction, alternate patching, and fully correcting base out prism. Only if all conservative approaches have been exhausted is additional surgery indicated.[23 p.441; 57 p.335]

(10) A spontaneous change from exotropia to esotropia in the absence of an obvious cause such as fifth nerve palsy is rare and has been reported only once.[17]

2.09

3 Advance LR or recess MR

2 Free passive ductions

4 Transpose SR and IR to LR insertion

Limited abduction

5 Restricted passive ductions

6 Recess MR

7 Recess MR and resect or advance LR

After muscle surgery

9 Wait!

Base out prisms

In patients with fusional potential

Full plus or least minus correction

Patch

Repeat surgery as needed after above

1 **Consecutive esotropia**

8 Normal abduction

In patients without fusional potential

Repeat surgery after waiting

No prior surgery

10 Spontaneous change from XT to ET

2.10   Acute Esotropia

(1) Acute esotropia is always a disturbing experience for the patient who, because of double vision, promptly seeks medical attention. Children may be less likely to complain about double vision, but this symptom is apparent when parents notice that a child closes one eye or assumes an abnormal head posture. On examination the first decision must be whether the deviation is comitant or incomitant.

(2) In the acute stage, patients with abducens paralysis or paresis have grossly incomitant esotropia. However, with time, and especially in mild pareses, the deviation becomes increasingly comitant. Thus even a comitant deviation does not rule out a paretic origin **(see 2.45).**

(3) This condition is limited to childhood and is often preceded by an upper respiratory infection of viral origin.[32] Its course is benign and full restoration of function occurs. In some instances, contracture of the ipsilateral medial rectus muscle causes a residual esotropia even after the abducens paralysis has recovered; in such cases, surgery is required. Recurrences have been described.[4]

(4) Acute comitant esotropia may occur without obvious cause.[7] It appears that such patients have lost the ability to fuse an underlying esophoria, perhaps because of stress or fatigue. Double vision is a prominent symptom. An underlying uncorrected hypermetropia should be corrected. If the patient is emmetropic and results of a neurologic examination are negative, surgery is indicated.

(5) Fusional amplitudes may rapidly deteriorate in some patients after only brief disruption of binocular vision, such as after wearing an occlusive patch over one eye for a few days after a corneal injury or after minor surgery (chalazion). An esophoria previously controlled by fusional divergence may become manifest when the patch is removed.[57 p.307] Correction of an underlying hypermetropia should be the first step in treating these patients; surgery must be considered if no other cause can be found. If patching is considered for amblyopia in children with uncorrected significant hypermetropia, it is advisable to warn the parents that patching may trigger a strabismus that had not been present before.

2.10

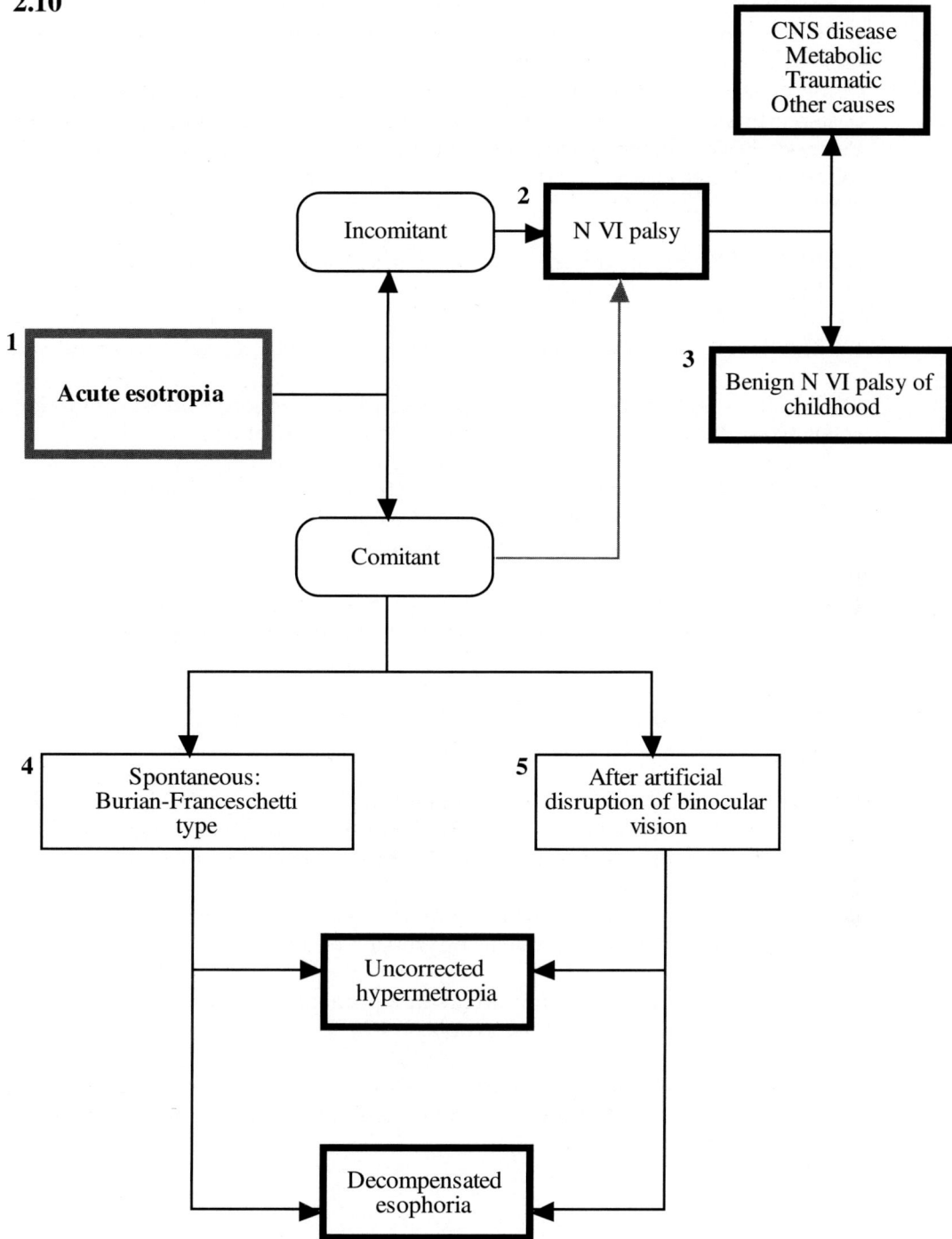

2.11   Microtropia and Subnormal Binocular Vision

(1) Ultrasmall angles of strabismus may escape diagnosis by conventional methods of examination and are easily overlooked. Whenever stereoacuity is reduced in the presence of apparent ocular alignment with a scotoma response on the 4$^\Delta$ base-out prism test,[57 p.309] the examiner must search for microtropia or other subtle anomalies of binocular vision. For the measurement of stereoacuity we prefer random dot stereo tests, such as the TNO, Randot, or Lang test. The Titmus stereotest may be used but has the disadvantage of providing monocular clues.

(2) The amblyopia in microtropia is, as a rule, mild and rarely deeper than 20/100.

(3) The Bagolini striated lens test[57 p.251] shows anomalous retinal correspondence.

(4) Fundus examination with a Visuscope[57 p.221] or a regular direct ophthalmoscope with a built-in fixation target shows parafoveal fixation.

(5) Absence of a shift on the cover test in the presence of eccentric fixation and anomalous correspondence is interpreted as an identity between the degree of eccentricity of fixation and the angle of anomaly.[27; 57 p.309]

(6) Because fixation is foveolar and there is a minute shift on the cover test, no identity exists between the fixation behavior and the state of retinal correspondence.

(7) Microtropia may occur as a primary anomaly of binocular vision[36] but is more common as a secondary microtropia.[60]

(8) Secondary microtropia occurs as an end stage of treatment of essential infantile esotropia[36,60] **(see 1.17, 1.18, and 1.19)** but may also be associated with anisometropic amblyopia or amblyopia with a history of anisometropia.[27]

(9) Reduced visual acuity of one eye when measured under binocular conditions with a polaroid test indicates foveal suppression of that eye.

(10) Subnormal binocular vision occurs in a primary form in family members of patients with essential infantile esotropia.[23 p.410]

(11) More frequent than the primary is the secondary form of subnormal binocular vision, which is seen as an ideal end stage of the treatment of essential infantile esotropia.[60]

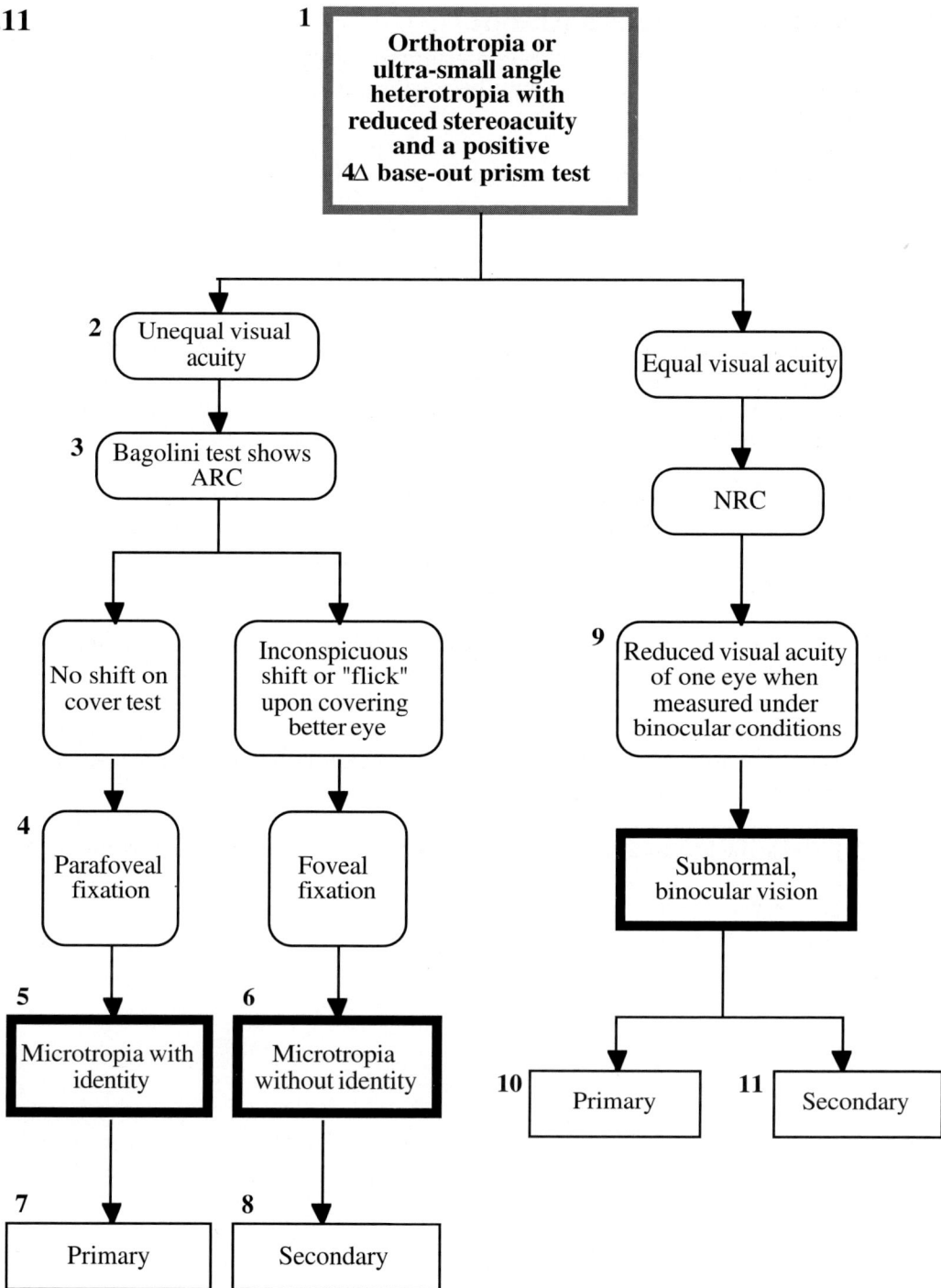

2.11

1 Orthotropia or ultra-small angle heterotropia with reduced stereoacuity and a positive 4Δ base-out prism test

2 Unequal visual acuity

Equal visual acuity

3 Bagolini test shows ARC

NRC

No shift on cover test

Inconspicuous shift or "flick" upon covering better eye

9 Reduced visual acuity of one eye when measured under binocular conditions

4 Parafoveal fixation

Foveal fixation

Subnormal, binocular vision

5 Microtropia with identity

6 Microtropia without identity

10 Primary

11 Secondary

7 Primary

8 Secondary

2.12   **Exodeviations: Treatment**

(1) A patient with an exophoria, intermittent or constant exotropia and with or without potential for fusion may be a candidate for medical or surgical treatment.[23 p.443; 57 p.323]

(2) The type of procedure selected depends on the nature of the underlying deviation **(see 1.22).**

(3) If unilateral surgery is performed, we prefer to operate on the nondominant eye.

(4) Patients with an exodeviation greater at near than at distance fixation may have a normal or remote near point of convergence. This condition must be distinguished from functional convergence insufficiency **(see 1.22 and 1.23),** which is rarely treated surgically.

(5) As in (3), the choice of the eye to be operated on depends on the fixation preference. Surgery on the dominant eye is considered only when maximal surgery has been performed on the nondominant eye. For larger exodeviations, three or even four muscles may be operated on.

(6) Most symptomatic exodeviations are treated surgically. If the angle is too small to be operated on, conservative measures should be considered.[57 p.330]

(7) Botulinum A-toxin (Botox) injection of the lateral rectus under electromyographic control is considered by some as an alternative to surgery. The injection may have to be repeated several times.

(8) The same formula for surgery may be used as listed in the algorithm at (3).

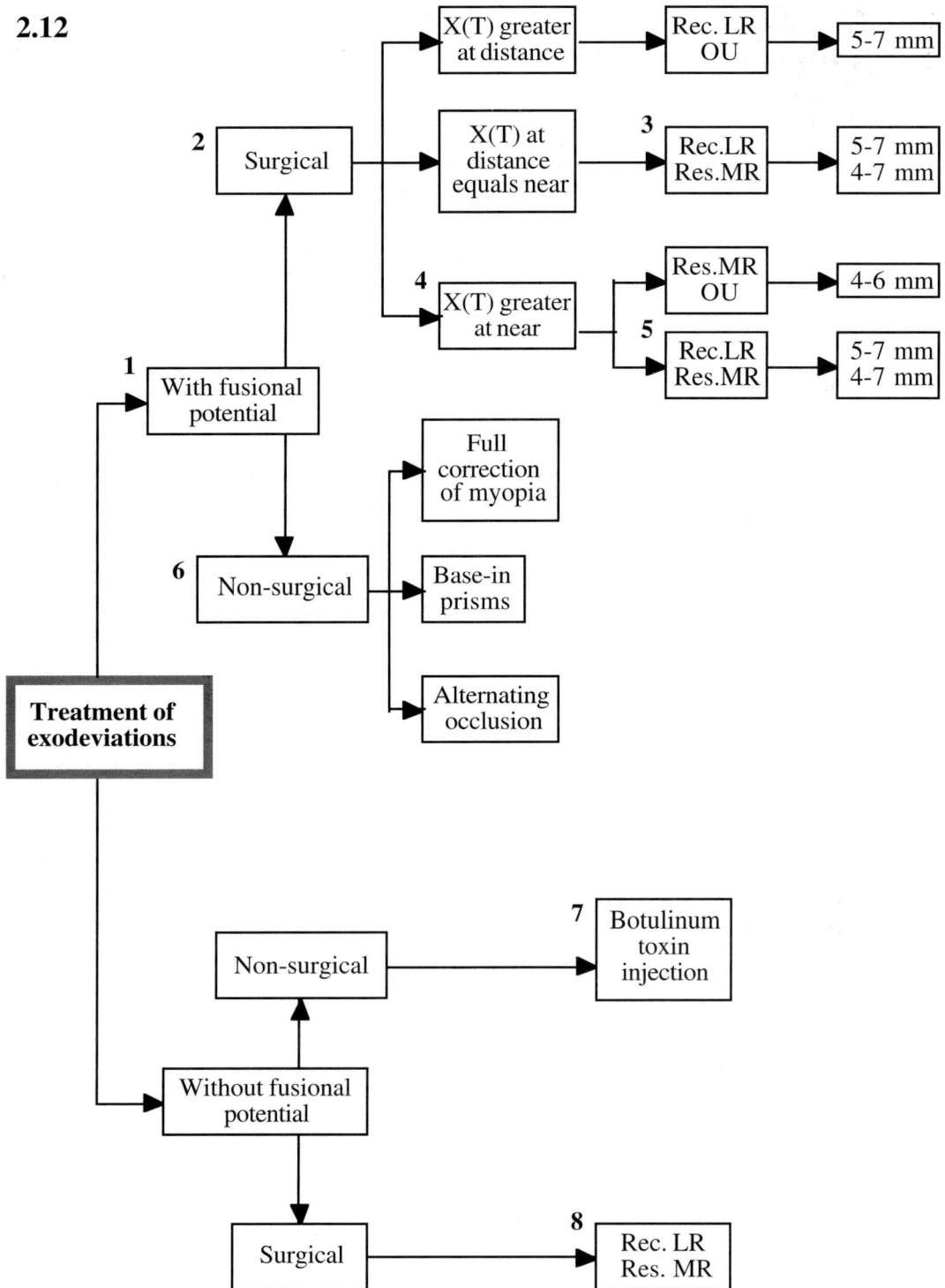

2.12

```
                                        ┌─────────────┐      ┌─────────┐      ┌──────────┐
                                        │ X(T) greater│─────▶│ Rec. LR │─────▶│ 5-7 mm   │
                                        │ at distance │      │   OU    │      └──────────┘
                                        └─────────────┘      └─────────┘
            ┌──────────┐                ┌─────────────┐    3 ┌─────────┐      ┌──────────┐
          2 │          │                │  X(T) at    │─────▶│ Rec.LR  │─────▶│ 5-7 mm   │
            │ Surgical │───────────────▶│  distance   │      │ Res.MR  │      │ 4-7 mm   │
            └──────────┘                │ equals near │      └─────────┘      └──────────┘
                 ▲                      └─────────────┘
                 │                                          ┌─────────┐      ┌──────────┐
                 │                    4 ┌─────────────┐   ┌▶│ Res.MR  │─────▶│ 4-6 mm   │
                 │                      │ X(T) greater│   │ │   OU    │      └──────────┘
                 │                      │  at near    │───┤ └─────────┘
                 │                      └─────────────┘ 5 │ ┌─────────┐      ┌──────────┐
        1 ┌──────────────┐                               └▶│ Rec.LR  │─────▶│ 5-7 mm   │
          │ With fusional │                                 │ Res.MR  │      │ 4-7 mm   │
          │  potential   │                                 └─────────┘      └──────────┘
          └──────────────┘
                 │                      ┌─────────────┐
                 │                      │    Full     │
                 │                   ┌─▶│ correction  │
                 │                   │  │  of myopia  │
                 ▼                   │  └─────────────┘
        6 ┌──────────────┐           │  ┌─────────────┐
          │ Non-surgical │───────────┼─▶│  Base-in    │
          └──────────────┘           │  │   prisms    │
                                     │  └─────────────┘
                                     │  ┌─────────────┐
                                     │  │ Alternating │
                                     └─▶│  occlusion  │
                                        └─────────────┘
```

Treatment of exodeviations

```
                ┌──────────────┐                      7 ┌──────────────┐
                │ Non-surgical │────────────────────────▶│  Botulinum   │
                └──────────────┘                         │    toxin     │
                       ▲                                 │  injection   │
                       │                                 └──────────────┘
        ┌──────────────────┐
        │ Without fusional │
        │    potential     │
        └──────────────────┘
                 │                                      8 ┌──────────┐
                 ▼                                        │ Rec. LR  │
          ┌──────────┐                                    │ Res. MR  │
          │ Surgical │───────────────────────────────────▶└──────────┘
          └──────────┘
```

2.13 Consecutive Exotropia

(1) Consecutive exotropia occurs either spontaneously in a formerly esotropic patient or from surgical overcorrection of an esodeviation.

(2) Limited adduction after surgery for esotropia may be caused by a tight lateral rectus muscle (excessive resection) or a weak medial rectus muscle (excessive recession).[23 p.425]

(3) Free passive ductions exclude a tight lateral rectus muscle as the cause of the exodeviation.

(4) Advancement of the previously recessed medial rectus muscle usually corrects most cases of consecutive exotropia. In larger deviations a recession of the lateral rectus may be added.[23 pp.291,324]

(5) If the medial rectus muscle cannot be located, a transfer of the inferior and superior rectus muscle insertions to the original insertion site of the medial rectus muscle may be indicated.[23 p.296]

(6) Restricted passive ductions indicate a tight lateral rectus muscle or scar formations involving the lateral aspects of the globe, conjunctiva, or Tenon's capsule.

(7) The lateral rectus muscle must be recessed, the scar tissue removed, and the medial rectus muscle may have to be advanced.

(8) In absence of any restriction of adduction, it is prudent to wait several months before the reoperation is considered. To lessen the cosmetic defect or complaints about diplopia, a reduction in hypermetropic spectacle correction may be considered.

(9) A spontaneous change from esotropia to exotropia may be associated with poor vision of the deviating eye (sensory exotropia) or with high hypermetropia.

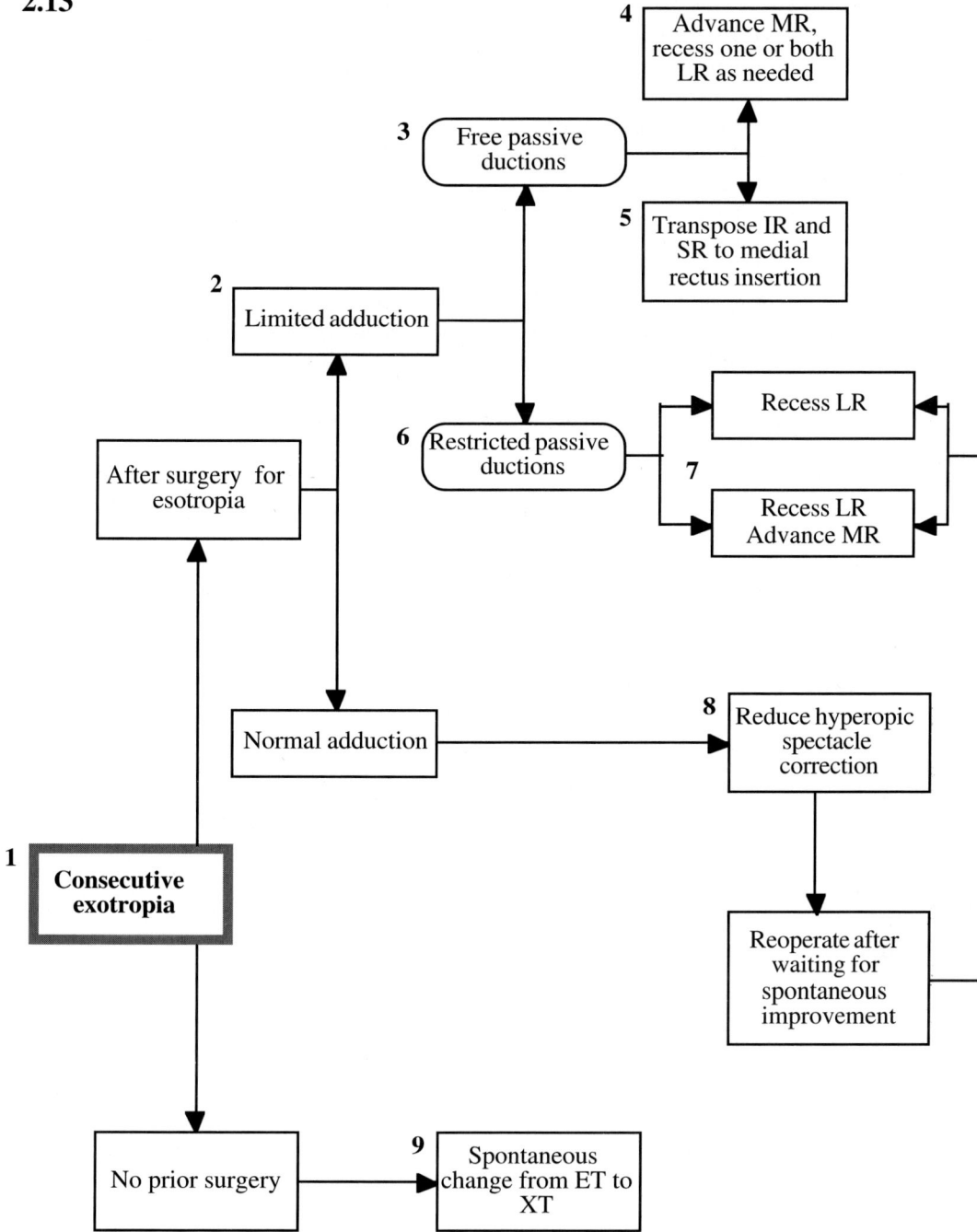

2.13

4 Advance MR, recess one or both LR as needed

3 Free passive ductions

5 Transpose IR and SR to medial rectus insertion

2 Limited adduction

6 Restricted passive ductions

7 Recess LR

Recess LR Advance MR

After surgery for esotropia

Normal adduction

8 Reduce hyperopic spectacle correction

1 **Consecutive exotropia**

Reoperate after waiting for spontaneous improvement

No prior surgery

9 Spontaneous change from ET to XT

2.14   Paralytic Cyclovertical Strabismus: Right Hypertropia

(1) Parks pointed out that the Bielschowsky head tilt test not only identifies paralyzed oblique muscles but is also useful in identifying paralyzed vertical rectus muscles.[44] He introduced the three-step test to determine a weak or paralyzed vertical rectus or oblique muscle. The test should be performed with the patient fixating on a distant object. The **first step** determines with the cover test whether the patient has a right or left hypertropia. A right hypertropia narrows the diagnostic possibilities to a paralysis of the right superior oblique (RSO), right inferior rectus (RIR), left superior rectus (LSR), or left inferior oblique (LIO).

(2) The **second step** identifies whether the right hypertropia increases in right or left gaze. If the deviation increases in right gaze the diagnostic possibilities are further narrowed to only two muscles, the RIR or LIO.

(3) A right hypertropia greater in left gaze is caused by weakness of either the RSO or the LSR.

(4) We now add the Bielschowsky maneuver as the **third step** and determine whether the deviation increases on tilting the head to the right or left shoulder. The lower boxes identify the paretic or paralyzed muscle.

(5) **See 2.40.**

(6) **See 2.26.**

(7) **See 2.42.**

(8) **See 2.25.**

2.14

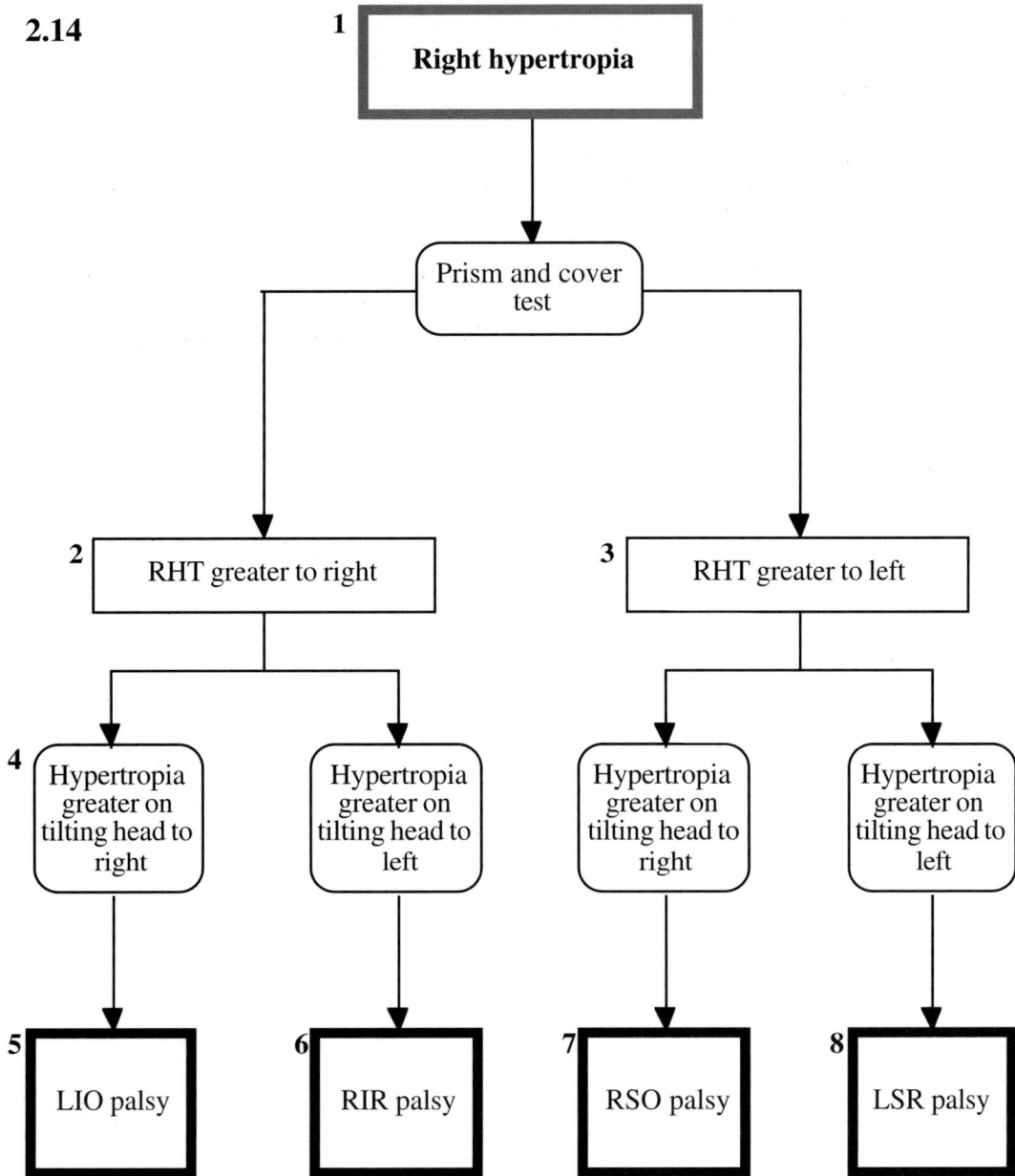

2.15   Paralytic Cyclovertical Strabismus: Left Hypertropia

(1) The cover test has determined that a left hypertropia is present (first step of the three-step test of Parks[44] **(see 2.14)**. This reduces the diagnostic possibilities to a paralysis of the RSR, RIO, LSO, and LIR muscles **(see 2.14)**.

(2) A left hypertropia greater to the right (second step) is caused by paralysis of the RSR or LSO muscles.

(3) A left hypertropia increasing in left gaze implicates the RIO or LIR muscles.

(4) The offending muscle is now identified by measuring the deviation with the head tilted to the right or left shoulder.

(5) **See 2.25.**

(6) **See 2.42.**

(7) **See 2.26.**

(8) **See 2.40.**

2.15

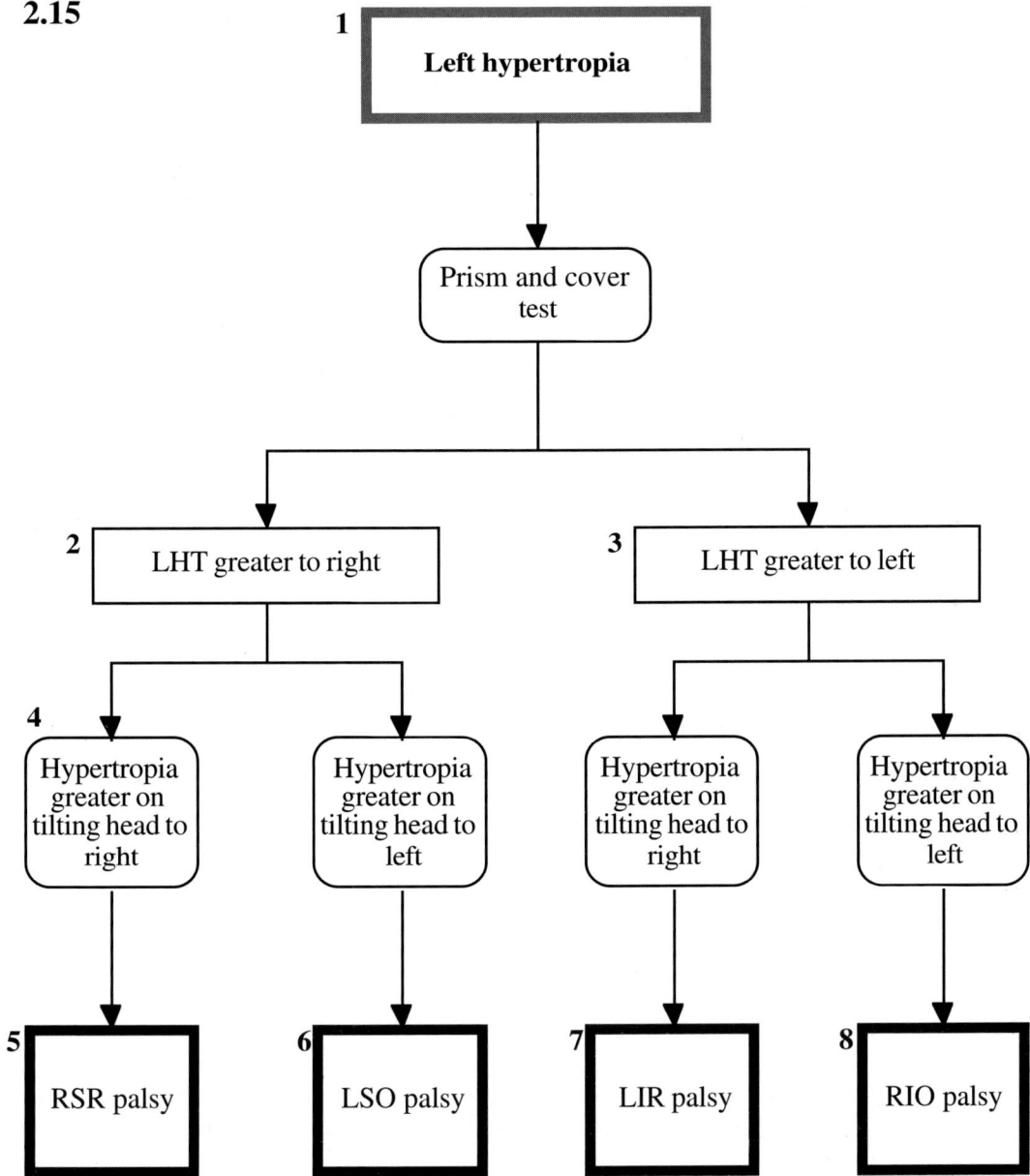

2.16 Dissociated Deviations

(1) The less experienced clinician may easily mistake a dissociated horizontal deviation (DHD) for exotropia or exophoria or a dissociated vertical deviation (DVD) for vertical strabismus. The entity most frequently confused with DVD is an upshoot in adduction **(see 2.17 and 2.18)** caused, for instance, by overaction of the inferior oblique muscle. The differential diagnosis, discussed elsewhere in detail,[57] p.343 is based on the cover-uncover test (objective) and the red glass (subjective) tests. In addition, there are other features listed on this flowchart that are characteristic for dissociated deviations and not seen in other forms of strabismus.

(2) The vertical refixation movements of either eye are of equal amplitude after removal of the cover.

(3) With bilateral DVD either eye moves down to refixate after removal of the cover. The condition is bilateral in most instances but most often asymmetric in magnitude.

(4) DHD may be associated with DVD or occur in isolated form.[73] In DHD (mostly an exodeviation) only one eye abducts under cover and refixates with a slow, tonic adduction movement. In contrast, in exophoria the just uncovered eye refixates with a brisk adduction saccade.

(5) Unlike in paralytic vertical strabismus, the degree of elevation of the dissociated eye is often the same, regardless of whether the eye elevates from adduction, primary position, or abduction.

(6) The dissociated eye not only elevates but excycloducts. When the fellow eye is covered, the dissociated eye returns to primary position with a corrective incycloduction movement.

(7) If a photometric neutral filter is placed before one eye while the other eye is occluded, the eye behind the cover makes a gradual *downward* movement as the density of the filter is increased in front of the fixating eye (Bielschowsky phenomenon).[57] p.187 A similar adduction movement of the dissociated eye occurs in DHD.

(8) Unlike the brisk saccadic refixation movement that occurs during the cover-uncover test in patients with horizontal and vertical heterotopias or heterophorias, the refixation movement in dissociated vertical and horizontal deviations is slow and tonic.

(9) Dissociated vertical and horizontal deviations may occur in a manifest or latent form. The latent form can only be observed by covering either eye; the manifest form occurs spontaneously, often with inattention or when the patient is tired.

(10) DVD may be associated with A and V patterns and oblique muscle overaction that may be true or simulated **(see 2.17).**

(11) The principal surgical treatment of DVD is large superior rectus recession that is usually bilateral. When DVD is associated with inferior oblique overaction, anterior transposition of the inferior oblique is effective.[57] p.431 Inferior rectus resection may be done as a secondary procedure.

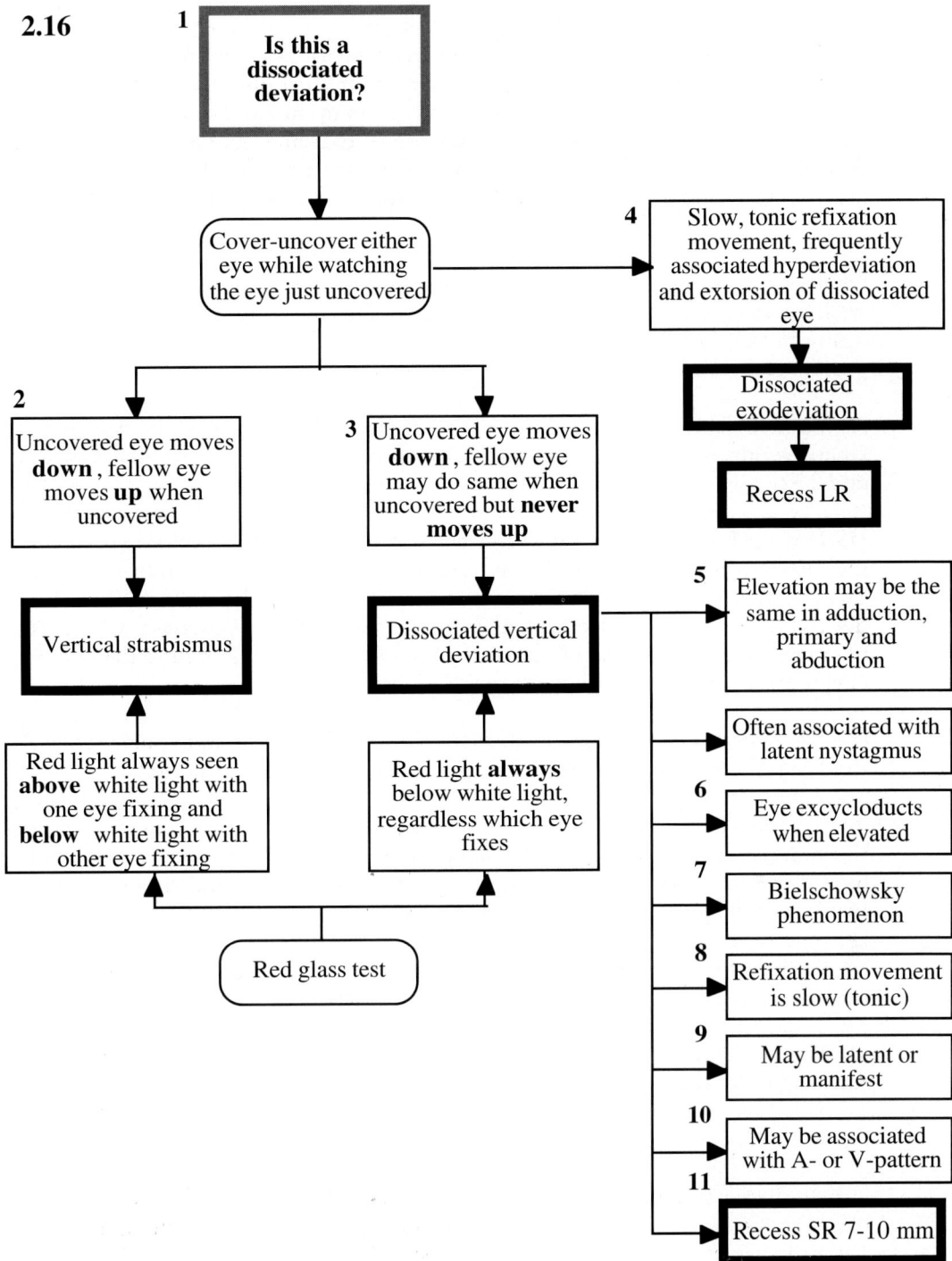

2.16

1 Is this a dissociated deviation?

Cover-uncover either eye while watching the eye just uncovered

4 Slow, tonic refixation movement, frequently associated hyperdeviation and extorsion of dissociated eye

Dissociated exodeviation

Recess LR

2 Uncovered eye moves **down**, fellow eye moves **up** when uncovered

3 Uncovered eye moves **down**, fellow eye may do same when uncovered but **never moves up**

Vertical strabismus

Dissociated vertical deviation

Red light always seen **above** white light with one eye fixing and **below** white light with other eye fixing

Red light **always** below white light, regardless which eye fixes

Red glass test

5 Elevation may be the same in adduction, primary and abduction

Often associated with latent nystagmus

6 Eye excycloducts when elevated

7 Bielschowsky phenomenon

8 Refixation movement is slow (tonic)

9 May be latent or manifest

10 May be associated with A- or V-pattern

11 Recess SR 7-10 mm

2.17   Upshoot in Adduction: Right Eye

(1) An elevation of the adducted eye in the absence of a significant hypertropia in primary position is commonly referred to as an upshoot in adduction. It is fallacious to believe that every apparent overaction in the field of action of the inferior oblique muscle is, in fact, an overaction of that muscle. Failure to recognize that a variety of different conditions may produce a similar clinical picture may lead to the wrong diagnosis and the wrong therapy.

(2) The first step in analyzing the problem is to observe and then to measure whether the elevation is limited to adduction or exists in other gaze positions as well. Special attention should be paid to any other overacting or, perhaps, underacting muscles as the patient maintains fixation with either eye in the diagnostic positions of gaze.

(3) Upshoot, downshoot, or both on attempted adduction may be a feature of Duane syndrome type I and, more commonly, of types II and III **(see 2.50, 2.51, and 2.52)**.

(4) This upshoot in adduction is caused by a primary or secondary overaction of the inferior oblique muscle. This muscle is unopposed by its paretic antagonist. The difference in vertical deviation on tilting the head to the right and left shoulder (Bielschowsky test, **see 2.14**) is measured with the prism cover test. During the measurement the base of the vertical prism must be held before the eye, parallel to the inferior orbital rim.

(5) The Bielschowsky test is positive for a right superior oblique palsy when the right hypertropia increases with the head tilted to the right shoulder.

(6) In primary overaction of the inferior oblique muscle, the function of the superior oblique is usually normal. The condition is often bilateral and accompanied by a V pattern esotropia in downward gaze. Unlike in bilateral superior oblique paralysis, the Bielschowsky test is negative.

(7) Because the secondary deviation is always greater than the primary deviation, the left eye must be the paretic eye **(see 1.08)**.

(8) The Bielschowsky head tilt test may be helpful in identifying paretic vertical rectus muscles **(see 2.14)**.

(9) **See 2.37.**

(10) In dissociated vertical deviation (DVD) **(see 2.16)**, elevation of the involved eye occurs from primary position, abduction, and adduction. Although this elevation is usually more pronounced in abduction, it may be present to an equal degree in adduction.

(11) Unlike in secondary inferior oblique overaction where underaction of the antagonist of the yoke muscle (LSR) is the rule, that muscle acts normally when a patient with DVD fixates with the involved eye in elevation and abduction.

(12) **See 2.16.**

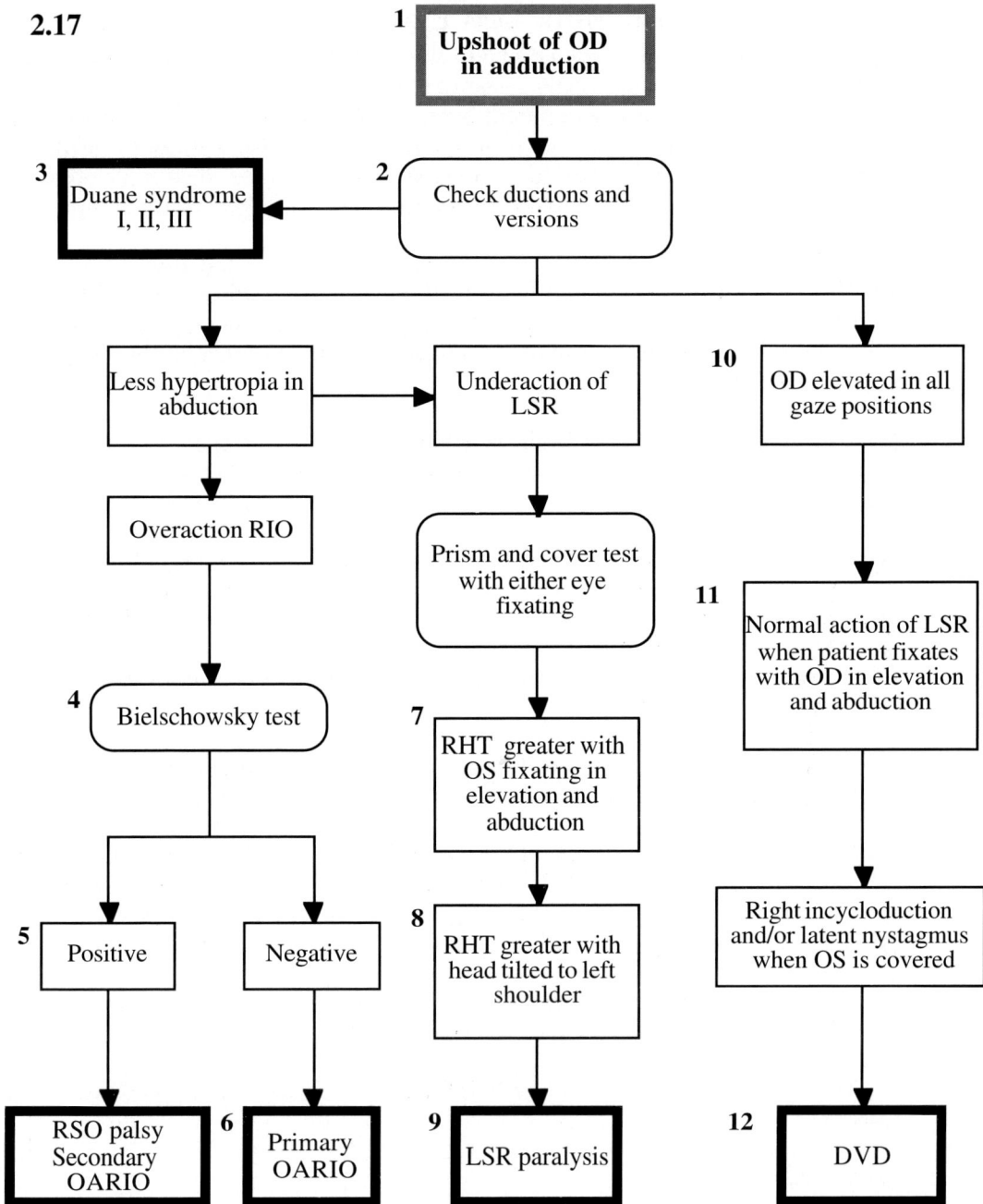

2.17

1 **Upshoot of OD in adduction**

2 Check ductions and versions

3 Duane syndrome I, II, III

Less hypertropia in abduction

Underaction of LSR

10 OD elevated in all gaze positions

Overaction RIO

Prism and cover test with either eye fixating

11 Normal action of LSR when patient fixates with OD in elevation and abduction

4 Bielschowsky test

7 RHT greater with OS fixating in elevation and abduction

8 RHT greater with head tilted to left shoulder

Right incycloduction and/or latent nystagmus when OS is covered

5 Positive

Negative

RSO palsy Secondary OARIO

6 Primary OARIO

9 LSR paralysis

12 DVD

2.18   Upshoot in Adduction: Left Eye

(1) An elevation of the adducted eye in the absence of a significant hypertropia in primary position is commonly referred to as an upshoot in adduction. It is fallacious to believe that every apparent overaction in the field of action of the inferior oblique muscle is, in fact, an overaction of that muscle. Failure to recognize that a variety of different conditions may produce a clinical picture of often remarkable similarity may lead to the wrong diagnosis and the wrong therapy.

(2) The first step in analyzing the problem is to observe and then to measure whether the elevation is limited to adduction or exists in other gaze positions as well. Special attention should be paid to any other overacting or, perhaps, underacting muscles as the patient maintains fixation with either eye in the diagnostic positions of gaze.

(3) Upshoot, downshoot, or both on attempted adduction may be a feature of Duane syndrome type I and, more commonly, of types II and III **(see 2.50, 2.51, and 2.52).**

(4) This upshoot in adduction is caused by a secondary overaction of the inferior oblique muscle. This muscle is unopposed by its paretic antagonist. The difference in vertical deviation on tilting the head to the right and left shoulder (Bielschowsky test, **see 2.14**) is measured with the prism cover test. During the measurement the base of the vertical prism must be held before the eye, parallel to the inferior orbital rim.

(5) The Bielschowsky test is positive for a left superior oblique palsy when the left hypertropia increases with the head tilted to the left shoulder.

(6) In primary overaction of the inferior oblique muscle, the function of the superior oblique is usually normal. The condition is often bilateral and accompanied by a V pattern esotropia in downward gaze. Unlike in bilateral superior oblique paralysis, the Bielschowsky test is negative.

(7) Because the secondary deviation is always greater than the primary deviation, the right eye must be the paretic eye **(see 1.08).**

(8) The Bielschowsky test may be helpful in identifying paretic vertical rectus muscles.

(9) **See 2.37.**

(10) In dissociated vertical deviation (DVD) **(see 2.16),** elevation of the involved eye occurs from primary position, abduction, and adduction. Although this elevation is usually more pronounced in abduction, it may be present to an equal degree in adduction.

(11) Unlike in secondary inferior oblique overaction where underaction of the antagonist of the yoke muscle (RSR) is the rule, that muscle acts normally when a patient with DVD fixates with the involved eye in elevation and abduction.

(12) **See 2.16.**

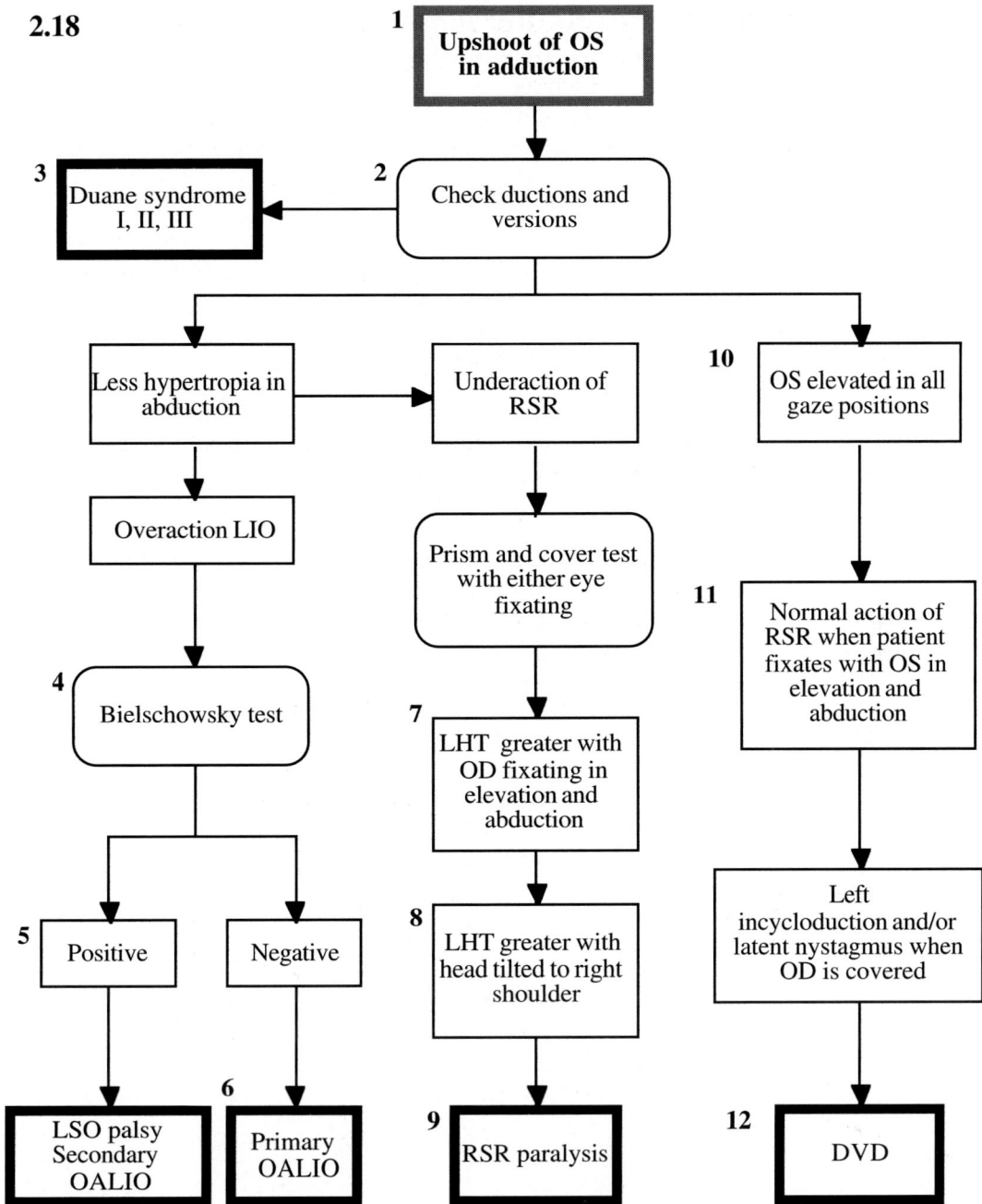

2.18

1 Upshoot of OS in adduction

3 Duane syndrome I, II, III ← **2** Check ductions and versions

Less hypertropia in abduction → Underaction of RSR

10 OS elevated in all gaze positions

Overaction LIO

Prism and cover test with either eye fixating

11 Normal action of RSR when patient fixates with OS in elevation and abduction

4 Bielschowsky test

7 LHT greater with OD fixating in elevation and abduction

Left incycloduction and/or latent nystagmus when OD is covered

5 Positive   Negative

8 LHT greater with head tilted to right shoulder

LSO palsy Secondary OALIO

6 Primary OALIO

9 RSR paralysis

12 DVD

2.19   Downshoot in Adduction: Right Eye

(1) Depression of the adducted eye has multiple causes but it occurs less frequently than upshoot in adduction.

(2) Downshoot of the adducted eye may be associated with Duane syndromes types I, II, and III **(see 2.50, 2.51, and 2.52).**

(3) Most patients with Brown syndrome **(see 2.53)** adduct the involved eye normally. However, with severe restriction of elevation the eye may actually depress on attempts to adduct from the primary position.[23 p.452]

(4) **See 2.40.**

(5) Downshoot in adduction may be caused by overaction of the superior oblique muscle. This is a secondary deviation, resulting from paralysis of the contralateral inferior rectus muscle, which is the yoke of the superior oblique.

(6) Patients with superior oblique paralysis **(see 2.41)** have overaction of the contralateral superior oblique muscle in 14% of cases.[70] This is produced by contracture of the ipsilateral superior rectus muscle. Excess innervation is required to depress the paralyzed eye in abduction, which causes downshoot of the adducted sound eye whenever the patient fixates with the paralyzed eye. Surgical weakening of the secondarily overacting superior oblique can result in an iatrogenic bilateral superior oblique palsy which can cause great problems for a potentially fusing patient.

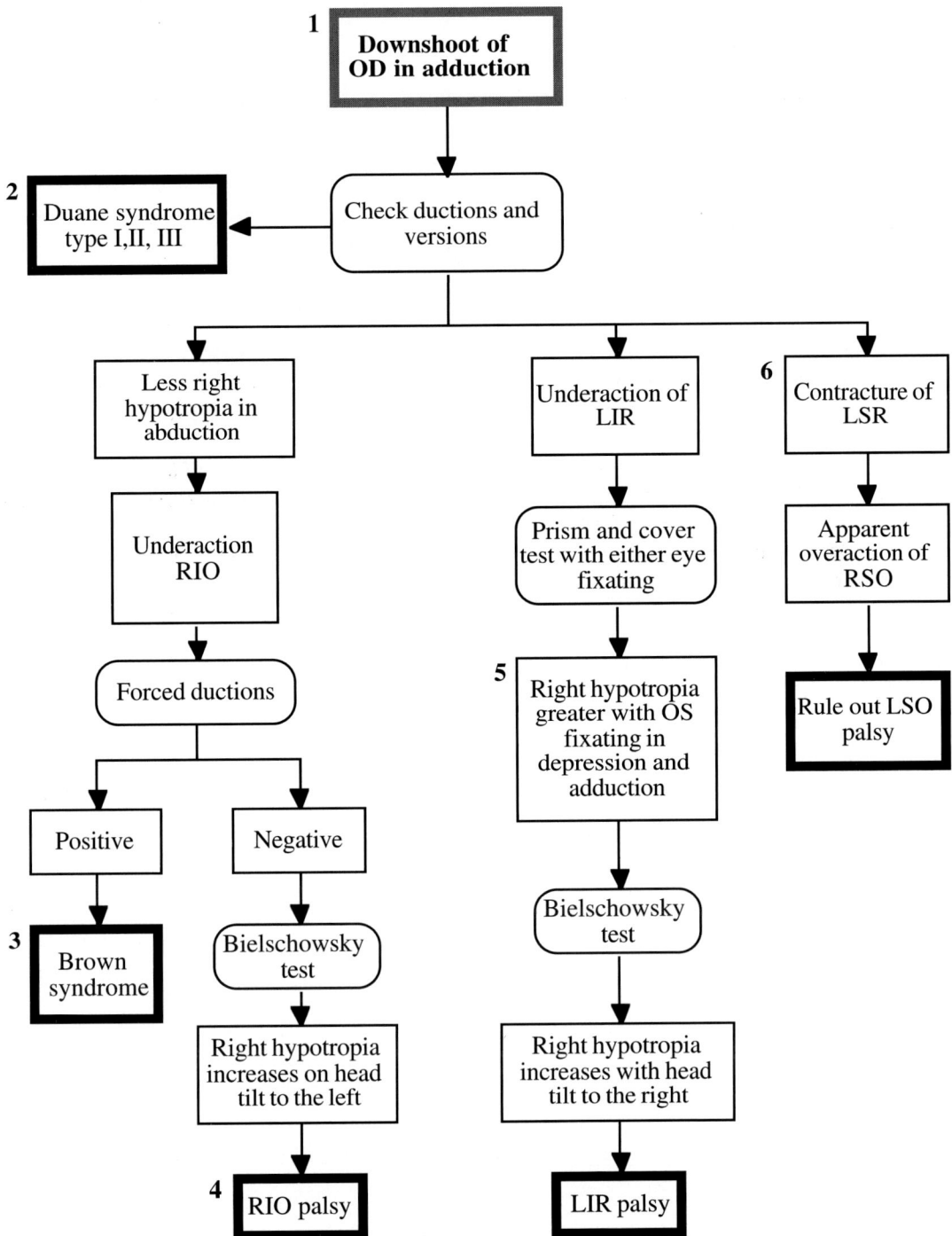

2.19

1 **Downshoot of OD in adduction**

↓

Check ductions and versions

2 Duane syndrome type I,II, III ←

Less right hypotropia in abduction

Underaction of LIR

6 Contracture of LSR

↓

Underaction RIO

Prism and cover test with either eye fixating

Apparent overaction of RSO

↓

Forced ductions

5 Right hypotropia greater with OS fixating in depression and adduction

Rule out LSO palsy

↓

Positive

Negative

Bielschowsky test

3 Brown syndrome

Bielschowsky test

Right hypotropia increases with head tilt to the right

Right hypotropia increases on head tilt to the left

LIR palsy

4 RIO palsy

2.20   Downshoot in Adduction: Left Eye

(1) Depression of the adducted eye has multiple causes but it occurs less frequently than upshoot in adduction.

(2) Downshoot of the adducted eye may be associated with Duane syndromes types I, II, and III **(see 2.50, 2.51, and 2.52)**.

(3) Most patients with Brown syndrome **(see 2.53)** adduct the involved eye normally. However, with severe restriction of elevation the eye may actually depress on attempts to adduct from the primary position.[23 p.452]

(4) **See 2.40.**

(5) Downshoot in adduction is caused by overaction of the superior oblique muscle. This is a secondary deviation, resulting from paralysis of the contralateral inferior rectus muscle, which is the yoke of the superior oblique.

(6) Patients with superior oblique paralysis **(see 2.41)** have overaction of the contralateral superior oblique muscle in 14% of cases.[70] This is produced by contracture of the ipsilateral superior rectus muscle. Excess innervation is required to depress the paralyzed eye, which causes downshoot of the adducted sound eye whenever the patient fixates with the paralyzed eye **(see 1.08, 2.43)**.

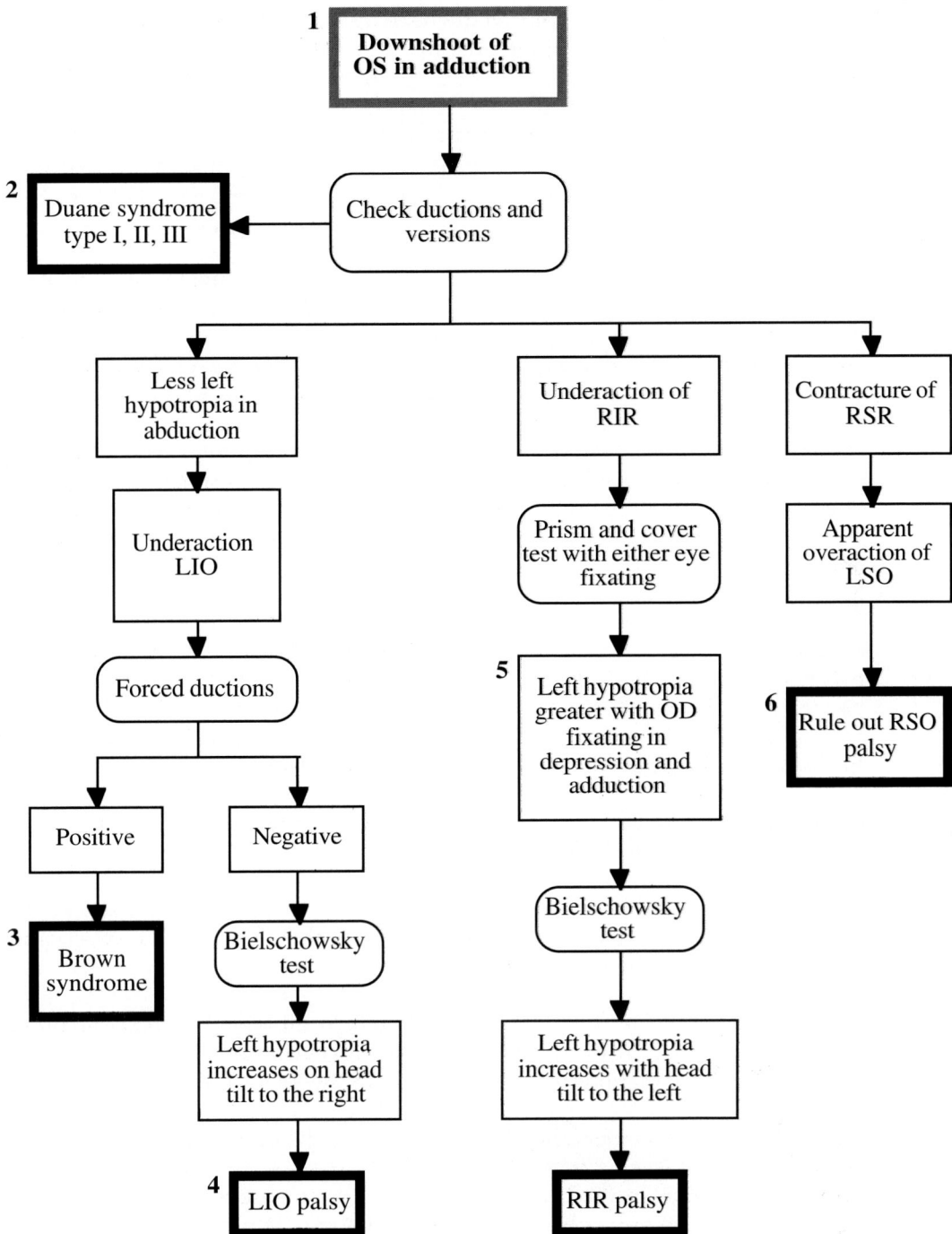

2.20

1 Downshoot of
OS in adduction

Check ductions and
versions

2 Duane syndrome
type I, II, III

Less left
hypotropia in
abduction

Underaction of
RIR

Contracture of
RSR

Underaction
LIO

Prism and cover
test with either eye
fixating

Apparent
overaction of
LSO

Forced ductions

5 Left hypotropia
greater with OD
fixating in
depression and
adduction

6 Rule out RSO
palsy

Positive

Negative

3 Brown
syndrome

Bielschowsky
test

Bielschowsky
test

Left hypotropia
increases on head
tilt to the right

Left hypotropia
increases with head
tilt to the left

4 LIO palsy

RIR palsy

2.21   Cyclotropia: Diagnosis

A workup for cyclotropia is indicated whenever a patient reports tilting of one or both double images, in the differential diagnosis of cyclovertical muscle pareses or paralyses, or when the patient is seen with a head tilt **(see 1.24, 1.27, and 1.33).**

(1) Cyclotropia may be symptomatic (i.e., causing image tilt) or asymptomatic. In either case the examiner must decide which eye is involved, whether incyclotropia or excyclotropia is present, and determine the amount of cyclotropia.[56 p.56]

(2) A patient's awareness of image tilt suggests a bilateral superior oblique palsy or other cyclotropia of recent onset.[19] In the case of a superior oblique paralysis, a neuroophthalmologic workup is rarely necessary, especially if trauma can be established as a cause. Noninnervational causes of cyclotropia of recent onset include orbital trauma and torsion of the globe after scleral buckling.

(3) Unawareness of image tilt does not rule out a cyclotropia. The patient may compensate for cyclotropia by cyclofusion, have acquired a sensorial adaptation of the vertical retinal meridian(s) or localize the visual environment correctly on the basis of experiential factors.[57 p.347] Such adaptations are the norm in cyclodeviations of long standing.

(4) Red and white Maddox rods are inserted in a trial frame. The orientation of the rods must be identical in both eyes and oriented toward 90°. A small vertical prism may be placed before one eye to separate the two lines seen by the patient.[56 p.56] The rod seen as tilted by the patient is adjusted until both lines are seen as parallel. This accurately indicates the amount of cyclotropia, but the Maddox rods dissociate the eyes and prevent cyclofusion.

(5) The cyclotropia can be measured with the Bagolini lenses in a trial frame without disrupting fusion.[46]

(6) Objective diagnosis of cyclotropia is possible by observing supraplacement or infraplacement of the macula with the indirect ophthalmoscope. This observation may be documented by fundus photography.[4]

(7) A subjective image tilt that produces torsional diplopia is usually accompanied by a head tilt. However, not all patients with cyclotropia have a head tilt because sensorial adaptations may compensate for the image tilt.[57 p.346]

(8) To determine whether a head tilt is caused by the cyclotropia or a coexisting vertical deviation **(see 1.27),** a patch is applied to either eye and the patient is observed for changes in the head position. The most common cause for spontaneous torsional diplopia is bilateral superior oblique palsy.

(9) Once it has been determined that the head tilt is caused by cyclotropia, the deviation is measured with the Maddox double rod. The offending eye is the eye that, when patched, causes the head to straighten.

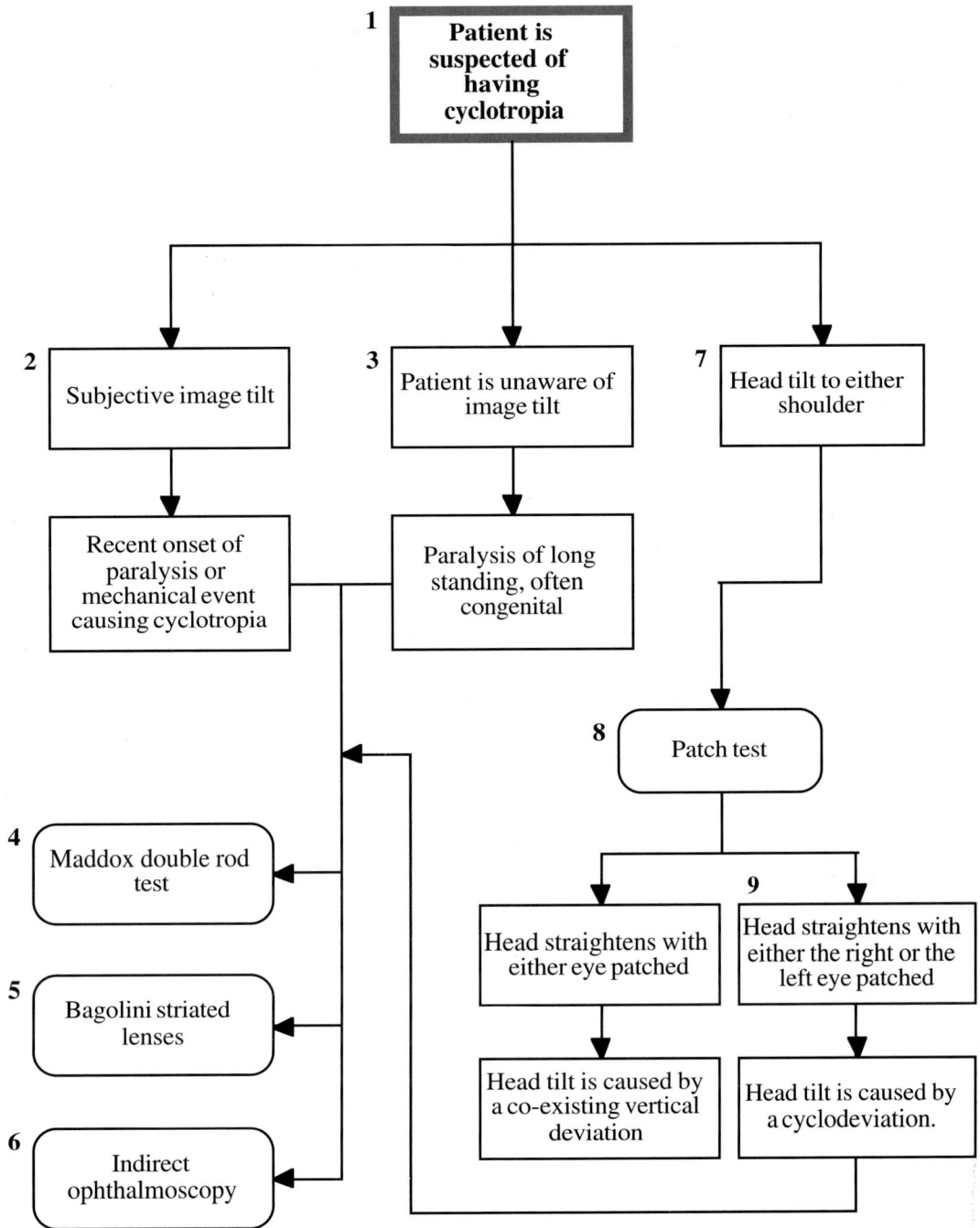

2.21

1   **Patient is suspected of having cyclotropia**

2   Subjective image tilt

3   Patient is unaware of image tilt

7   Head tilt to either shoulder

Recent onset of paralysis or mechanical event causing cyclotropia

Paralysis of long standing, often congenital

8   Patch test

4   Maddox double rod test

9   Head straightens with either eye patched

Head straightens with either the right or the left eye patched

5   Bagolini striated lenses

Head tilt is caused by a co-existing vertical deviation

Head tilt is caused by a cyclodeviation.

6   Indirect ophthalmoscopy

2.22 Cyclotropia: Treatment

(1) Cyclodeviations occur more commonly in association with vertical strabismus (especially superior oblique palsy) than in an isolated form.

(2) Surgical correction of the vertical deviation usually also corrects the cyclotropia. For instance, most patients with superior oblique paralysis have a hypertropia and excyclotropia of the involved eye. A myectomy of the ipsilateral inferior oblique and/or tucking of the paretic superior oblique muscle corrects both the hypertropia and the excyclotropia (see 2.43).

(3) Pure cyclotropia (i.e., a cyclotropia without a coexisting hyperdeviation) is infrequent and requires a surgical technique that selectively affects cyclorotation of the eyes without inducing other forms of strabismus. For instance, tucking of the superior oblique tendon in a patient with a trochlear paresis and excyclotropia without coexisting hypertropia corrects for the excyclotropia but at the same time induces an undesirable hypotropia of the operated eye in a patient without vertical tropia.

(4) The Harada-Ito operation[23 p.234; 57 p.515] is effective in correcting excyclotropia. However, it may cause undercorrection of the excyclotropia and cannot be performed in cases of congenital absence of the superior oblique muscle or after the tendon has been previously tenectomized. For such cases effective surgical alternatives exist; these consist of horizontal transposition of the vertical rectus[23 p.194; 38; 65; 67] or vertical transposition of the horizontal rectus muscles. Horizontal transposition of the vertical rectus muscles can be modified depending on the gaze direction in which the deviation is most pronounced. For instance, if excyclotropia is limited to downward gaze, nasal transposition of the inferior rectus muscle alone suffices.

(5) An isolated incyclotropia occurs much less frequently than an excyclotropia. Although operations on the insertions of the oblique muscles comparable to the Harada-Ito procedure exist, displacing the insertions of the vertical rectus muscles has been shown to be as effective and is technically simpler.[67]

2.22

```
                    ┌─────────────────────┐
                    │   Treatment of      │
                    │   cyclotropia       │
                    └─────────────────────┘
```

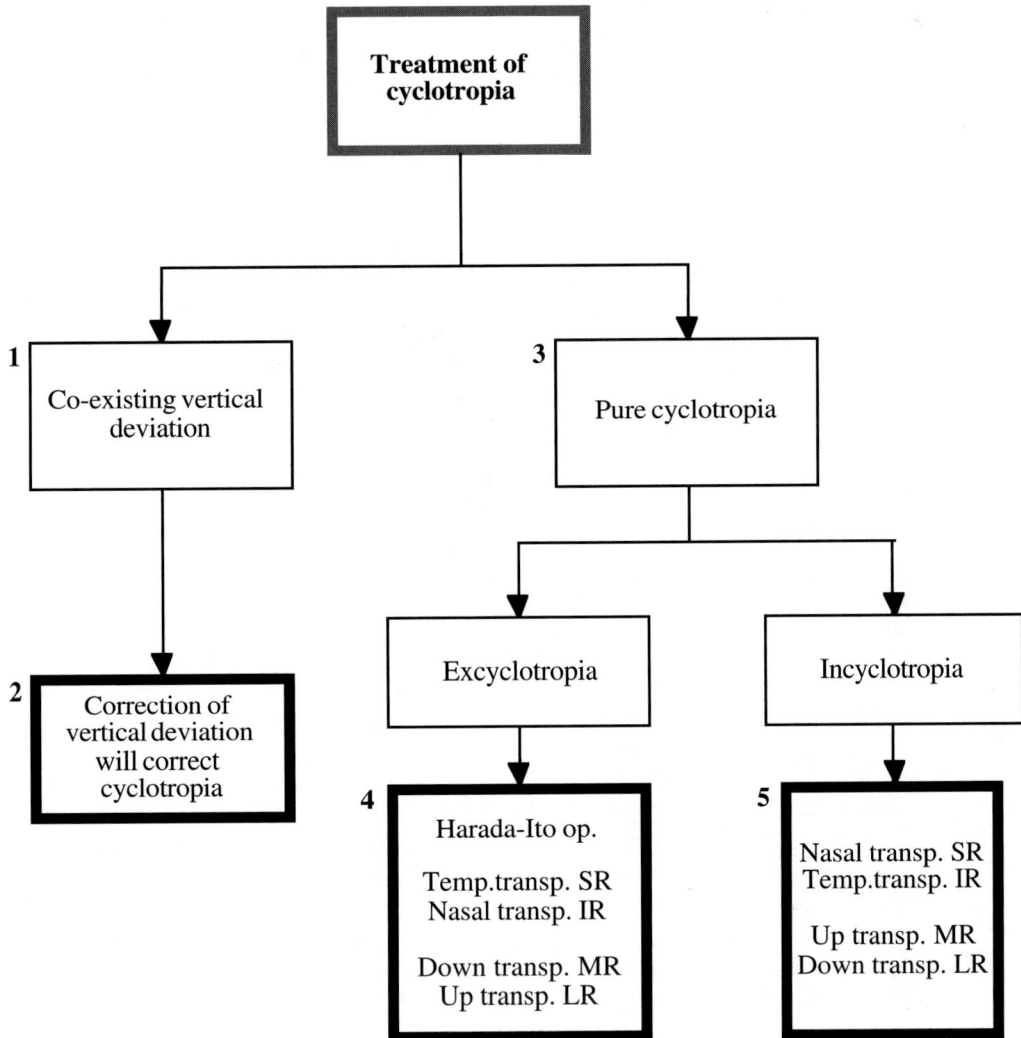

1 Co-existing vertical deviation

3 Pure cyclotropia

2 Correction of vertical deviation will correct cyclotropia

Excyclotropia

Incyclotropia

4 Harada-Ito op.

Temp.transp. SR
Nasal transp. IR

Down transp. MR
Up transp. LR

5 Nasal transp. SR
Temp.transp. IR

Up transp. MR
Down transp. LR

2.23 A Pattern Strabismus: Treatment

(1) A horizontal strabismus (esotropia or exotropia) whose angle changes more than 10$^\Delta$ between 30° upward and 30° downward gaze has an A pattern. These measurements are usually taken at distance fixation. The horizontal incomitance in vertical gaze may not be functionally significant and not require treatment in all cases.

(2) In addition to the various forms of A patterns listed in this algorithm additional variations exist. For instance, an exotropia may be present exclusively in downward gaze (inverted Y or lambda pattern). In such cases, the surgery is limited to superior oblique tenectomies if these muscles are overacting. If they are not, nasal transpositions of the inferior recti without recession or resection of the transposed muscle should be done.

(3) Depending on the difference of the angle of strabismus in upward and downward gaze, the amount of transposition of the horizontal rectus muscles is varied. For more than 15$^\Delta$ difference, we transpose one full muscle width, for lesser differences the transposition varies between one half and three fourths of the muscle width. When vertical transposition of the horizontal recti are performed to treat A pattern strabismus the medial recti are moved upward (toward the closed end) and the lateral recti are moved down (toward the open end).[56, p. 189] Temporal transposition of the superior rectus muscles is equally effective in counteracting the A pattern with esotropia in upgaze but is less frequently performed. The amount of temporal transposition is graded in a manner similar to vertical transpositions.

(4) Whether to do symmetric horizontal surgery or to perform a recess-resect operation on one eye depends on the individual clinician's preference. In most instances we prefer symmetric surgery but limit the horizontal surgery to one eye when the other eye has already been operated on or when the patient is amblyopic.

(5) An A pattern with normally acting superior oblique muscles is an unusual finding. Repeated testing is essential to exclude the possibility that an overaction may have been overlooked.

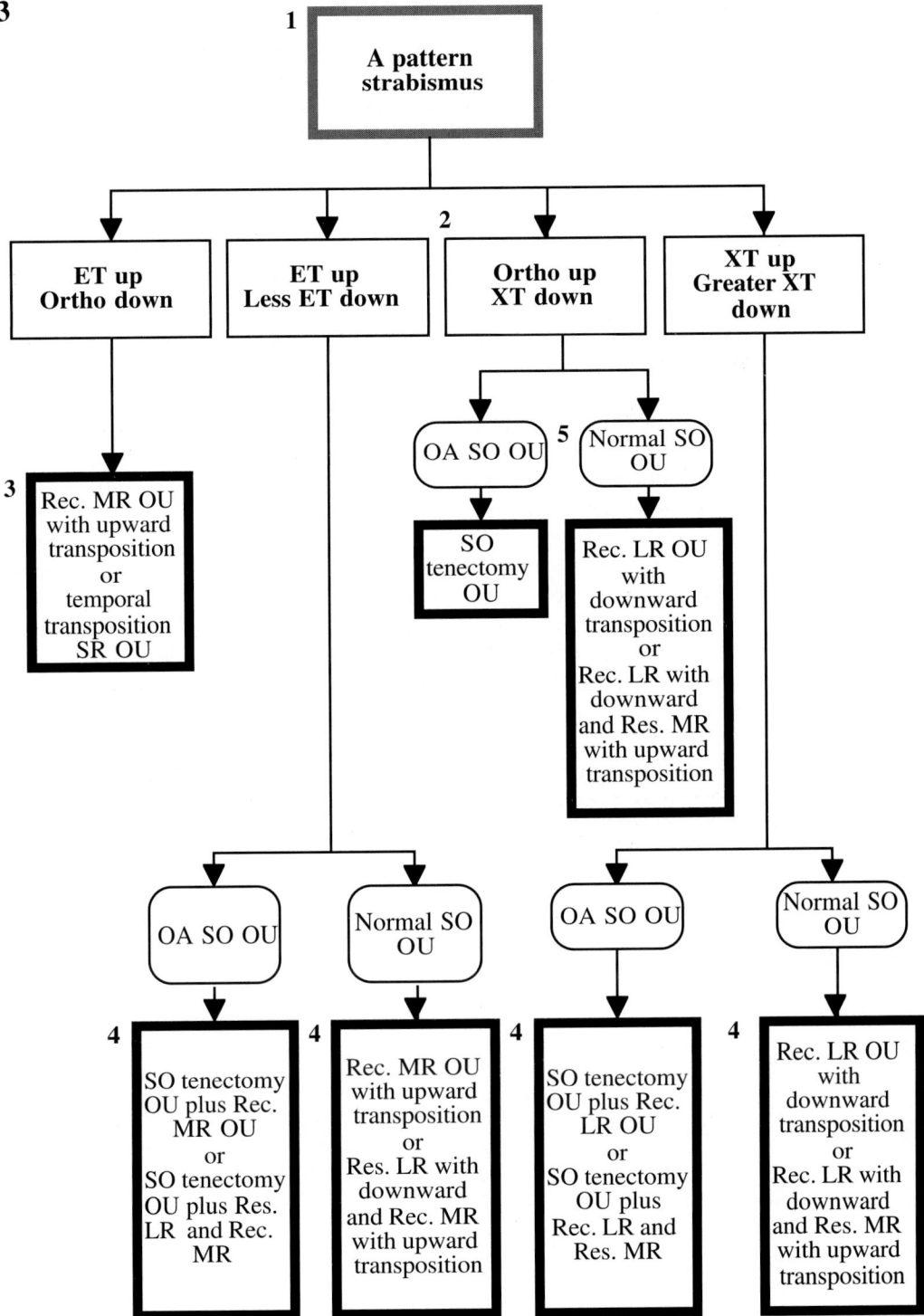

2.23

1
```
A pattern
strabismus
```

2

ET up
Ortho down

ET up
Less ET down

Ortho up
XT down

XT up
Greater XT
down

OA SO OU   5   Normal SO
OU

3
Rec. MR OU
with upward
transposition
or
temporal
transposition
SR OU

SO
tenectomy
OU

Rec. LR OU
with
downward
transposition
or
Rec. LR with
downward
and Res. MR
with upward
transposition

OA SO OU

Normal SO
OU

OA SO OU

Normal SO
OU

4
SO tenectomy
OU plus Rec.
MR OU
or
SO tenectomy
OU plus Res.
LR and Rec.
MR

4
Rec. MR OU
with upward
transposition
or
Res. LR with
downward
and Rec. MR
with upward
transposition

4
SO tenectomy
OU plus Rec.
LR OU
or
SO tenectomy
OU plus
Rec. LR and
Res. MR

4
Rec. LR OU
with
downward
transposition
or
Rec. LR with
downward
and Res. MR
with upward
transposition

2.24   V Pattern Strabismus: Treatment

(1) A horizontal strabismus (esotropia or exotropia) whose angle changes more than 15△ between 30° upward and 30° downward gaze has a V pattern. These measurements are usually taken at distance fixation. This horizontal incomitance in vertical gaze may not be functionally significant and not require treatment in all cases.

(2) Additional variations exist in addition to the V patterns listed in this algorithm. For instance, orthotropia may be present in downward gaze and in primary position and the exotropia limited to upward gaze. This is called a Y pattern. In that case the surgery is limited to inferior oblique myectomies if these muscles are overacting. If they are not, vertical muscle transpositions without recession or resection of the transposed muscle should be done.

(3) Another variation is an exotropia significantly larger in upward gaze than in primary position. An exotropia greater in upward and downward gaze than in the primary position is called an X pattern exotropia. Horizontal surgery usually suffices to eliminate the X pattern.

(4) As in the treatment of A pattern strabismus, the amount of transposition depends on the difference between measurements in upward and downward gaze. Temporal transposition of the inferior rectus muscles is less frequently performed but remains a viable alternative for the treatment of V pattern esotropia. The amount of temporal transposition is graded in a manner similar to vertical transpositions.

(5) As in A pattern strabismus, the choice whether to do symmetric surgery or limit the operation to one eye depends on previous surgery and on our preference to limit surgery to the amblyopic eye, if possible.

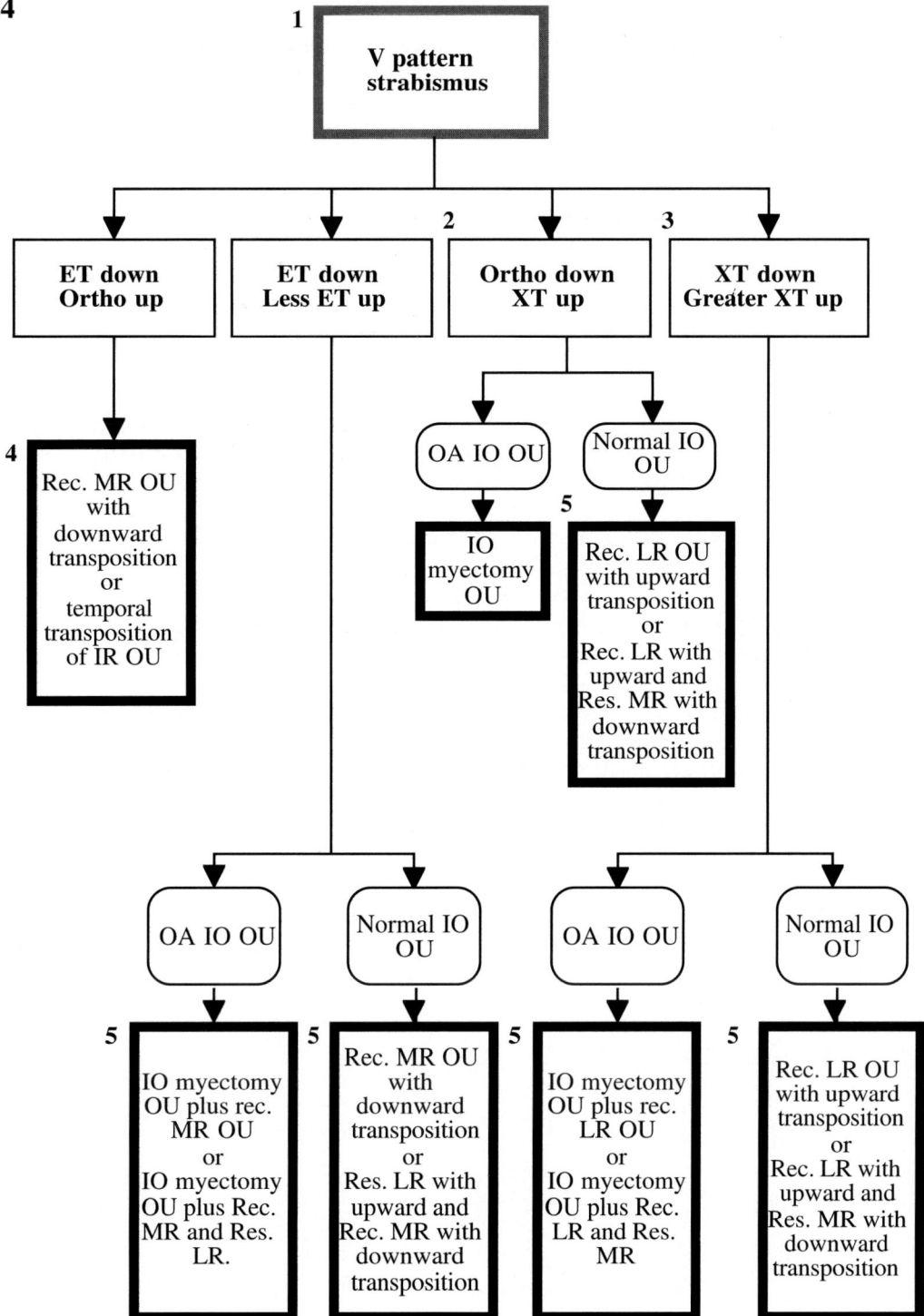

2.24

1 V pattern strabismus

ET down Ortho up

ET down Less ET up

2 Ortho down XT up

3 XT down Greater XT up

4 Rec. MR OU with downward transposition or temporal transposition of IR OU

OA IO OU

Normal IO OU

IO myectomy OU

5 Rec. LR OU with upward transposition or Rec. LR with upward and Res. MR with downward transposition

OA IO OU

Normal IO OU

OA IO OU

Normal IO OU

5 IO myectomy OU plus rec. MR OU or IO myectomy OU plus Rec. MR and Res. LR.

5 Rec. MR OU with downward transposition or Res. LR with upward and Rec. MR with downward transposition

5 IO myectomy OU plus rec. LR OU or IO myectomy OU plus Rec. LR and Res. MR

5 Rec. LR OU with upward transposition or Rec. LR with upward and Res. MR with downward transposition

2.25   Limitation of Elevation of One Eye

(1) In a recently acquired superior rectus paralysis a forced duction test would be negative. In superior rectus paralysis (see 2.37) of longer standing this test may become positive because of contracture of the ipsilateral inferior rectus muscle.

(2) It is debatable whether true double elevator paralysis (i.e., paralysis of a superior rectus associated with paralysis of the ipsilateral inferior oblique) exists. It is possible that double elevator paralysis with ptosis is a misnomer and that the generalized weakness of elevation is caused by long-standing superior rectus and levator palpebrae palsy. Depending on the state of contracture of the ipsilateral inferior rectus muscle in such cases, the forced duction test may be negative or positive.

(3) An intact Bell's phenomenon suggests a supranuclear cause for limited elevation and helps to explain weakness of muscles supplied by different branches of the third nerve.

(4) Myasthenia gravis may mimic paralysis of any individual muscle or muscle groups (see 2.56).

(5) Paralysis of the inferior oblique muscle does not affect elevation from the abducted position (see 2.40).

(6) The excessive recession of the superior rectus muscle "loss" of this muscle during surgery or denervation results in severe limitation of elevation from adduction, primary position, and abduction.

(7) See 2.53.

(8) See 1.28.

(9) See 2.55.

(10) See 2.54.

(11) See 2.32.

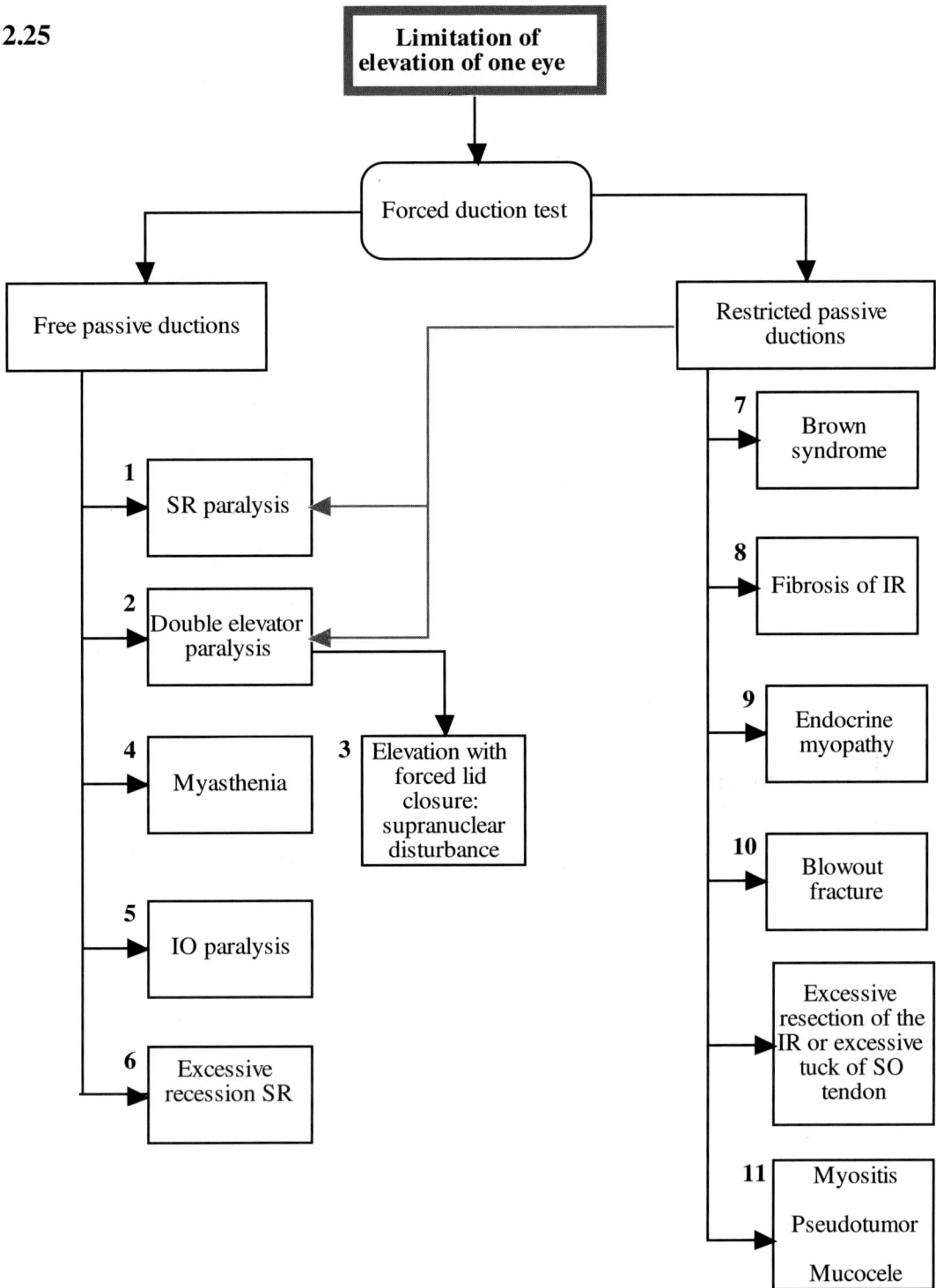

2.25

```
┌─────────────────────────┐
│   Limitation of         │
│   elevation of one eye  │
└─────────────────────────┘
            │
            ▼
     ┌──────────────────┐
     │ Forced duction test │
     └──────────────────┘
      │                  │
      ▼                  ▼
┌──────────────┐   ┌──────────────┐
│ Free passive │   │ Restricted   │
│ ductions     │   │ passive      │
│              │   │ ductions     │
└──────────────┘   └──────────────┘
```

1 SR paralysis

2 Double elevator paralysis

3 Elevation with forced lid closure: supranuclear disturbance

4 Myasthenia

5 IO paralysis

6 Excessive recession SR

7 Brown syndrome

8 Fibrosis of IR

9 Endocrine myopathy

10 Blowout fracture

Excessive resection of the IR or excessive tuck of SO tendon

11 Myositis

Pseudotumor

Mucocele

2.26   Limited Depression of One Eye

(1) The forced duction test is negative in inferior rectus paralysis **(see 2.38)** of recent onset. However, with a long-standing paralysis, contracture of the ipsilateral superior rectus muscle restricts passive infraduction.

(2) Paralysis of both depressor muscles of one eye (inferior rectus and superior oblique muscles) is rare. Only a congenital form is known; as with double elevator paralysis, the cause of double depressor paralysis is obscure and difficult to explain neuroanatomically. Therefore we suspect that so-called double depressor paralyses are caused by long-standing inferior rectus paralyses, in which case the forced duction test has become positive.

(3) Myasthenia gravis may mimic paralysis of any muscle or muscle group **(see 2.56)**.

(4) Limitation of depression in superior oblique paralysis is more pronounced in adduction and primary position but is extreme only in case of absence of the superior oblique **(see 2.42)**.

(5) Severe limitation of depression from all gaze positions may result if the inferior rectus muscle is "lost" during surgery or denervated traumatically or, iatrogenically, during repair of a blowout fracture. This may also occur after inferior rectus recession for endocrine myopathy **(see 2.55)**.[23 p.515]

(6) Most blowout fractures **(see 2.54)** cause limitation of elevation. However, when the fracture involves the posterior orbit, depression of the eye may become restricted. Limited depression in such cases may also be caused by a coexisting inferior rectus paralysis of traumatic or iatrogenic (during surgical repair of the fracture) origin. The estimation of generated muscle force[23 pp.260,266; 57 p.375] is helpful in distinguishing between restrictive or paralytic strabismus in such cases **(see 1.30)**.

2.26

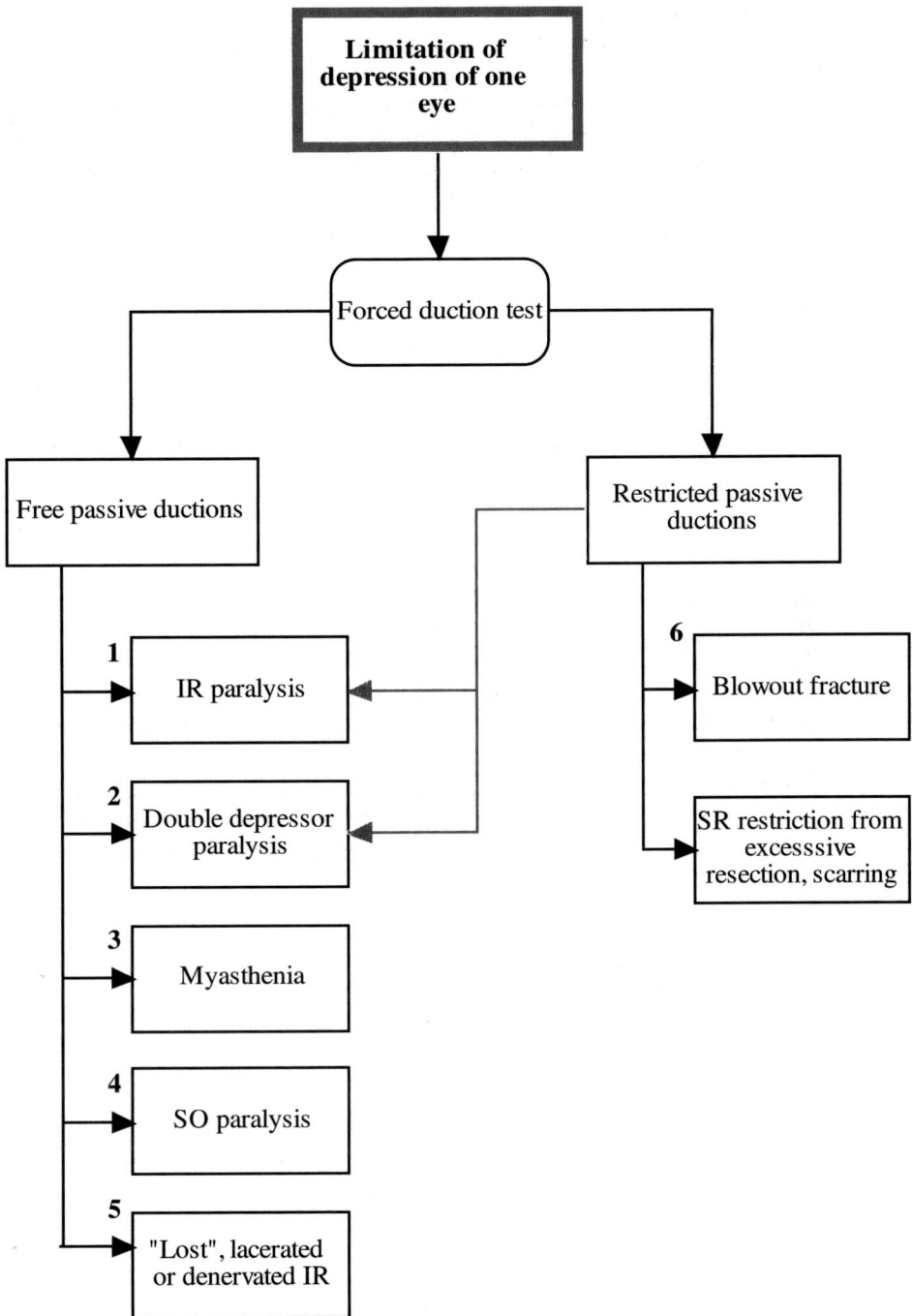

2.27   **Limitation of Abduction**

(1) Acute sixth nerve paralysis may occur after trauma, from an intracranial lesion, vascular disease, or as a benign transient form during childhood.[4; 23 p.495; 32]

(2) Limitation of abduction after surgery on the lateral rectus muscle in the presence of free forced ductions is caused by excessive recession or a slipped lateral rectus muscle. This condition is accompanied by a floating saccade and decreased or absent generated muscle force on attempted abduction.

(3) **See 2.50 and 2.52.**

(4) Limited abduction after a resection of the medial rectus muscle is caused by tightness of this muscle. Usually, this is only a temporary problem during the immediate postoperative phase. It is treated by patching the fellow eye and abduction exercises to stretch the medial rectus muscle of the involved eye. Occasionally if time and exercise fail, the tight muscle needs to be recessed.

(5) An often overlooked consequence of orbital trauma is a fracture of the medial orbital wall. Entrapment of tissue may result in limited abduction with restricted passive ductions.

(6) Infantile esotropia **(see 1.17)** and nystagmus blockage by convergence **(see 2.33)** are often accompanied by apparent limitation of abduction. The doll's head maneuver or patching of one eye distinguishes pseudoabducens paralysis from a true paralysis in these cases by uncovering normal abduction.

(7) Möbius syndrome is a bilateral congenital paralysis of the abducens and facial nerves resulting in esotropia and an expressionless facial appearance. There is also atrophy of the distal third of the tongue with a history of poor feeding.[23 p.519]

(8) The medial rectus muscle(s) is the second most commonly involved of the extraocular muscles in endocrine myopathy. The inferior rectus muscle is most frequently involved.

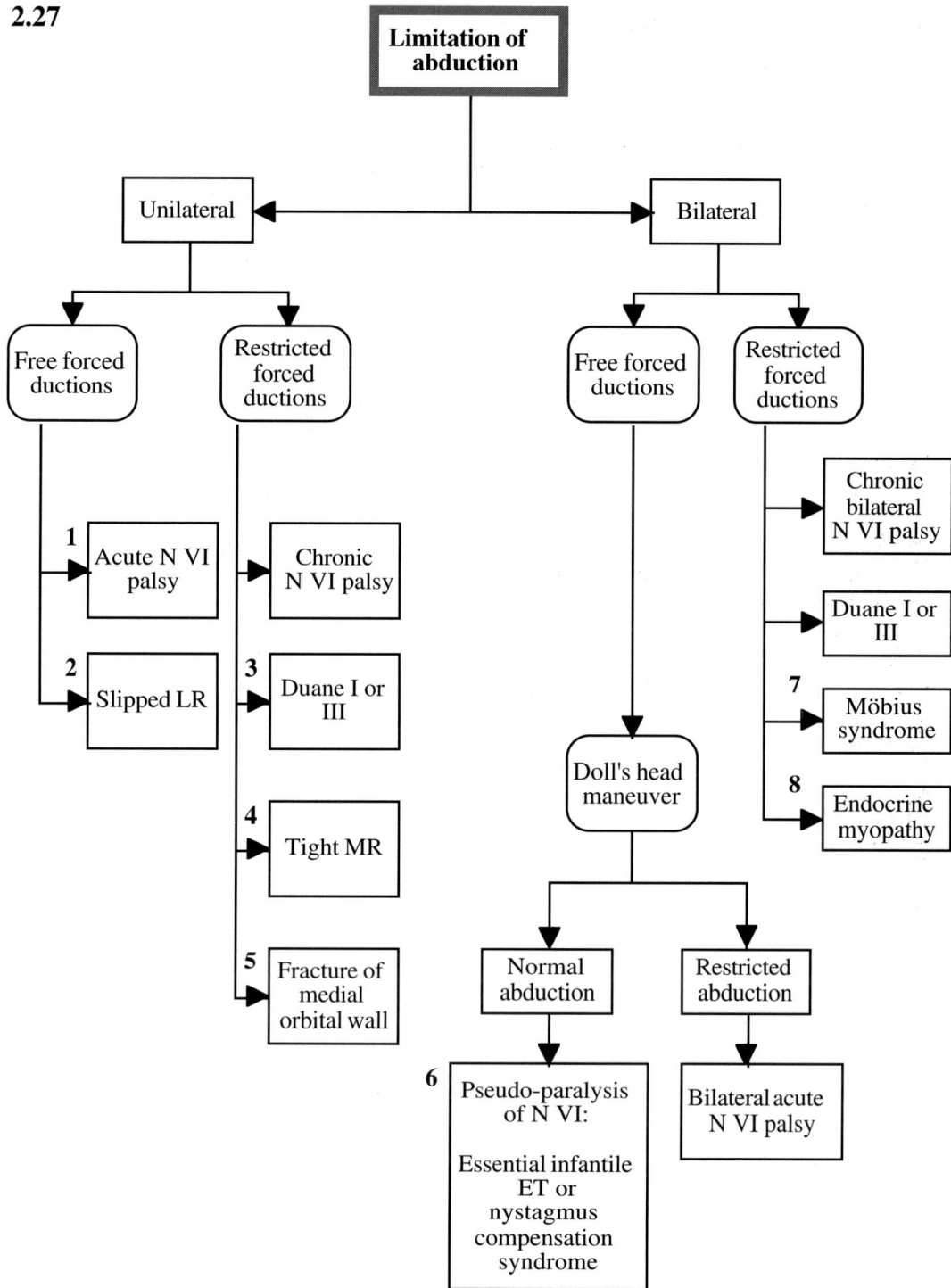

2.27

```
                        ┌─────────────────┐
                        │  Limitation of  │
                        │    abduction    │
                        └─────────────────┘
```

Unilateral ← → Bilateral

Unilateral branch:

Free forced ductions:
- **1** Acute N VI palsy
- **2** Slipped LR

Restricted forced ductions:
- Chronic N VI palsy
- **3** Duane I or III
- **4** Tight MR
- **5** Fracture of medial orbital wall

Bilateral branch:

Free forced ductions → Doll's head maneuver

Restricted forced ductions:
- Chronic bilateral N VI palsy
- Duane I or III
- **7** Möbius syndrome
- **8** Endocrine myopathy

Doll's head maneuver:
- Normal abduction → **6** Pseudo-paralysis of N VI: Essential infantile ET or nystagmus compensation syndrome
- Restricted abduction → Bilateral acute N VI palsy

2.28   Limitation of Adduction

(1) **See 2.36.**

(2) Internuclear ophthalmoplegia is caused by a lesion in the medial longitudinal fasciculus and causes limited adduction on attempted gaze to either side with abduction nystagmus in the other eye. Convergence may be spared because this is a supranuclear function.

(3) Myasthenia gravis may affect any extraocular muscle or muscle groups **(see 2.56).**

(4) **See 2.51 and 2.52.**

(5) Endocrine myopathy involving the lateral rectus muscle causes limitation of adduction with restricted passive ductions. However, other extraocular muscles, such as the inferior or medial rectus muscles, are more frequently involved, and isolated involvement of the lateral rectus muscle is rare **(see 2.55).**

(6) Limitation of adduction after surgery on the medial rectus muscle may be caused by a slipped or excessively recessed muscle. This may be accompanied by a floating saccade, reduction or absence of generated muscle force and a widened palpebral fissure.[23 p.427]

(7) Limitation of adduction after resection of the lateral rectus muscle(s) is caused by tightness of the operated muscle. The resected muscle(s) may stretch with time, and alternating occlusion with adduction exercises may be helpful. However, if this overeffect of surgery persists recession of the lateral rectus muscle(s) may be necessary.

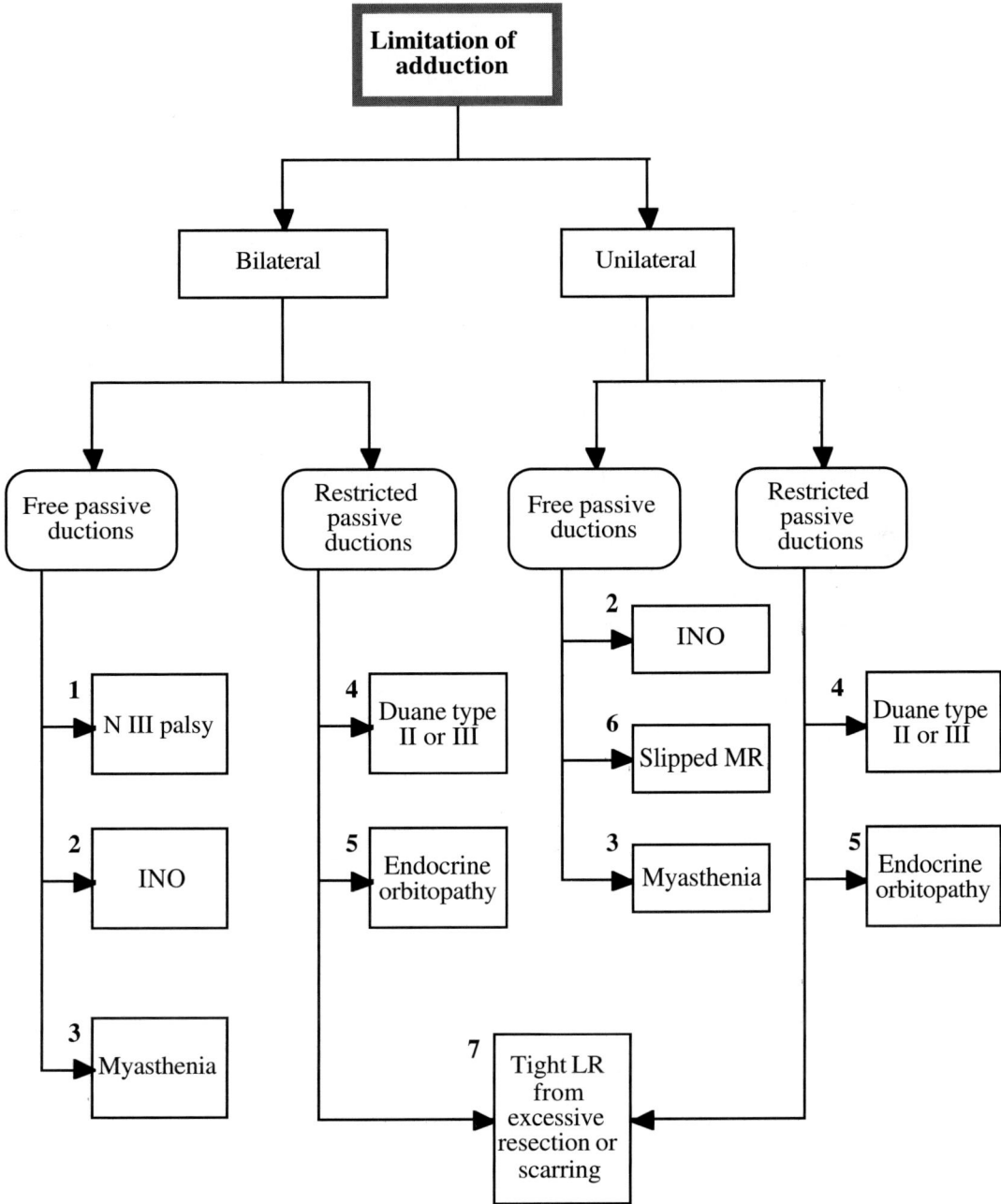

2.28

```
                    ┌─────────────────┐
                    │  Limitation of  │
                    │    adduction    │
                    └─────────────────┘
                   ┌──────────┴──────────┐
              ┌─────────┐           ┌──────────┐
              │Bilateral│           │Unilateral│
              └─────────┘           └──────────┘
```

Free passive ductions

Restricted passive ductions

Free passive ductions

Restricted passive ductions

1 N III palsy

4 Duane type II or III

2 INO

4 Duane type II or III

2 INO

6 Slipped MR

5 Endocrine orbitopathy

5 Endocrine orbitopathy

3 Myasthenia

3 Myasthenia

7 Tight LR from excessive resection or scarring

2.29   Limitation of Vertical Gaze of Both Eyes

(1) Only a few conditions cause a symmetric restriction of upward or downward gaze, or both, in both eyes while horizontal excursions remain normal.

(2) **See 2.55.**

(3) **See 1.28.**

(4) A blowout fracture of both orbits is rare but has occurred. A history of blunt trauma to both orbits immediately separates this rare cause of vertical gaze restriction from others. Surgical decompression of the orbits may cause a clinically similar picture.

(5) Supranuclear palsy of elevation may eventually also involve depression of the eyes. Impaired convergence, lid retraction, convergence-retraction nystagmus, and large pupils with light/near dissociation may be associated findings. A tumor of the pineal region is the most common cause.[23 p.541]

(6) This entity occurs only in the older age group, is characterized by supranuclear palsy of vertical gaze, especially of downward gaze, and may advance to cause total ophthalmoplegia.[57 p.419]

(7) Limitation of upward gaze occurs as an age-related normal phenomenon without clinical significance.[10]

(8) **See 2.31.**

2.29

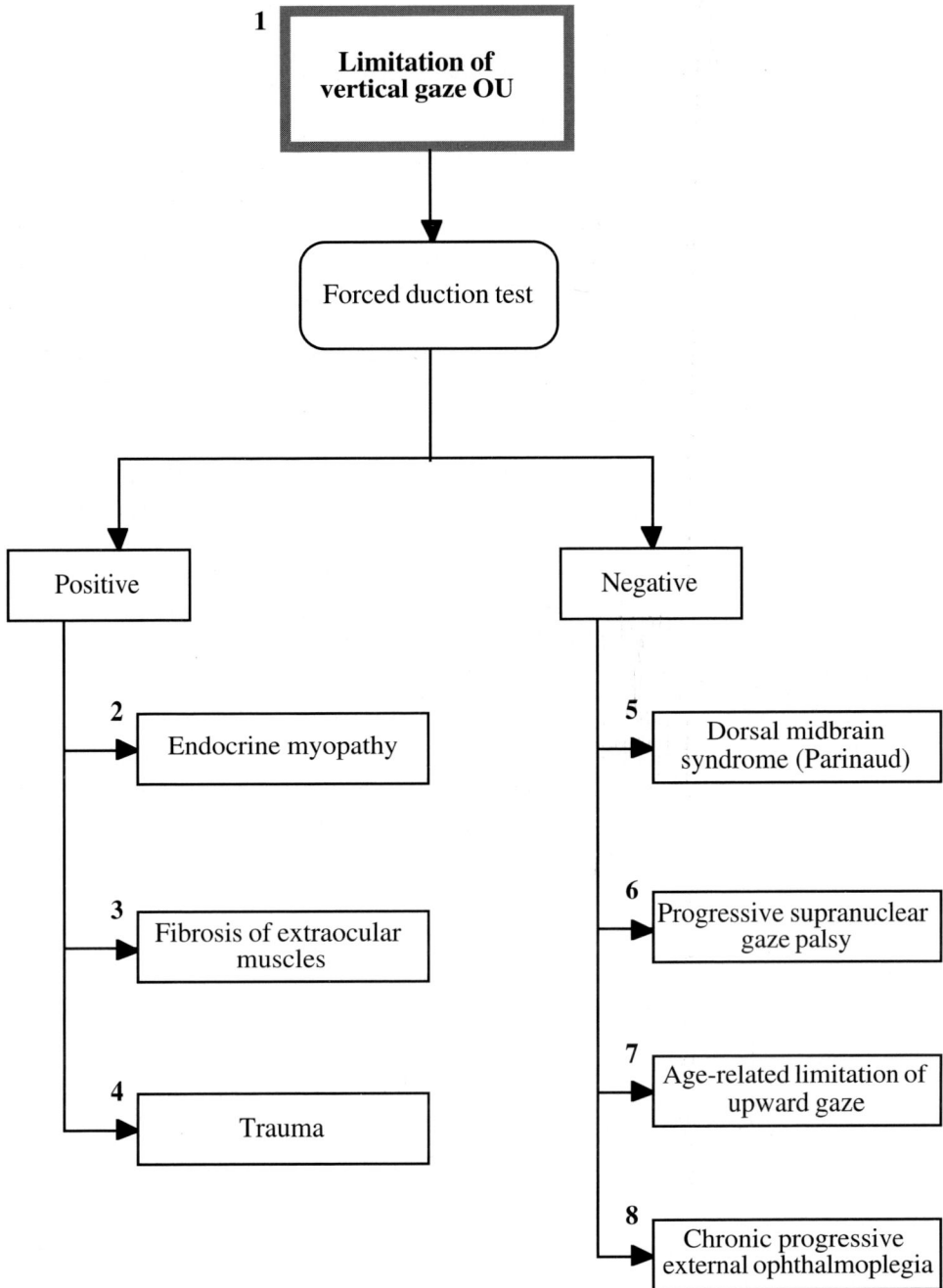

2.30 Acquired Vertical Deviation With Diplopia

(1) Acquired vertical strabismus in the adult, especially if acute, is easy to recognize because it is usually associated with diplopia and preceded by ocular surgery, trauma, or a neurologic event. However, the neurologic event may be subtle, mild, and transient. The angle of strabismus may be small requiring the use of red glass dissociation to appreciate the diplopia fields.[23] p.366; 56 p.60

(2) If the deviation is incomitant, the usual diagnostic workup for cyclovertical strabismus is done. This includes evaluation of ductions and versions, prism cover testing in the diagnostic positions, estimation of generated muscle force, forced duction testing, the Bielschowsky head tilt test, and tests for cyclotropia which usually establish the diagnosis **(see 2.36, 2.37, 2.38, 2.40, and 2.42).**

(3) A comitant or nearly comitant acquired vertical deviation can be caused by a long-standing unilateral fourth nerve palsy. The patient may have lost the ability to fuse and the deviation has now become manifest.[23] p.468

(4) A recently acquired comitant vertical deviation without an apparently offending cyclovertical muscle, associated with free passive ductions and normal generated muscle force, is called a skew deviation.[57] p.387 Vertical divergence drives one eye upward and the other downward. Although the eyes are "driven apart" vertically, because one eye is required to take up fixation, the deviation appears to be either a right hypertropia or left hypertropia at any given time. The association of skew deviation with acute neurologic disease and symptoms, usually with brainstem or cerebellar signs, and the absence of preceding trauma distinguish this condition from ordinary comitant cyclovertical strabismus.[23] p.168 The deviation is often small, occurring in an older individual and successfully treated with prisms **(see 2.49).** The term skew deviation is rejected by some in favor of the more descriptive "acquired comitant vertical deviation."

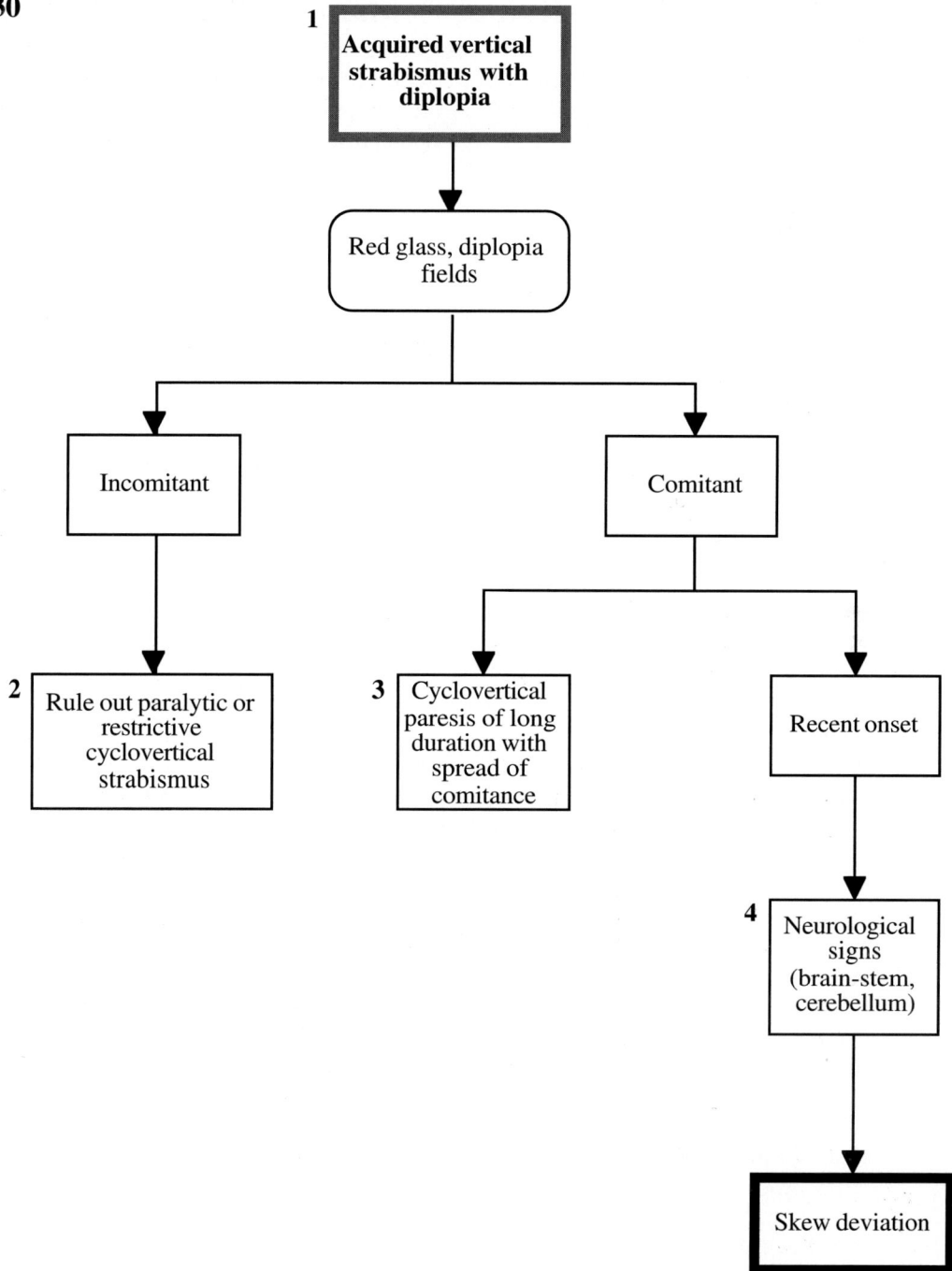

2.30

1 **Acquired vertical strabismus with diplopia**

Red glass, diplopia fields

Incomitant

Comitant

2 Rule out paralytic or restrictive cyclovertical strabismus

3 Cyclovertical paresis of long duration with spread of comitance

Recent onset

4 Neurological signs (brain-stem, cerebellum)

Skew deviation

2.31   **Generalized Limitation of Ocular Motility of Both Eyes**

(1) Restriction of motility of both eyes in all gaze positions can be a confounding diagnostic problem. This limitation may be symmetric or asymmetric. However, because all conditions listed in this algorithm can cause both symmetric or asymmetric limitation of motility in both eyes, symmetry or the lack thereof is not a helpful differentiating sign.

(2) When the forced duction test shows restriction of motility in all fields of gaze, neuroimaging is indicated, unless associated signs and symptoms are diagnostic so that no further workup is required.

(3) Endocrine myopathy may affect multiple extraocular muscles and is often bilateral. CT scanning shows thickening of the muscle bellies in the posterior aspects of the orbit **(see 2.55).**

(4) Generalized restriction of ocular motility in all gaze positions may be caused by axial elongation of the globe in the case of severe myopia. The globe "collides" with the orbital walls during its excursions. Axial length measurements in such cases may exceed 30 mm.[12]

(5) Chronic progressive external ophthalmoplegia (CPEO) of long standing may cause fibrosis of the extraocular muscles, causing the forced duction test to become positive.[23 p.524]

(6) **See 1.28.**

(7) False-positive reactions to Tensilon are infrequent but have been reported in patients with dermatomyositis and botulism.[18]

(8) A false-negative Tensilon test result is not uncommon. When myasthenia is suspected, the test should be repeated while carefully monitoring ocular motility during and immediately after the injection.

(9) CPEO may be difficult to distinguish from myasthenia gravis when the Tensilon test result is negative. Both conditions may lead to total external ophthalmoplegia, bilateral ptosis, and facial weakness. However, CPEO is often familial and characterized by a slow, progressive course, whereas remissions and fluctuations of the disease are common in myasthenia. In cases of suspected CPEO, an EKG should be obtained to rule out (or in) CPEO with heart block (Kearns-Sayre syndrome).[23 p.524]

(10) **See 2.29.**

(11) Myotonic dystrophy may mimic CPEO but has other ocular signs, such as cataracts and pigment degeneration of the retina, in addition to the typical myotonic reaction of skeletal muscles and muscle groups.

(12) Oculomotor apraxia is characterized by an inability to perform voluntary eye movements. The doll's head maneuver (oculocephalic reflex) which is normal quickly distinguishes this condition from true restriction of ocular motility.[57 p.71]

2.31

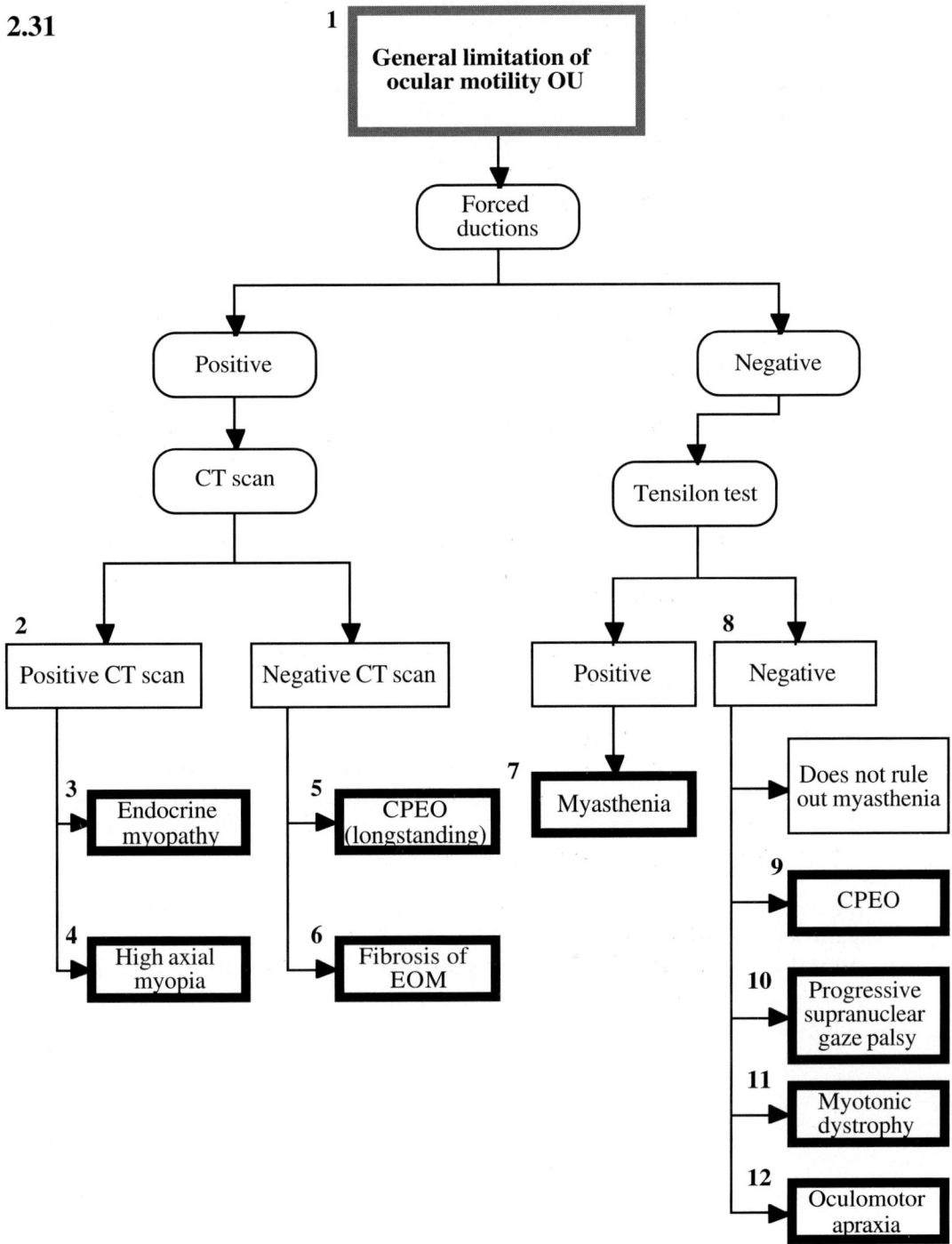

2.32   Painful Ophthalmoplegia

(1) Restriction of ocular motility associated with pain and diplopia usually has an acute or subacute onset. The patient is seen in acute distress, and the examiner must distinguish between several conditions that produce clinically similar pictures. None of these occur frequently. Orbital cellulitis, mucormycosis, orbital tumors, and the parasellar syndrome are not included in this consideration, but each of these conditions may at some stage mimic one of the entities listed in this table.

(2) Ocular myositis (inflammatory pseudotumor of the orbit) is a nonspecific inflammatory condition that involves one or several of the extraocular muscles. The cause is unknown but autoimmune disease has been implicated. Unlike in endocrine ophthalmopathy, which shows predilection for some but not all orbital tissues, any or all orbital structures may become involved in the inflammatory process of pseudotumor. Restriction of gaze may occur in the field of action of an involved muscle; this is in contrast to endocrine orbitopathy, where the limitation is in the opposite field of gaze.[57 p.410]

(3) An acquired Brown syndrome (see 2.53) caused by inflammation of the peritrochlear region may cause pain to local palpation and when elevation of the involved eye is attempted.[20,23 p.454]

(4) With the advent of antibacterial therapy, Gradenigo syndrome has become rare in developed countries.

(5) The distinction between the superior orbital fissure syndrome, in which the third, fourth, and sixth nerves may become involved in any combination,[18] and orbital pseudotumor is not always easy. The clinical manifestations (pain, exophthalmos, and ophthalmoplegia) are the same. It has been suggested that both entities are different presentations of the same disease.[57 p.413]

(6) Trichinosis has become a rare disorder in developed countries. The first stage, characterized by diarrhea, vomiting, and fever, the history, and bilateral orbital involvement clearly distinguish this condition from other forms of painful ophthalmoplegia.[57 p.413]

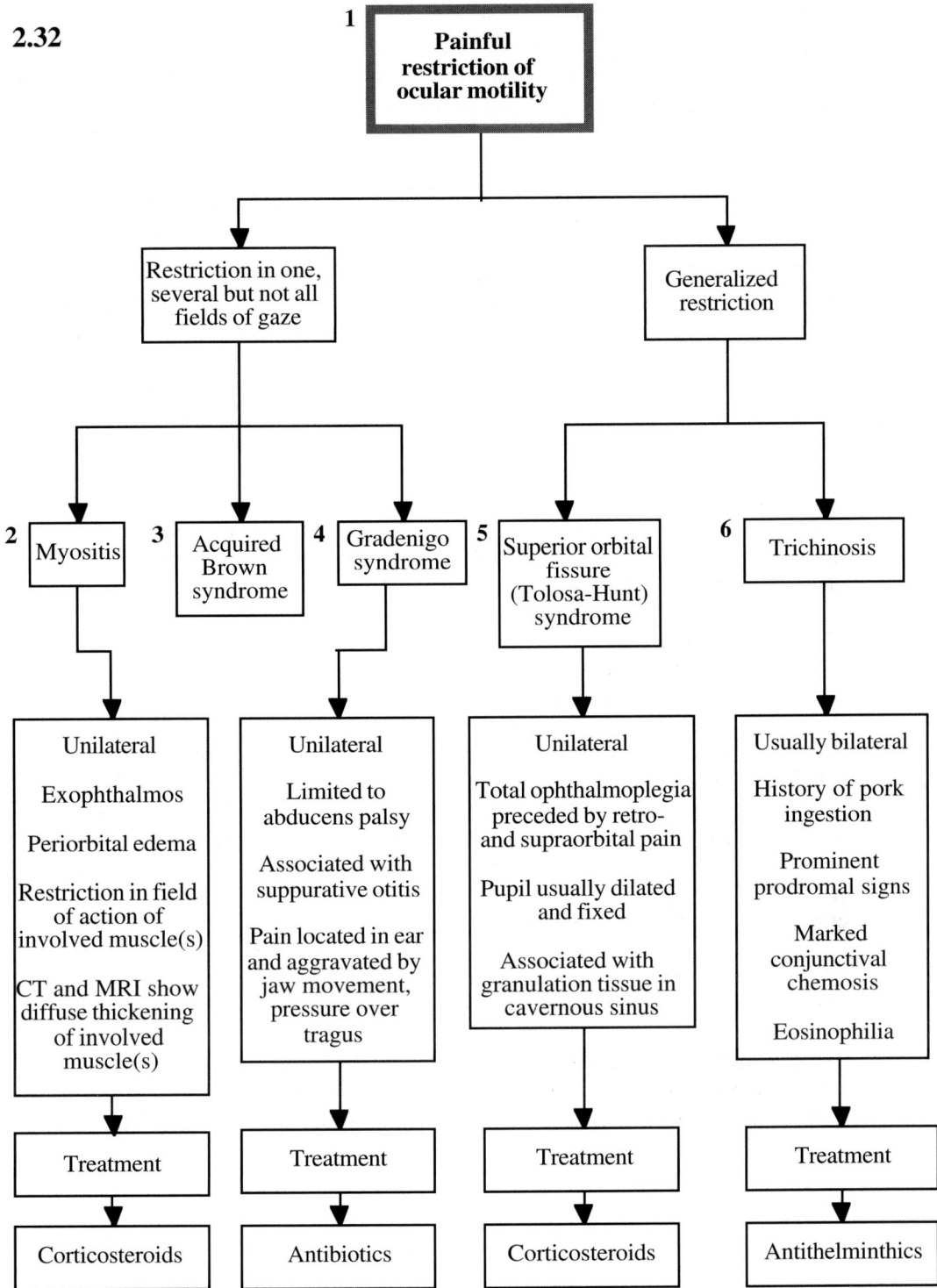

2.32

```
                          1  ┌─────────────────┐
                             │     Painful     │
                             │  restriction of │
                             │ ocular motility │
                             └─────────────────┘
                                      │
              ┌───────────────────────┴───────────────────────┐
   ┌──────────────────┐                          ┌──────────────────┐
   │ Restriction in one, │                        │   Generalized    │
   │ several but not all │                        │   restriction    │
   │   fields of gaze    │                        └──────────────────┘
   └──────────────────┘
```

2 Myositis	3 Acquired Brown syndrome	4 Gradenigo syndrome	5 Superior orbital fissure (Tolosa-Hunt) syndrome	6 Trichinosis

Unilateral	Unilateral	Unilateral	Usually bilateral
Exophthalmos	Limited to abducens palsy	Total ophthalmoplegia preceded by retro- and supraorbital pain	History of pork ingestion
Periorbital edema	Associated with suppurative otitis	Pupil usually dilated and fixed	Prominent prodromal signs
Restriction in field of action of involved muscle(s)	Pain located in ear and aggravated by jaw movement, pressure over tragus	Associated with granulation tissue in cavernous sinus	Marked conjunctival chemosis
CT and MRI show diffuse thickening of involved muscle(s)			Eosinophilia

Treatment	Treatment	Treatment	Treatment
Corticosteroids	Antibiotics	Corticosteroids	Antithelminthics

2.33   Compensation Strategies in Manifest Congenital Nystagmus

Patients with congenital motor nystagmus may use several strategies to decrease nystagmus intensity and thus improve visual acuity.[23 p.542; 69]

(1) Convergence innervation superimposed on any type of nystagmus dampens nystagmus intensity; thus patients with congenital nystagmus frequently have better vision at near than at distance fixation.[23 p.422]

(2) Sustained convergence in an effort to dampen nystagmus may cause hypertonicity of the medial rectus muscles and esotropia (nystagmus compensation or blocking syndrome, i.e., NBS)[57 p.438] **(see 1.17).**

(3) Treatment of nystagmus blockage syndrome (NBS) consists of recession of the medial rectus muscles, posterior fixation of the medial recti, or a combination of both.[23 p.422]

(4) Some patients have a null zone or neutral point in right or left gaze where the nystagmus is least pronounced and where vision is best. Such patients assume a compensatory head turn to the right or left to place the eyes in the position of least nystagmus especially during tasks where better vision is required.[69]

(5) To normalize the head turn, both eyes are moved into the direction of the head turn or away from the preferred gaze position by the appropriate recession and resection surgery on the extraocular muscles.[23 p.542; 57 p.448]

(6) In some patients the neutral zone is in upward or downward gaze, which may cause chin elevation or depression.

(7) Both superior rectus muscles are resected and the inferior rectus muscles are recessed to move the eye upward in cases of a neutral zone in downward gaze with chin elevation. For chin depression the superior rectus muscles are recessed and the inferior rectus muscles are resected.[23 p.541; 57 p.448]

(8) Less frequently the neutral zone is in a tertiary gaze position and the patient assumes a head tilt to the right or left shoulder.[69]

(9) The vertical recti are transposed horizontally to cause excycloduction or incycloduction of the eye(s). This causes tilting of the subjective visual horizon, which the patient must overcome by straightening the head[69] **(see 2.21 and 2.22).**

2.33

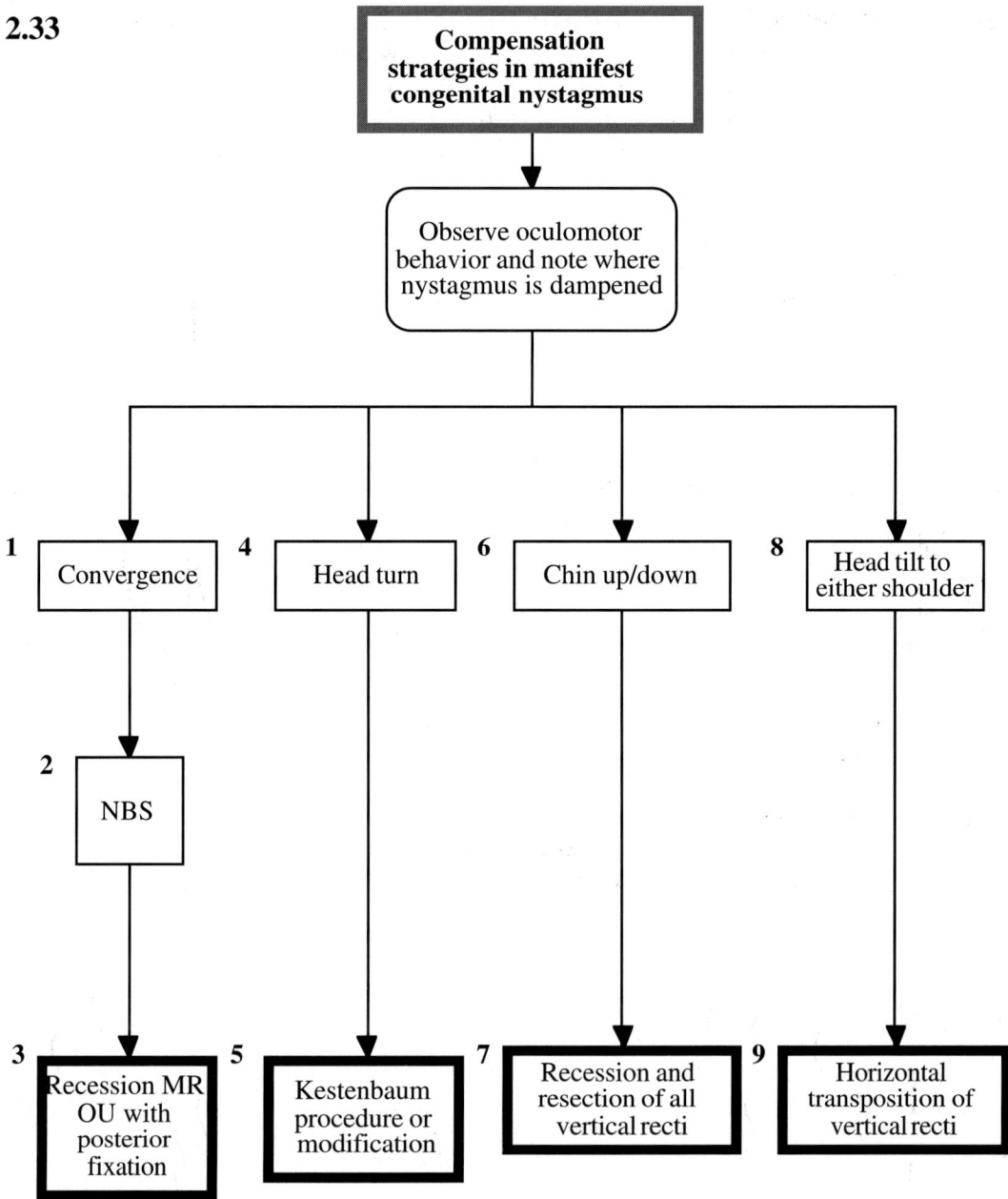

2.34   Compensation Strategies of Manifest-Latent Nystagmus

(1) About 10% to 20% of patients with essential infantile esotropia have manifest-latent nystagmus.[57,60] It is essential to understand this oxymoronic term. True latent nystagmus occurs only when one eye is occluded. Manifest-latent nystagmus occurs with both eyes open but intensifies when one eye is covered or suppressed.

(2) In most patients with manifest-latent nystagmus, the fixating eye assumes a position of adduction because the nystagmus is least pronounced in that position. Nystagmus increases and visual acuity usually decreases as the eye moves from adduction toward primary position and abduction.[69] Fixation preference in abduction with a decrease of nystagmus in that position may also occur but is unusual.[23 p.422]

(3) In the presence of strong ocular preference the preferred eye is in a position of adduction and the patient turns the head toward the side of the fixating eye. The nonfixating eye frequently becomes amblyopic.

(4) Surgery for esotropia should be limited to the fixating eye.

(5) With alternating fixation the patient may have an alternating head turn, and surgery may be performed on both eyes.

(6) Manifest-latent nystagmus may occur in orthotropic patients without history of previous strabismus.

(7) Binocular vision "blocks" the nystagmus completely (pure latent nystagmus) or dampens its intensity (manifest-latent nystagmus). After disruption of binocular vision the nystagmus increases.

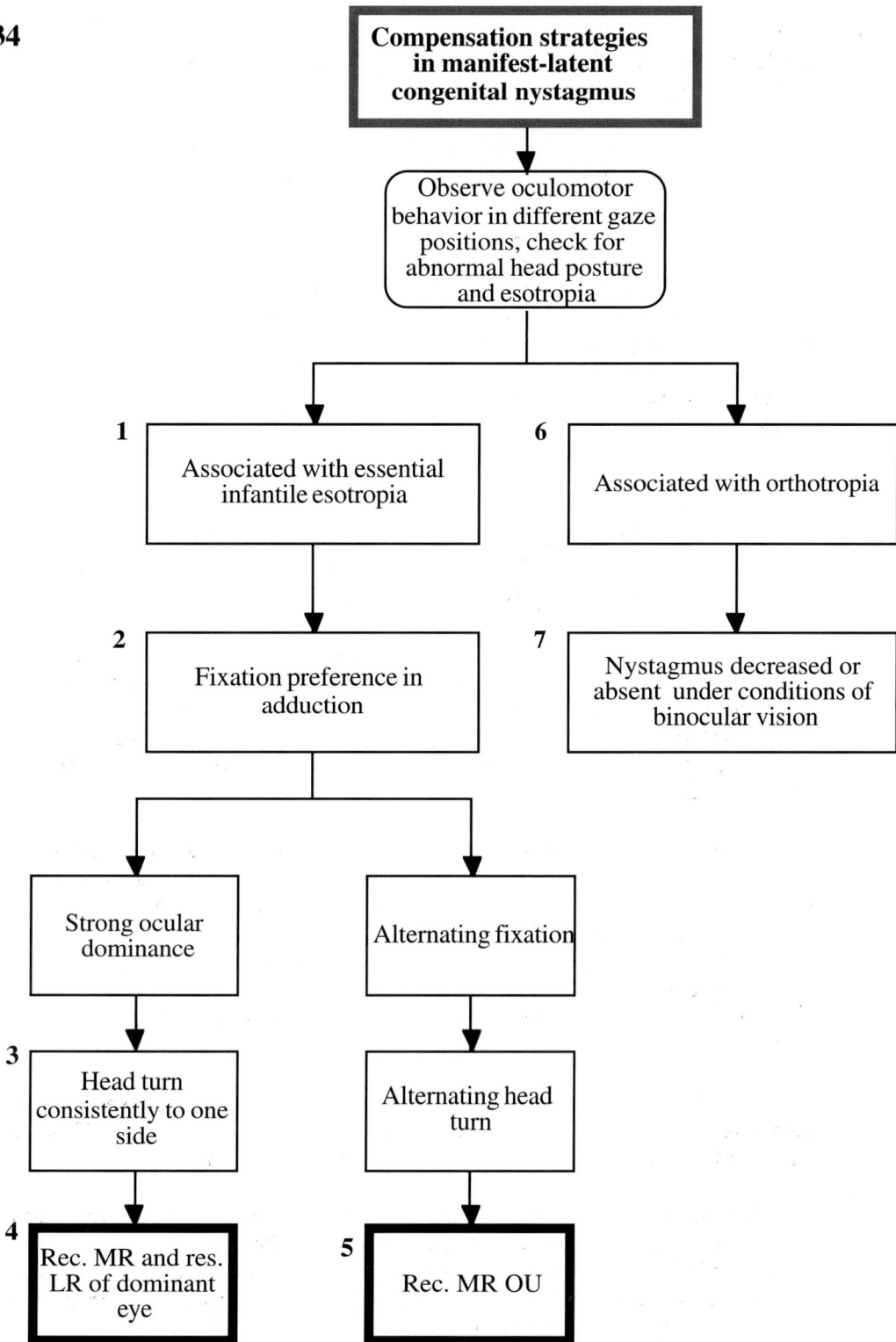

2.34

Compensation strategies in manifest-latent congenital nystagmus

Observe oculomotor behavior in different gaze positions, check for abnormal head posture and esotropia

1 Associated with essential infantile esotropia

6 Associated with orthotropia

2 Fixation preference in adduction

7 Nystagmus decreased or absent under conditions of binocular vision

Strong ocular dominance

Alternating fixation

3 Head turn consistently to one side

Alternating head turn

4 Rec. MR and res. LR of dominant eye

5 Rec. MR OU

2.35 Treatment of Nystagmus

(1) Most patients with manifest congenital nystagmus do not require treatment. However, occasionally treatment may be indicated for functional reasons. Before treatment is started the distinction between treatment directed at the nystagmus per se or at the anomalous head posture must be made. In this algorithm only treatment directed at the nystagmus is considered.

(2) In pure motor nystagmus the eyes are structurally normal and variations of visual acuity depend on the motor stability of the eyes. Stability is enhanced in certain gaze positions or under the influence of superimposed innervation. The less pronounced the nystagmus, the better the visual acuity. A prime example of motor type nystagmus is a patient whose visual acuity improves or even normalizes under the influence of convergence at near fixation compared with distance fixation. Treatment of motor nystagmus is directed at improving stabilization of the eyes.

(3) A significant refractive error must be fully corrected to create conditions for optimal visual acuity. Prisms before both eyes with the base in the same direction as the head turn shifts a lateral gaze neutral point, obviating the need for a compensatory head turn. Artificial stimulation of convergence by base-out prism spectacles may decrease nystagmus and thus improve distance vision.

(4) In sensory nystagmus visual acuity remains poor, regardless of ocular stability. The nystagmus occurs as a result of poor vision, which is often caused by retinal dysfunction. Treatment results in little if any functional improvement in acuity but some patients may benefit from the effect of decreasing nystagmus amplitude by means of improved eye contact and thereby derive functional benefit after surgery.

(5) Retroequatorial recession of all four horizontal rectus muscles has been shown to be effective in reducing the nystagmus amplitude in some cases.[25,71] In some but not all cases of motor-type nystagmus there may also be a moderate improvement of visual acuity. Such improvement cannot be expected in sensory type nystagmus. Because equal amounts of recession of the medial and lateral rectus muscles may cause a consecutive exodeviation, we recess the medial recti 2 mm less than the lateral recti. The amounts of recession may be further modified in the presence of coexisting esodeviations or exodeviations.

(6) A surgically induced exotropia causes a convergence impulse to regain fusion and avoid diplopia, provided the patient has the ability to fuse. This method must undergo additional study before it can be recommended.

Although there is no difference in treatment techniques for sensory and motor manifest congenital nystagmus, outcomes are different. Visual improvement from stabilizing eye movements cannot exceed the eye's inherent visual potential, which is reduced in sensory nystagmus from albinism, congenital cataract, optic nerve hypoplasia, and so on.

2.35

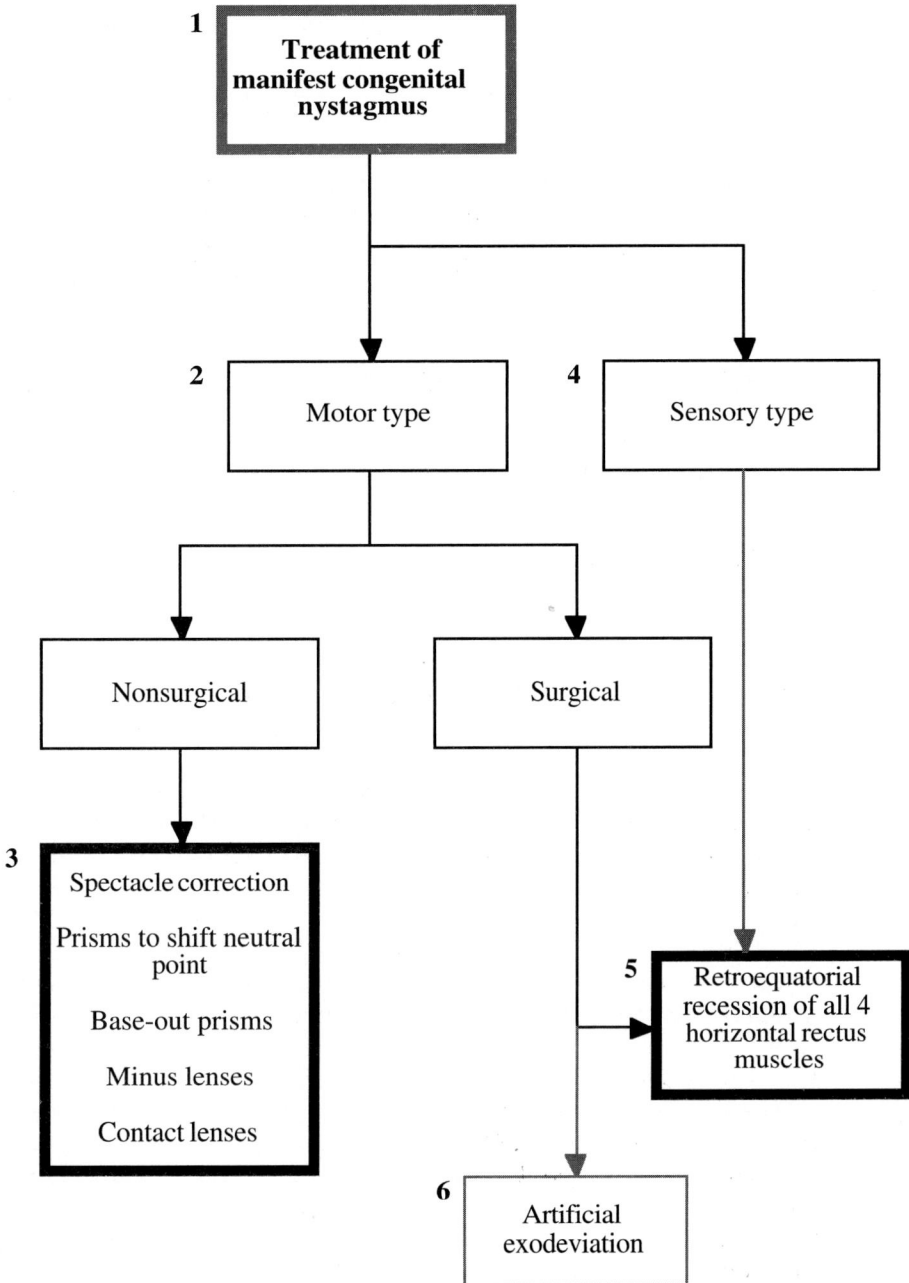

2.36   Complete Third Nerve Palsy

(1) The combination of exotropia, hypotropia, limitation of adduction, elevation, and depression in association with ptosis is diagnostic for a third nerve paralysis. Abduction and incycloduction are the only remaining oculomotor functions. Depending on the degree of ptosis, the patient may or may not see double.

(2) Congenital paralysis may be unilateral or bilateral. The unilateral form is the more common one.

(3) Lid elevation on attempted adduction and depression with or without constriction of the pupil are signs of aberrant regeneration of the third nerve. Aberrant regeneration is seen in about two thirds of congenital third nerve paralyses. It is a common finding in third nerve paralysis acquired early in life.

(4) The pupil reaction may be normal or the pupil is fixed and dilated. In congenital third nerve palsy, the pupil may be constricted.

(5) Occasionally patients with a congenital third nerve paralysis fixate with the paralyzed eye. This causes a large combined exodeviation and hyperdeviation of the normal eye, which may become deeply amblyopic.

(6) Associated ocular or systemic abnormalities may be associated with congenital third nerve paralysis and should be searched for, including neuroimaging.

(7) A leading cause of nontraumatic third nerve paralysis is diabetes. The pupil is spared and no aberrant regeneration occurs. The condition is usually self-limiting and associated with diplopia unless ptosis is complete.

(8) Third nerve paralysis can occur from extrinsic fascicular defects, caused by pressure, vascular lesions, or nerve interruptions. This may be related to systemic disease or trauma. Aberrant regeneration is common and occurs in two thirds of patients.

(9) Traumatic third nerve paralysis is usually associated with a fixed and dilated pupil. Aberrant regeneration may occur and diplopia is frequent unless visual acuity is decreased by associated ocular injuries or ptosis.

(10) The surgical treatment of third nerve paralysis presents a formidable challenge to the ophthalmic surgeon. A complete third nerve paralysis with complete ptosis is best left untreated. When the paralysis is partial, especially when some adduction is preserved, the patient may benefit from a maximal recession of the lateral and resection of the medial rectus muscles. This may be combined with upward transposition of the muscle insertions to counteract the hypotropia. Transfer of the superior oblique muscle to the insertion of the medial rectus muscle with or without fracture of the trochlea has also been recommended.[23 p.300] Ptosis surgery is postponed until alignment of the eyes has been achieved by surgery. Caution with regard to ptosis surgery is advised if elevation is impaired because of exposure problems.

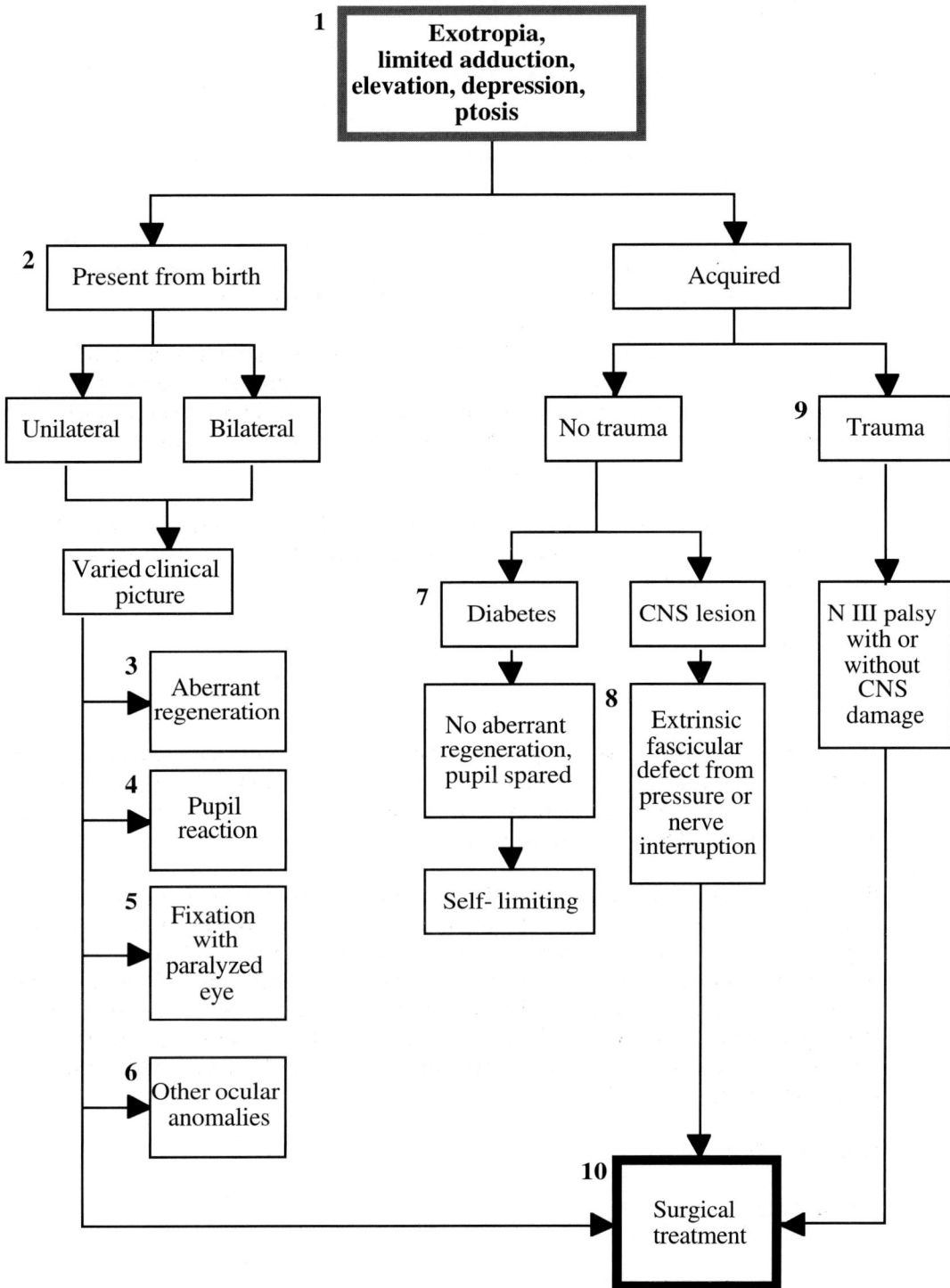

2.36

1 Exotropia, limited adduction, elevation, depression, ptosis

2 Present from birth

Acquired

Unilateral

Bilateral

No trauma

9 Trauma

Varied clinical picture

7 Diabetes

CNS lesion

N III palsy with or without CNS damage

3 Aberrant regeneration

No aberrant regeneration, pupil spared

8 Extrinsic fascicular defect from pressure or nerve interruption

4 Pupil reaction

Self- limiting

5 Fixation with paralyzed eye

6 Other ocular anomalies

10 Surgical treatment

2.37 Superior Rectus Muscle Paralysis

(1) Initial decision making in a patient with hypertropia has identified paralysis of a superior rectus muscle. Further diagnostic and differential diagnostic maneuvers are now required to confirm the diagnosis and exclude similar conditions.

(2) The head tilt test **(see 2.42)** is less consistent in vertical rectus paralyses than in oblique muscle paralyses.

(3) Measuring the deviation with either eye fixing may be useful. The contralateral inferior oblique muscle overacts when the patient fixates with the paralyzed eye in elevation and abduction (secondary deviation) **(see 1.08).**

(4) Superior rectus paralysis may be associated with weakness of the ipsilateral levator palpebrae muscle, in which case a true ptosis is present. In other cases, levator function may be essentially normal and pseudoptosis is present, caused by the depressed position of the paretic eye. In that case the upper lid elevates normally when the sound eye is covered.

(5) A superior rectus paralysis frequently causes a head tilt with chin elevation. However, the direction of the head tilt (i.e., to the right or left shoulder) is inconsistent and therefore of no diagnostic value.

(6) **See 2.56.**

(7) **See 2.25.**

(8) Patients with trochlear palsy who habitually fixate with their paralyzed eye have a pseudoparalysis of the contralateral superior rectus muscle (inhibitional palsy of the contralateral antagonist).[57 p.367] The Bielschowsky head tilt test distinguishes between these two conditions **(see 2.47).**

(9) Depending on the comitance of the deviation and on whether secondary contracture of the ipsilateral inferior rectus muscle has developed, resection of the superior rectus is combined with recession of its antagonist.[57 p.393] In paralysis of both elevator muscles (double elevator paralysis), the insertions of both horizontal rectus muscles are transposed to the insertion of the superior rectus muscle (Knapp procedure), provided the forced duction test is negative. In other cases, resection of the paretic superior rectus may be combined with recession of the contralateral superior rectus.

(10) **See 1.28 and 2.25.**

(11) **See 2.54.**

2.37

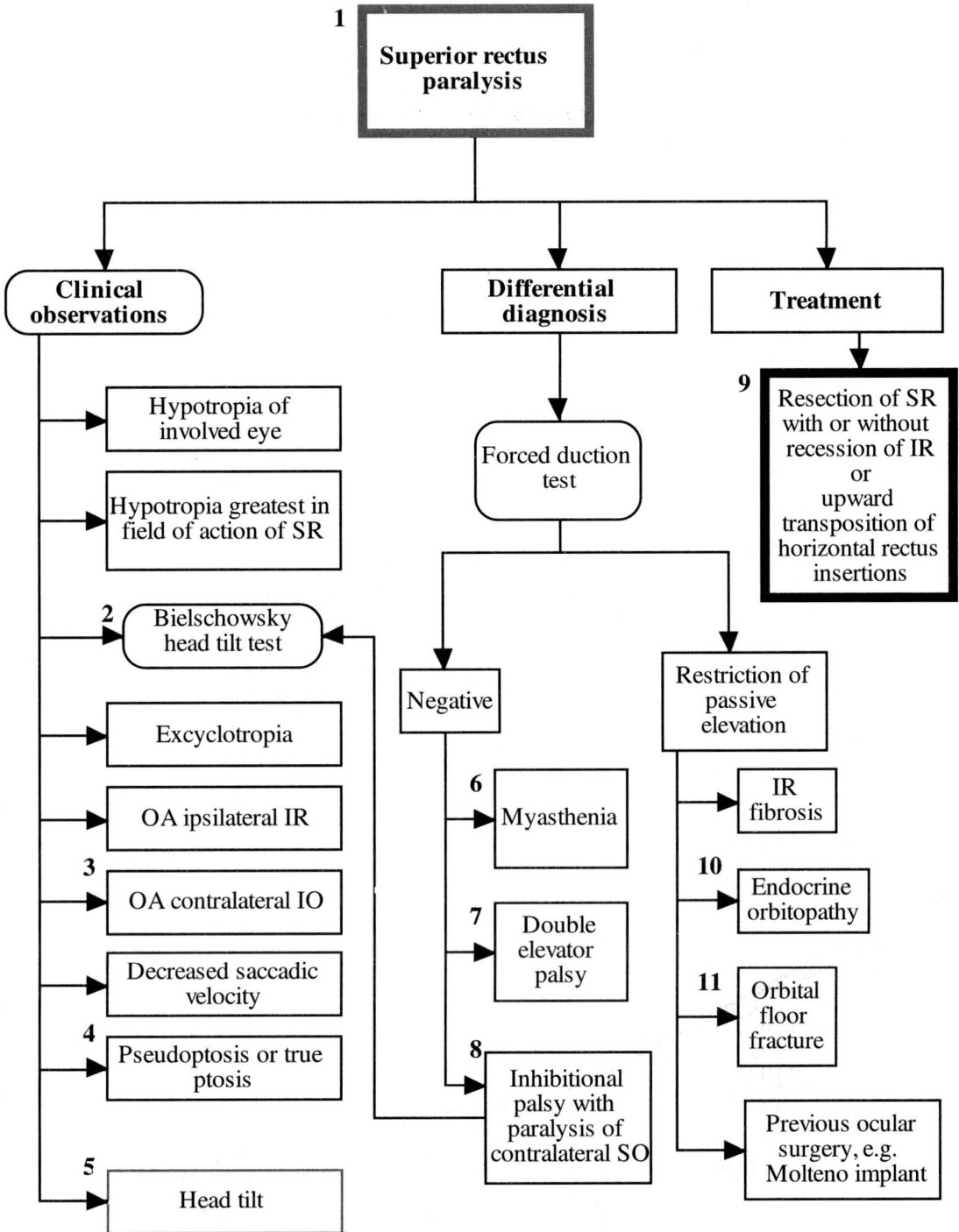

1 Superior rectus paralysis

Clinical observations

Hypotropia of involved eye

Hypotropia greatest in field of action of SR

2 Bielschowsky head tilt test

Excyclotropia

OA ipsilateral IR

3 OA contralateral IO

Decreased saccadic velocity

4 Pseudoptosis or true ptosis

5 Head tilt

Differential diagnosis

Forced duction test

Negative

6 Myasthenia

7 Double elevator palsy

8 Inhibitional palsy with paralysis of contralateral SO

Treatment

9 Resection of SR with or without recession of IR or upward transposition of horizontal rectus insertions

Restriction of passive elevation

IR fibrosis

10 Endocrine orbitopathy

11 Orbital floor fracture

Previous ocular surgery, e.g. Molteno implant

2.38   **Inferior Rectus Muscle Paralysis**

(1) Initial decision making has identified paralysis of an inferior rectus muscle. The diagnosis needs confirmation and clinically similar conditions must be distinguished.

(2) Long-standing paralysis of the inferior rectus muscle may cause contracture of the ipsilateral superior rectus muscle. In such cases, depression is limited not only in abduction but also in adduction.

(3) The head tilt test is more reliable in paralyses of the oblique muscles than of the vertical rectus muscles **(see 2.42).**

(4) Measuring the deviation with either eye fixing may be useful. The contralateral superior oblique muscle overacts when the patient fixates with the paralyzed eye in depression and abduction (secondary deviation) **(see 1.08).**

(5) When the patient fixates with the paralyzed eye in primary position, excessive innervation flows to the depressor muscles of the normal eye (Hering's law), which becomes hypotropic. Because the upper lid follows the vertical movements of the eye, a pseudoptosis may occur in the sound eye and confound the diagnosis.

(6) An ocular head tilt may be present but neither its presence nor its direction are diagnostic for inferior rectus palsy.[66] In the presence of fusion a chin depression is usually found **(see 1.29).**

(7) **See 2.56.**

(8) **See 2.26.**

(9) **See 2.55.**

(10) **See 2.54.**

(11) **See 2.54.**

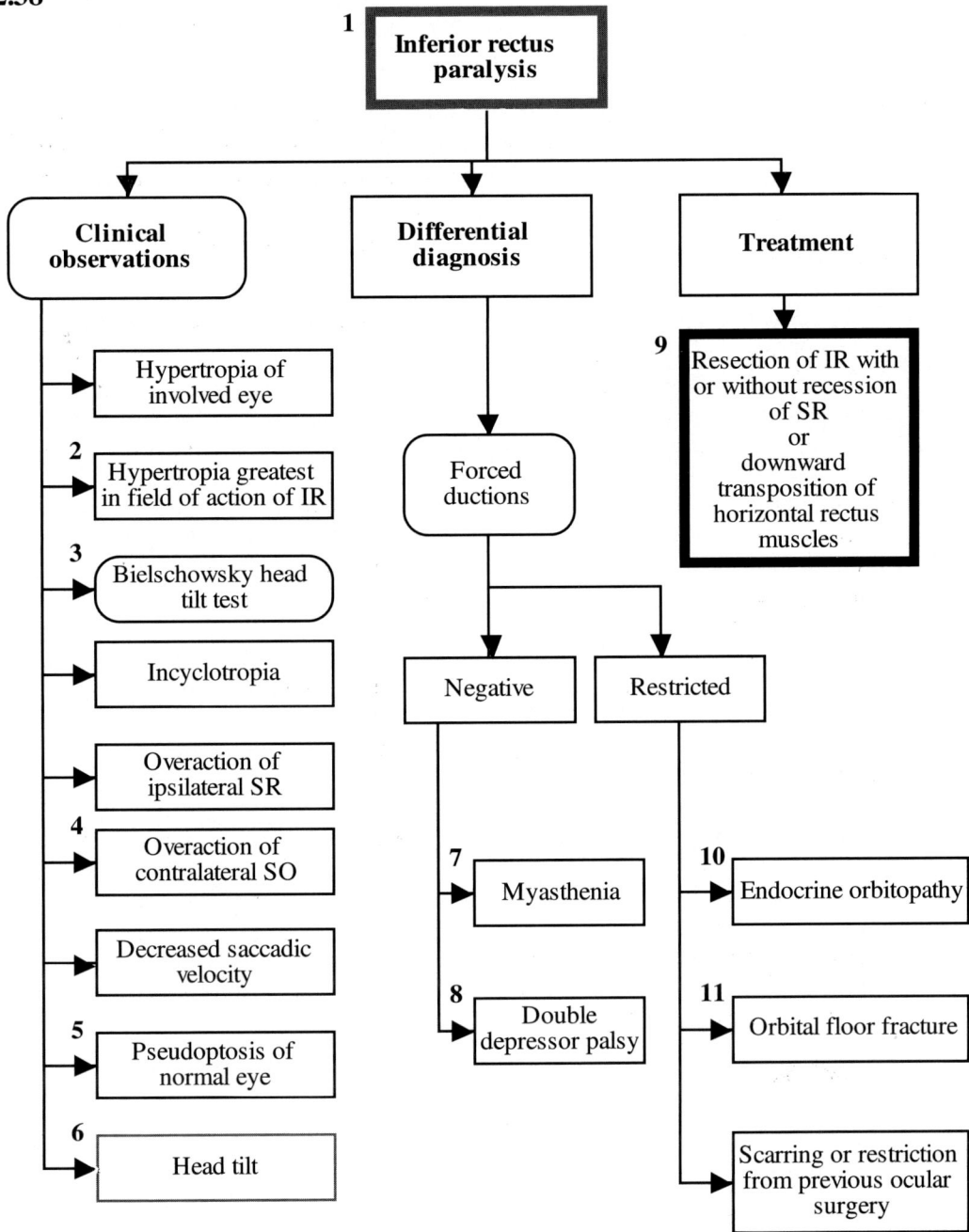

2.38

1 **Inferior rectus paralysis**

Clinical observations

Differential diagnosis

Treatment

Hypertropia of involved eye

2 Hypertropia greatest in field of action of IR

3 Bielschowsky head tilt test

Incyclotropia

Overaction of ipsilateral SR

4 Overaction of contralateral SO

Decreased saccadic velocity

5 Pseudoptosis of normal eye

6 Head tilt

Forced ductions

9 Resection of IR with or without recession of SR or downward transposition of horizontal rectus muscles

Negative

Restricted

7 Myasthenia

8 Double depressor palsy

10 Endocrine orbitopathy

11 Orbital floor fracture

Scarring or restriction from previous ocular surgery

2.39   Medial Rectus Muscle Paralysis

(1) Isolated medial rectus paralysis without involvement of other muscles supplied by the third nerve is rare.

(2) In the foreground of diagnostic features is a variable exotropia that decreases or may be completely absent when the affected eye is in abduction and increases exponentially as the paralyzed eye attempts adduction (secondary deviation).

(3) A head turn toward the nonparetic side may allow the patient to attain single binocular vision.

(4) Isolated medial rectus paralysis may be associated with ptosis and upper lid retraction on attempted adduction (aberrant regeneration) in patients with partial third nerve paralysis **(see 2.36).** A ptosis with aberrant regeneration, causing the lid to lift when the paralyzed eye attempts to adduct, is treated by resecting the contralateral medial and recessing the contralateral lateral rectus muscles.[41]

(5) Medial rectus paralysis must be distinguished from internuclear ophthalmoplegia (INO), caused by lesions in the medial longitudinal fasciculus. In this condition unilateral or bilateral limitation of adduction is associated with nystagmus of the abducting eye. Convergence may be or may not be normal.

(6) A clinical picture similar to INO or medial rectus paralysis may be simulated by myasthenia gravis. A Tensilon test may be indicated **(see 2.56).**

(7) Postoperative medial rectus paralysis after surgery on the medial rectus muscle may be caused by a "slipped" or "lost" muscle.[23 p.426]

(8) Surgery may be done on the affected eye or may be divided between the paralyzed and the sound eye and consists of resection of the paralyzed medial rectus and recession of its yoke muscle, the lateral rectus of the sound eye, or recession of the ipsilateral lateral rectus muscle. In case of complete paralysis with exotropia in the primary position and with the head passively straightened, or when a "lost" muscle cannot be located, a full tendon transfer of the vertical recti to the insertion of the medial rectus muscle may be indicated.

(9) **See 2.55.**

(10) Restriction of adduction may be caused by an excessively resected lateral rectus muscle.

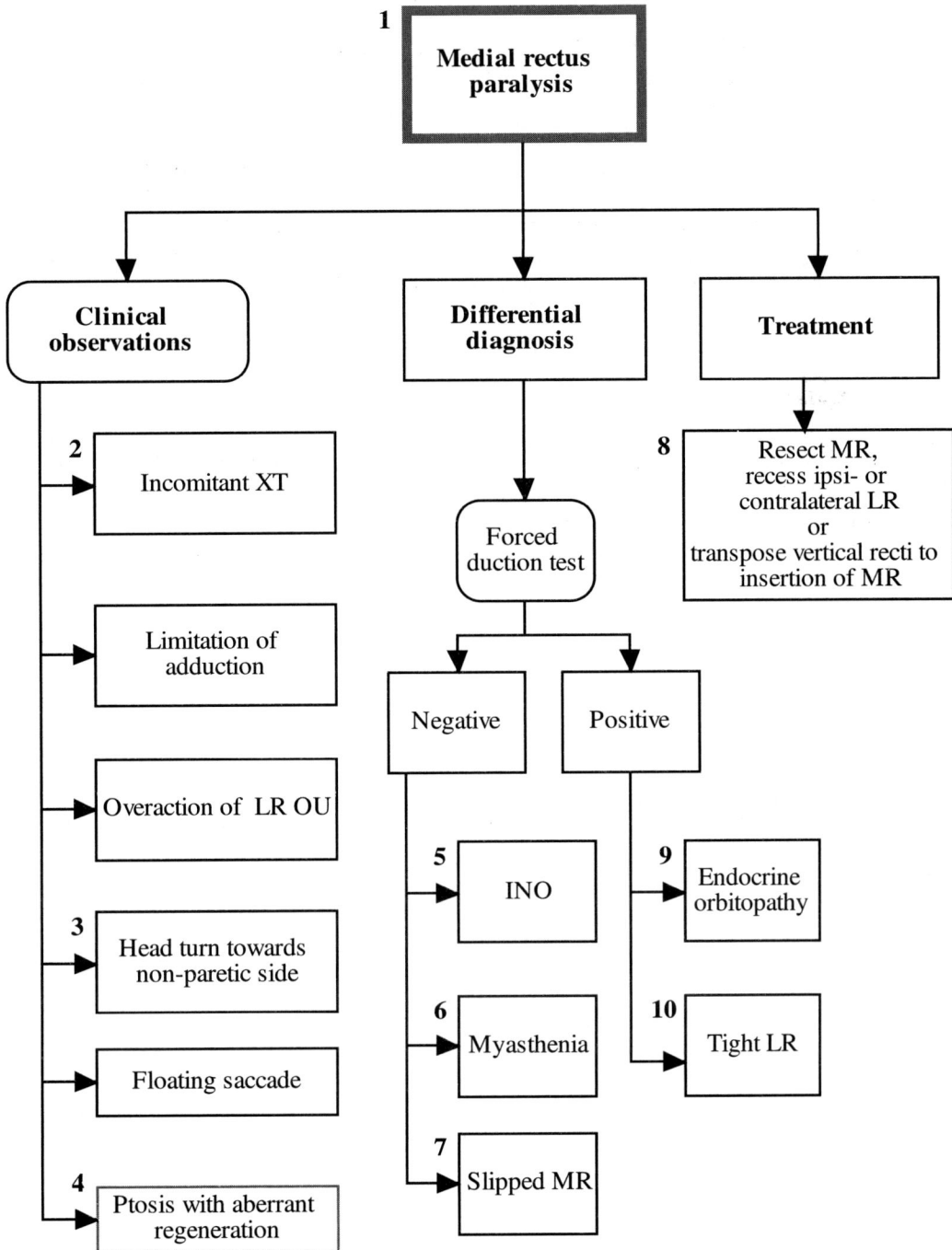

2.39

1 **Medial rectus paralysis**

Clinical observations

Differential diagnosis

Treatment

2 Incomitant XT

Limitation of adduction

Overaction of LR OU

3 Head turn towards non-paretic side

Floating saccade

4 Ptosis with aberrant regeneration

Forced duction test

Negative

Positive

8 Resect MR, recess ipsi- or contralateral LR or transpose vertical recti to insertion of MR

5 INO

6 Myasthenia

7 Slipped MR

9 Endocrine orbitopathy

10 Tight LR

2.40   Inferior Oblique Muscle Paralysis

(1) Among the extraocular muscles, the inferior oblique is the least likely to become paralyzed. The onset usually is congenital and treatment is surgical.

(2) The Bielschowsky head tilt test is fairly consistent and shows an increase of the vertical deviation on tilting the head toward the side opposite the paretic eye **(see 2.42).**[56 p.146]

(3) Measuring the deviation with either eye fixing may be helpful in identifying the offending muscle. The contralateral superior rectus overacts when the patient fixates with the paralyzed eye in elevation and adduction (secondary deviation). The hypotropia under these conditions is greater than when the patient fixates with the normal eye (primary deviation) **(see 1.08).**

(4) A head tilt toward the paralyzed side with chin elevation is present.

(5) **See 2.53.**

(6) Tenectomy of the ipsilateral superior oblique muscle is an effective procedure in this condition. However, it may cause an iatrogenic superior oblique paralysis and require additional surgery.[43] An alternative approach, surgery on the contralateral vertical recti, is also effective and safer but has little effect on the incyclotropia.

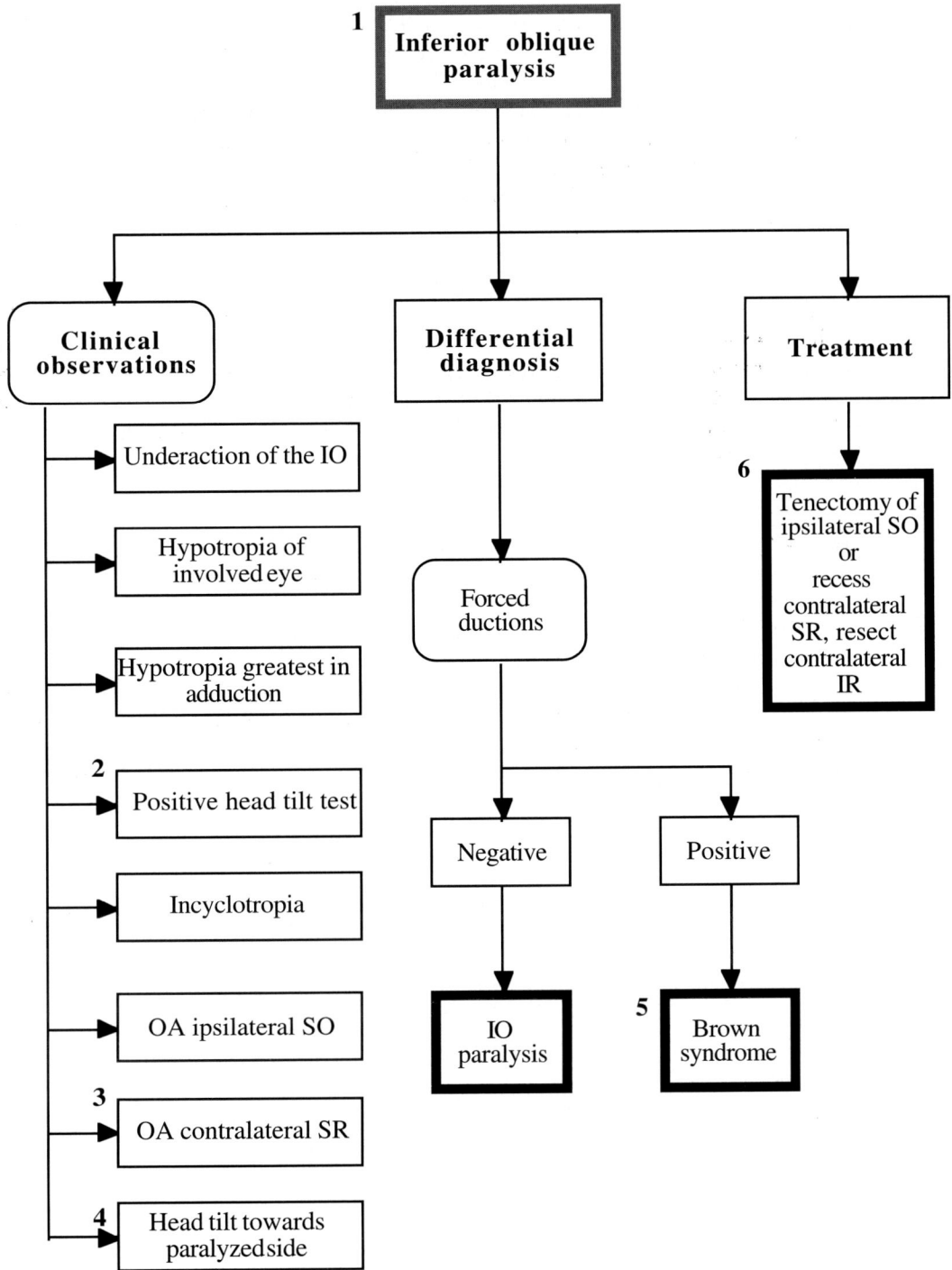

2.40

1 **Inferior oblique paralysis**

Clinical observations

Differential diagnosis

Treatment

Underaction of the IO

Hypotropia of involved eye

Hypotropia greatest in adduction

2 Positive head tilt test

Incyclotropia

OA ipsilateral SO

3 OA contralateral SR

4 Head tilt towards paralyzed side

Forced ductions

Negative

Positive

IO paralysis

5 Brown syndrome

6 Tenectomy of ipsilateral SO or recess contralateral SR, resect contralateral IR

2.41   Fourth Nerve Paralysis: Classification

(1) Congenital superior oblique palsy is commonly associated with an anomalously loose tendon or misdirection of the superior oblique muscle.[23 p.468; 26] It can also occur on an innervational basis with a normal tendon.

(2) Class I palsy is characterized by a loose, redundant reflected tendon of the superior oblique. When a loose tendon is found in a patient with congenital superior oblique palsy, the patient is ideally suited for superior oblique tendon tuck or resection. This can be done safely in most cases without producing an iatrogenic Brown syndrome.

(3) Class II congenital superior oblique palsy is characterized by a nasally displaced insertion of the superior oblique tendon. In this case, the temporal border of the insertion of the superior oblique tendon is located at the *nasal* border of the superior rectus muscle. This anomalous insertion is also usually associated with a redundant tendon. The torsional effect of the superior oblique tendon is theoretically reduced more than the vertical action with this anomalous insertion. This anomaly is treated with resection, temporal transposition of the superior oblique tendon or both.

(4) In Class III congenital superior oblique palsy, an attenuated superior oblique tendon fails to insert into the sclera but instead inserts into the undersurface of posterior Tenon's capsule. In such a case, the superior oblique is profoundly underacting. Surgery is directed to the antagonist ipsilateral inferior rectus and yoke contralateral inferior oblique muscles.

(5) Class IV congenital superior oblique palsy is absence of the reflected tendon of the superior oblique **(see 2.44).** Surgery is directed to the antagonist ipsilateral inferior oblique, ipsilateral superior rectus, and yoke contralateral inferior rectus.

(6) **See 2.42.**

2.41

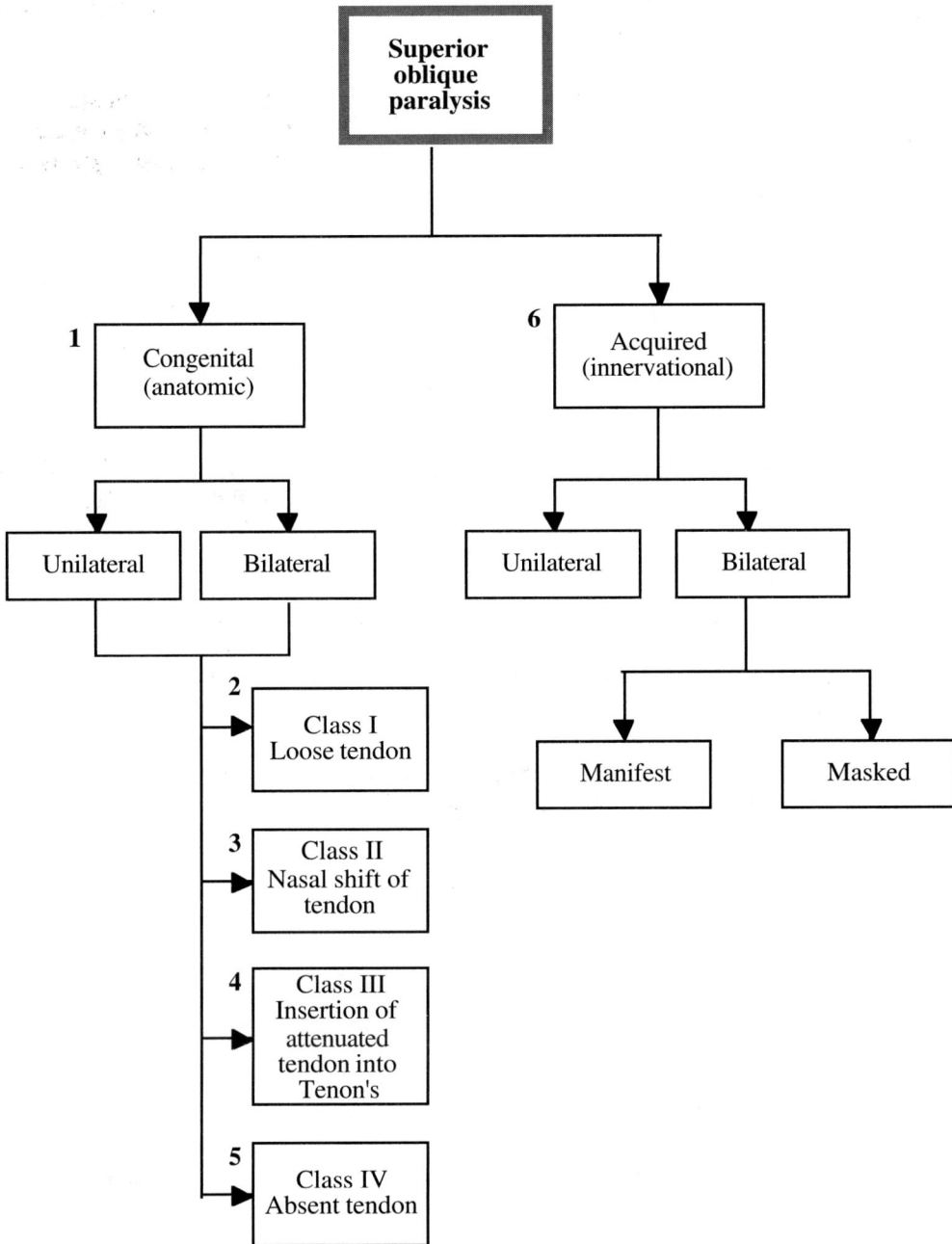

```
                        ┌──────────────┐
                        │   Superior   │
                        │   oblique    │
                        │   paralysis  │
                        └──────────────┘
                   ┌───────────┴────────────┐
              1 ┌──────────┐          6 ┌──────────────┐
                │ Congenital│            │  Acquired    │
                │(anatomic) │            │(innervational)│
                └──────────┘            └──────────────┘
             ┌──────┴──────┐          ┌──────┴──────┐
         ┌──────────┐ ┌──────────┐ ┌──────────┐ ┌──────────┐
         │Unilateral│ │ Bilateral│ │Unilateral│ │ Bilateral│
         └──────────┘ └──────────┘ └──────────┘ └──────────┘
```

1 Congenital (anatomic)

6 Acquired (innervational)

Unilateral Bilateral

Unilateral Bilateral

2 Class I
Loose tendon

3 Class II
Nasal shift of tendon

4 Class III
Insertion of attenuated tendon into Tenon's

5 Class IV
Absent tendon

Manifest

Masked

2.42 Superior Oblique Muscle Paralysis: Diagnosis

(1 to 3) Patients with superior oblique paralysis usually are seen with a head tilt to the opposite shoulder. Vertical diplopia, torsional diplopia, or a combination of these factors are also common findings. The diagnosis is usually made on the basis of the combination of the findings listed in 1 to 3 in the highlighted boxes. These features are consistently associated with superior oblique paralysis. The remaining features listed in 4 to 10 are variable.[23 p.469]

(4) Underaction of the involved superior oblique muscle may be subtle and escape detection on examining ductions and versions. In fact, the overaction of the ipsilateral inferior oblique is usually the most prominent finding on examining the ocular motility.

(5) The superior oblique muscle of the sound eye may be overacting. This is a secondary deviation, caused by contracture of the ipsilateral superior rectus muscle in cases of superior oblique paralysis with a large hypertropia.[28,53,70] The increased innervational effort to depress the paralyzed eye causes excessive depression of the normal eye, especially in adduction, causing overaction of the contralateral superior oblique.

(6) Examination with the ophthalmoscope and the Maddox double-rod test[56 p.54] shows excyclotropia of the involved eye. When the patient fixates habitually with the paralyzed eye, the excyclotropia may occur in the sound eye (paradoxic excyclotropia).[42]

(7) A head tilt toward the uninvolved side occurs in about 70% of the patients with superior oblique paralysis. In nearly 30% of such cases the head position is normal or the head may actually be tilted toward the paralyzed side (paradoxic head tilt).[70]

(8) Vertical diplopia, especially in the reading position, is frequently reported in patients with superior oblique paralysis.

(9) Torsional diplopia occurs only in recently acquired cases and is never seen in congenital superior oblique paralysis.

(10) Patients with head tilt from early infancy often develop facial asymmetry. This is a valuable sign to date the onset of the strabismus problem. The fuller facial features are always on the side of the abnormal superior oblique except in cases of brachiocephaly.

(11) If a patient habitually fixates with the paralyzed eye, the contralateral superior rectus muscle appears to be paretic or paralyzed. This is called "inhibitional palsy of the contralateral antagonist"[57 p.367] and may confound the correct diagnosis of superior oblique paralysis. This condition also produces a pseudoptosis in the sound eye.

(12) The Bielschowsky head tilt test determines the correct diagnosis **(see 2.42).**

(13) Bilateral involvement must be suspected in traumatic cases. The paralysis frequently is more pronounced on one than on the other side. In fact, the paralysis on one side may be obscured and not become manifest until the other eye has been operated on. Several diagnostic features are listed whose presence strongly suggests bilateral involvement.

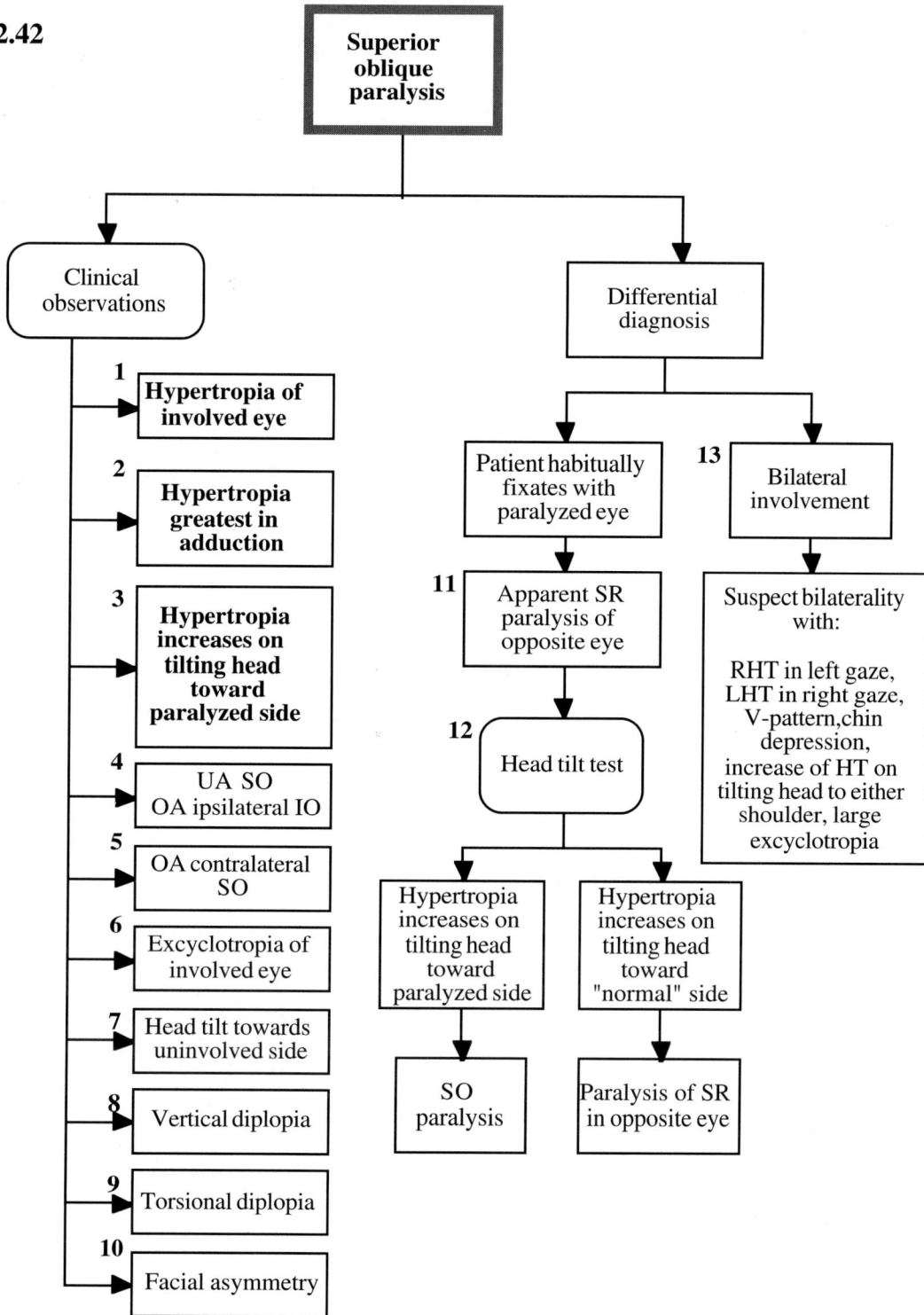

2.42

Superior oblique paralysis

Clinical observations

1 **Hypertropia of involved eye**

2 **Hypertropia greatest in adduction**

3 **Hypertropia increases on tilting head toward paralyzed side**

4 UA SO
OA ipsilateral IO

5 OA contralateral SO

6 Excyclotropia of involved eye

7 Head tilt towards uninvolved side

8 Vertical diplopia

9 Torsional diplopia

10 Facial asymmetry

Differential diagnosis

Patient habitually fixates with paralyzed eye

13 Bilateral involvement

11 Apparent SR paralysis of opposite eye

Suspect bilaterality with:

RHT in left gaze, LHT in right gaze, V-pattern, chin depression, increase of HT on tilting head to either shoulder, large excyclotropia

12 Head tilt test

Hypertropia increases on tilting head toward paralyzed side

Hypertropia increases on tilting head toward "normal" side

SO paralysis

Paralysis of SR in opposite eye

2.43   **Superior Oblique Muscle Paralysis: Treatment**

(1) Most patients with superior oblique paralysis require surgery. This should not detract from the fact that a small number do well with nonsurgical treatment with prisms or occlusion which should also be considered while waiting for recovery of an acquired paralysis.[23 p.465]

(2) Patients with a mild paresis of the superior oblique muscle (10^Δ or less), especially older persons who are used to wearing glasses, often do well with a prismatic correction. Although this treatment is not likely to eliminate diplopia in all fields of gaze, the patient may acquire sufficient visual comfort to avert surgery **(see 2.49).**

(3) Sector occlusion (translucent adhesive tape) of the lower segment may relieve diplopia that is limited to the reading position without interfering with single binocular vision in primary position.

(4) Surgical indications include diplopia, asthenopia a cosmetically disturbing hypertropia, and anomalous head position.

(5) **See 2.21 and 2.22.**

(6) To decide which of the various surgical options to consider, the deviation must be measured in the diagnostic positions of gaze. We have adopted the classification of Knapp[30,31] to categorize the different clinical manifestations. In the figure below the nine-section box indicates the gaze direction in which the hypertropia is greatest, taking the right eye as an example. In our experience, 90% of all patients are in classes 1 to 3.[70]

(7) A maximal tuck (10 to 12 mm or occasionally more with a redundant tendon) is reserved for congenital paralysis where the tendon is usually floppy and redundant.[23 pp.334,456; 26] In acquired paralysis much less of the tendon should be tucked to avoid causing postoperative restriction of elevation (iatrogenic Brown's syndrome, **see 2.53**). Contralateral inferior rectus recession is reserved as a secondary procedure after undercorrection with a tucking procedure.

(8) Class 4 and 5: A large hypertropia of long duration may cause contracture of the ipsilateral superior rectus muscle,[28,53] overaction of the contralateral depressor muscles, and a positive forced duction test. In that case, a recession of the ipsilateral superior rectus muscle is added. If the forced duction test is negative, the contralateral inferior rectus muscle is recessed.

(9) Trauma to the trochlea, for instance a dog bite, may cause generalized limitation of depression **(see 2.53).**[23 p.485] Surgery should be avoided in most cases.

Class 1*   Class 2*   Class 3*   Class 4*

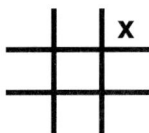   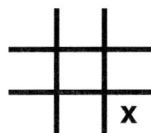   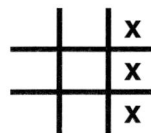   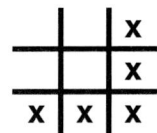

*Assumes right superior oblique palsy

2.43

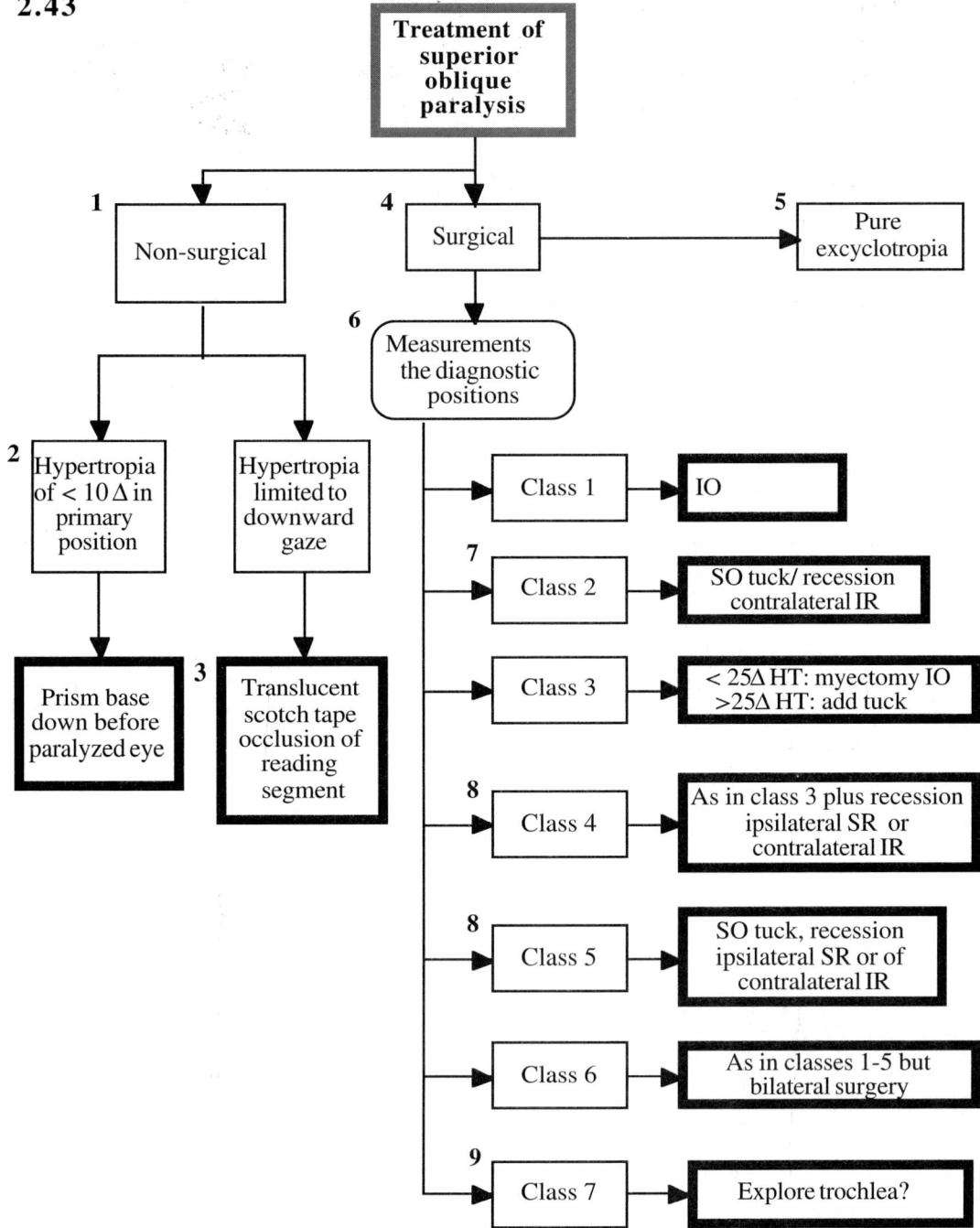

Treatment of superior oblique paralysis

1 → Non-surgical

4 → Surgical

5 → Pure excyclotropia

6 → Measurements the diagnostic positions

2 → Hypertropia of < 10 Δ in primary position

→ Hypertropia limited to downward gaze

→ Prism base down before paralyzed eye

3 → Translucent scotch tape occlusion of reading segment

Class 1 → IO

7 → Class 2 → SO tuck/ recession contralateral IR

→ Class 3 → < 25Δ HT: myectomy IO
>25Δ HT: add tuck

8 → Class 4 → As in class 3 plus recession ipsilateral SR or contralateral IR

8 → Class 5 → SO tuck, recession ipsilateral SR or of contralateral IR

→ Class 6 → As in classes 1-5 but bilateral surgery

9 → Class 7 → Explore trochlea?

Class 5*

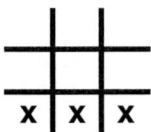

x | x | x

Class 6

Bilateral

Class 7*

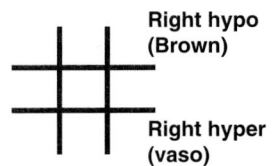

Right hypo (Brown)

Right hyper (vaso)

2.44   Congenital Absence of Superior Oblique Tendon

(1) This unexpected finding, which can also occur at the time of intended surgery on the superior oblique tendon (Harada-Ito procedure or tuck) can be suspected by observing marked to moderate facial asymmetry, associated horizontal strabismus, amblyopia, and underaction of the superior oblique muscle; however, it cannot be predicted reliably on the basis of preoperative findings and occurs infrequently as a real surprise! Nevertheless, the surgeon must be prepared to encounter it and to consider alternative procedures if surgery on the superior oblique tendon is planned but the tendon cannot be located.[23 p.487]

(2) The primary procedure for superior oblique underaction is inferior oblique weakening, but this alone is usually insufficient treatment.

(3) Restricted passive infraduction is associated with apparent overaction of the contralateral superior oblique and is caused by contracture of the ipsilateral superior rectus muscle.[70] If present, this sign calls for recession of the tight superior rectus.

(4) Inferior oblique overaction is one of the hallmarks of superior oblique paralysis or absence. If this muscle has been weakened by previous surgery, the only alternative is to recess the contralateral inferior rectus muscle.

(5) Pure excyclotropia without vertical misalignment is infrequently encountered in connection with congenital absence of a superior oblique but has been observed by one of us (GKvN). If the patient is symptomatic, horizontal transposition of the vertical rectus muscles should be considered.[67]

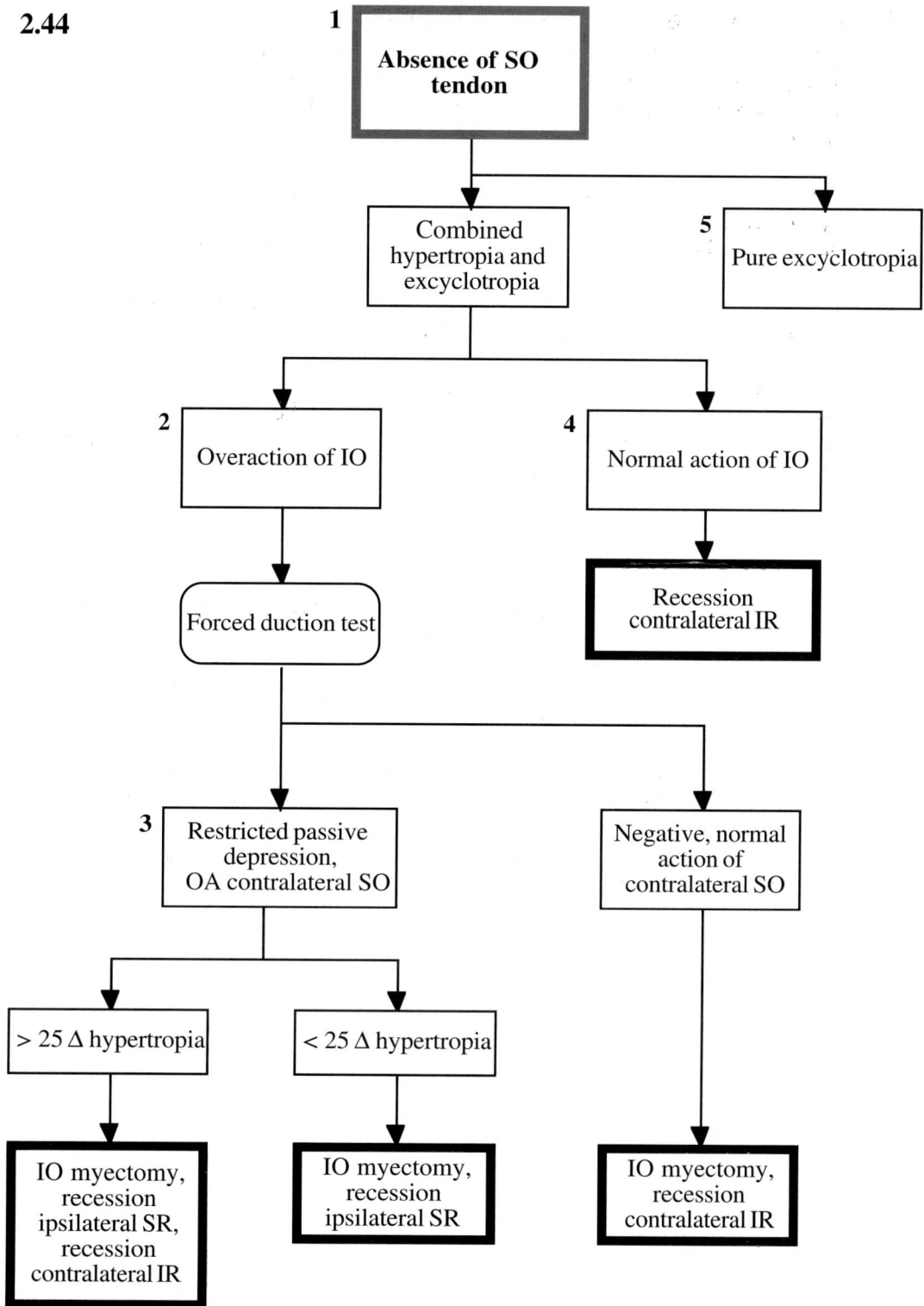

2.44

1 Absence of SO tendon

5 Pure excyclotropia

Combined hypertropia and excyclotropia

2 Overaction of IO

4 Normal action of IO

Forced duction test

Recession contralateral IR

3 Restricted passive depression, OA contralateral SO

Negative, normal action of contralateral SO

> 25 Δ hypertropia

< 25 Δ hypertropia

IO myectomy, recession ipsilateral SR, recession contralateral IR

IO myectomy, recession ipsilateral SR

IO myectomy, recession contralateral IR

2.45   Sixth Nerve Paralysis: Diagnosis

(1) In a patient who has esotropia and limited abduction of one or both eyes, the examiner should suspect abducens nerve palsy, but a differential diagnosis is always mandated. The onset of the esotropia should be established by the patient's history **(see 1.02).**

(2) Congenital sixth nerve paralysis occurs infrequently. On further testing, most apparent sixth nerve paralysis in infants is found to be pseudoabducens paralysis. Acquired sixth nerve palsy is more common and is usually self-limiting.

(3) The doll's head or the oculocephalic maneuver confirms the presence or absence of full abduction in infants. To assess abduction, **see 1.09 and 1.10.**

(4) In many cases of infantile esotropia, especially those associated with manifest-latent nystagmus in infants who prefer to use the fixating eye in adduction or with cross-fixation, there is apparent underaction of the lateral rectus muscle(s). Typically this reflects the infant's reluctance to fully abduct the eyes.

(5) **See 2.33.**

(6) Limited abduction with the doll's head maneuver should make the examiner suspect Duane syndrome types I or III or, if associated with facial paralysis, Möbius syndrome.[23 p.519]

(7) The forced duction test[23 p.262; 49; 57 p.375] determines whether there is restriction of passive abduction **(see 1.30).**

(8) With acquired sixth nerve paralysis it is essential to determine whether the restriction of abduction is caused by paralysis of the lateral rectus muscle, contracture of the medial rectus muscle or a combination of both conditions. The estimation of generated muscle force[23 p.266; 49; 56 p.375] determines whether residual lateral rectus muscle function is present **(see 1.30).**

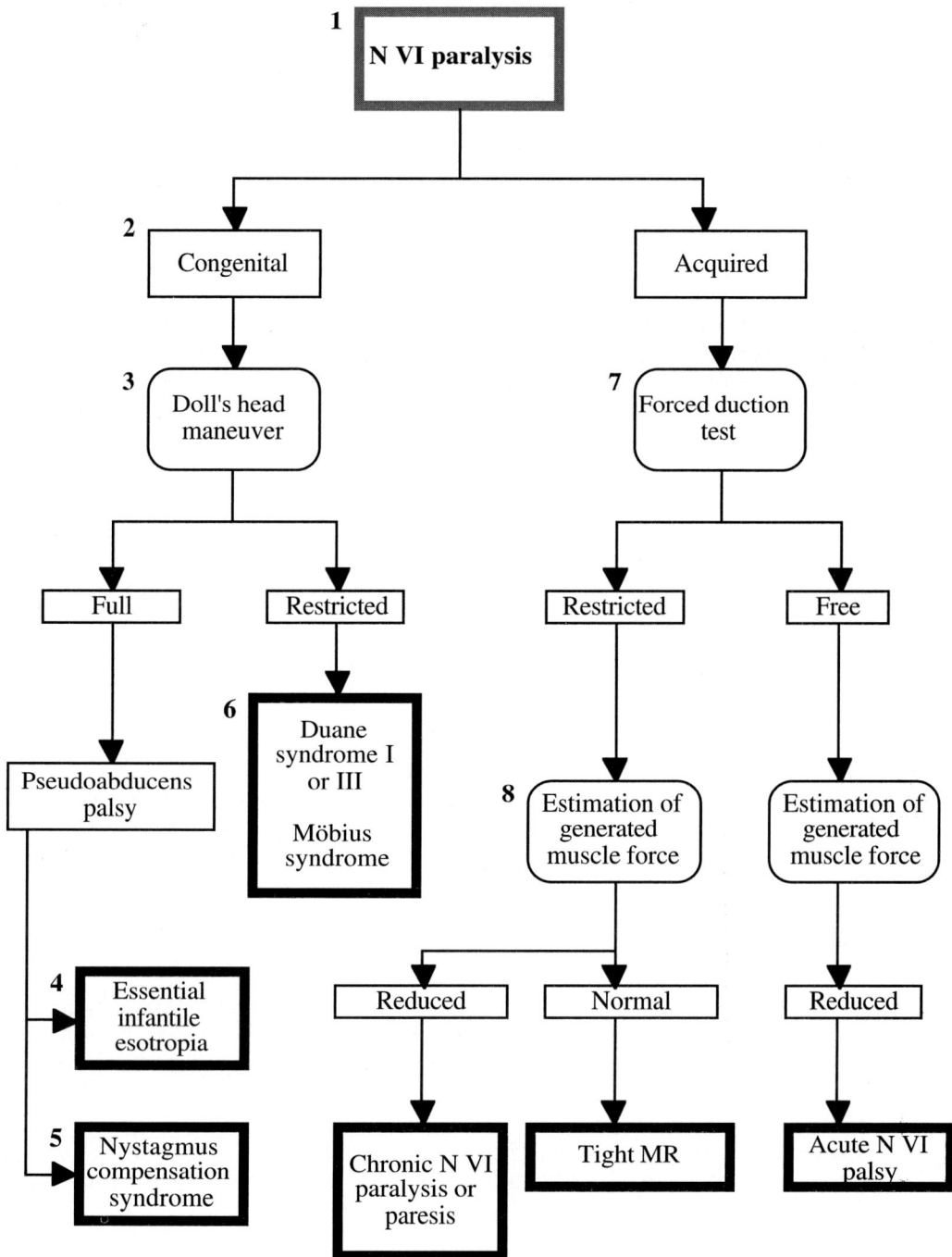

2.45

```
                              1  ┌──────────────┐
                                 │ N VI paralysis│
                                 └──────┬───────┘
                     ┌──────────────────┴──────────────────┐
                 2 ┌─┴────────┐                        ┌────┴─────┐
                   │Congenital│                        │ Acquired │
                   └─┬────────┘                        └────┬─────┘
                 3 ┌─┴────────┐                        7 ┌──┴───────┐
                   │Doll's head│                         │Forced duction│
                   │ maneuver │                          │   test    │
                   └──────────┘                          └──────────┘
```

| Full | | Restricted | | Restricted | | Free |

6
Duane syndrome I or III

Möbius syndrome

Pseudoabducens palsy

8
Estimation of generated muscle force

Estimation of generated muscle force

| Reduced | | Normal | | Reduced |

4
Essential infantile esotropia

5
Nystagmus compensation syndrome

Chronic N VI paralysis or paresis

Tight MR

Acute N VI palsy

2.46   Sixth Nerve Paralysis: Treatment

(1) A waiting period is advisable in all patients with acquired abducens palsy. During this interval the patient should be repeatedly examined, the deviation measured, and the field of single binocular vision determined.[57 p.392]

(2) Sector occlusion with translucent adhesive tape is helpful in relieving diplopia in the paretic field of gaze. The segment of the lens to be occluded is individually determined. According to the patient's preference, we occlude the temporal segment of the lens before the paretic eye and the nasal segment before the sound eye. In bilateral paresis bitemporal occlusion may be effective in relieving symptoms.

(3) Chemodenervation of the medial rectus muscle has been advocated by several authors. Although a difference in the recovery rate between treated and nontreated patients has yet to be established, the subjective benefit from having the face turn improved, at least temporarily, establishes the value of this symptomatic therapy.[23 p.345]

(4) Before surgery is planned, it is mandatory to determine to what extent limited abduction is caused by the paralysis and how much this limitation is caused by secondary contracture of the medial rectus muscle. The forced duction test is indispensable in providing this answer. When this test is positive, an estimation of muscle force generated by the lateral rectus, as the adducted eye moves toward primary position, informs the surgeon whether release of a restricted medial rectus muscle alone will improve abduction.[23 p.257; 57 p.375]

(5) In the presence of a complete paralysis, surgical expectations must be guarded. At best, the paralyzed eye can be moved to or just beyond the primary position while, at the same time, sacrificing some adduction. This will decrease diplopia and improve the head position. We combine a muscle transposition of the vertical recti or a union of these muscles with the lateral rectus, as described by Jensen, with recession of the medial rectus muscle. Chemodenervation of the medial rectus muscle instead of recession may be used with the theoretical advantage of decreasing the risk of anterior segment ischemia.*[23 p.327]

(6) When residual lateral rectus function can be demonstrated, a maximal recession of the medial and resection of the lateral rectus muscles are effective in enlarging the field of single binocular vision with alignment in the primary position.

---

*As an anecdotal report, one of us (EMH) has seen two cases of anterior segment ischemia in patients who have had the only remaining muscle, the medial rectus, treated by chemodenervation with Botulinum A-toxin.

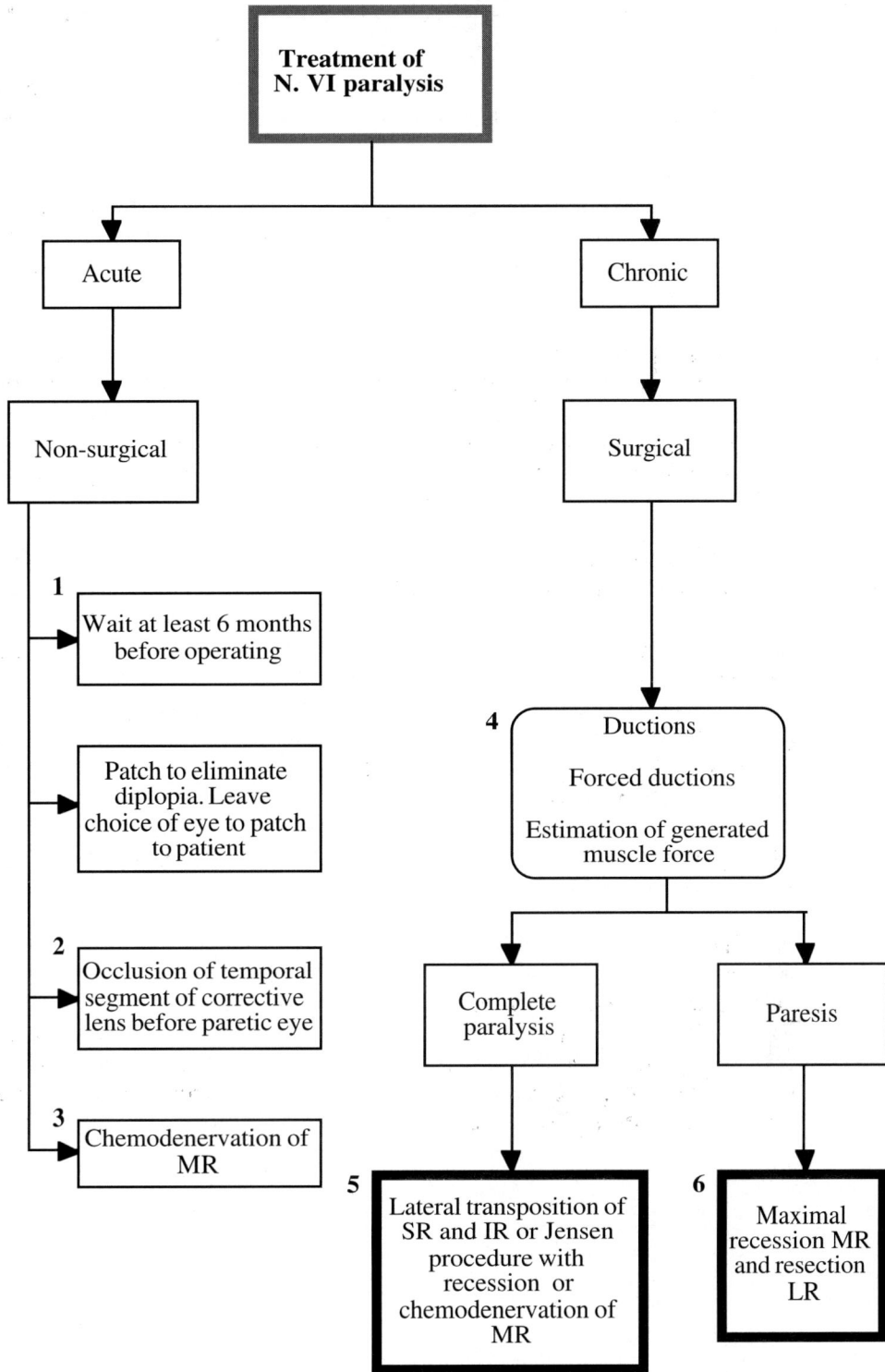

2.46

```
            ┌─────────────────┐
            │   Treatment of  │
            │  N. VI paralysis│
            └─────────────────┘
```

Acute

Chronic

Non-surgical

Surgical

1 Wait at least 6 months before operating

Patch to eliminate diplopia. Leave choice of eye to patch to patient

2 Occlusion of temporal segment of corrective lens before paretic eye

3 Chemodenervation of MR

4 Ductions

Forced ductions

Estimation of generated muscle force

Complete paralysis

Paresis

5 Lateral transposition of SR and IR or Jensen procedure with recession or chemodenervation of MR

6 Maximal recession MR and resection LR

2.47   Divergence Insufficiency Versus Bilateral Abducens Paresis

(1) This condition generally occurs in older patients and has a gradual onset. It is necessary to differentiate between divergence insufficiency and bilateral sixth nerve palsy.[57 p.432]

(2) The esotropia should be measured with a prism cover test at distance fixation with the eyes in primary position and in maximal dextroversion and levoversion. A difference of 5^Δ or more increase in distance esodeviation is considered significant.

(3) Special attention should be paid to limitation of abduction of either eye. The limitation may be subtle and not more than 1 on a scale of 1 to 4 **(see 1.09)**.

(4) Saccadic velocities may decrease in abduction. This difference in abduction versus adduction velocity may be too subtle for detection by gross observation and may require electrooculographic recording of the saccades.

(5) A **V** pattern esotropia at distance fixation with a chin depression may be present in some but not in all cases of bilateral sixth nerve palsy.

(6) Fusional amplitudes are measured in free space with a rotary prism, or the prism bar or on the major amblyoscope **(see 1.36)**.

(7) Spectacles with base-out prisms for distance correction relieve the symptoms in many patients, regardless of whether they have a bilateral sixth nerve paresis or divergence insufficiency **(see 2.49)**.

(8) If prisms are not tolerated, a small (4 mm) resection of both lateral rectus muscles is necessary.

(9) The differentiation between divergence insufficiency and paralysis is not an easy one. In the absence of neurologic anomalies divergence insufficiency is assumed. In the presence of neurologic anomalies, some of which may be associated with papilledema, divergence paralysis is assumed. Divergence paralysis may be difficult to distinguish from the initial stage of a bilateral abducens paresis; electrooculographically recorded decreased saccadic velocities may be the only distinguishing factor between these two conditions.

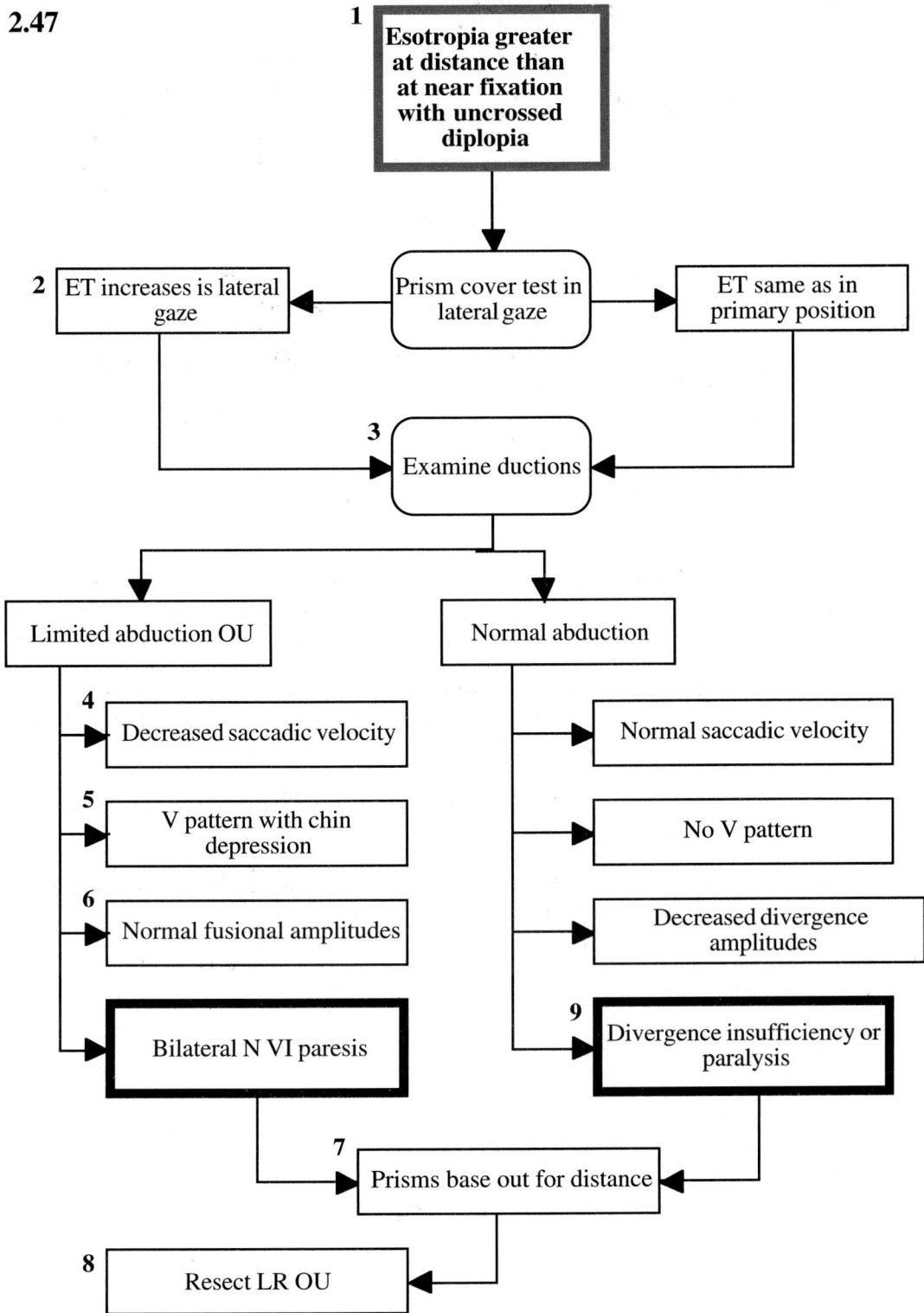

2.47

1 **Esotropia greater at distance than at near fixation with uncrossed diplopia**

Prism cover test in lateral gaze

2 ET increases is lateral gaze

ET same as in primary position

3 Examine ductions

Limited abduction OU

Normal abduction

4 Decreased saccadic velocity

5 V pattern with chin depression

6 Normal fusional amplitudes

Bilateral N VI paresis

Normal saccadic velocity

No V pattern

Decreased divergence amplitudes

9 Divergence insufficiency or paralysis

7 Prisms base out for distance

8 Resect LR OU

2.48   Convergence Insufficiency

(1) Asthenopia may have many causes **(see 1.32).** We distinguish between "muscular" and "refractive" asthenopia. The first is caused by an oculomotor imbalance such as heterophoria and the patient's sustained effort to overcome this imbalance. In the second case, asthenopia is caused by an uncorrected refractive error. When there is uncertainty whether asthenopia is muscular or refractive, we ask the patient to wear a patch while reading. If symptoms disappear the asthenopia clearly is of muscular origin.

(2) Convergence insufficiency may occur in the presence of exophoria, orthotropia, or esophoria. However, symptoms are exacerbated in patients with exophoria because the basic exodeviation must be overcome by fusion before the eyes can begin to converge. True convergence insufficiency should not be confused with "convergence insufficiency type" intermittent exotropia **(see 1.22).** Convergence insufficiency is the most common cause of muscular asthenopia. It is reversible by the appropriate therapy.

(3) The treatment, orthoptic exercises, in most instances provides long-lasting relief from symptoms.[57 p.465]

(4) In rare instances, when the patient has a significant exophoria at near fixation, surgery is indicated.[62] The operation may be followed by temporary overcorrection at distance fixation, which may require base-out prisms.

(5) Convergence insufficiency combined with subnormal accommodation[57 p.430] may follow diphtheria, mononucleosis, encephalitis, and upper respiratory infections.

(6) Orthoptic treatment is rarely successful; some patients find relief from their symptoms with bifocals and base-in prisms.

(7) Surgery may become necessary and is followed with a prescription of plus lenses to correct for the subnormal accommodation.

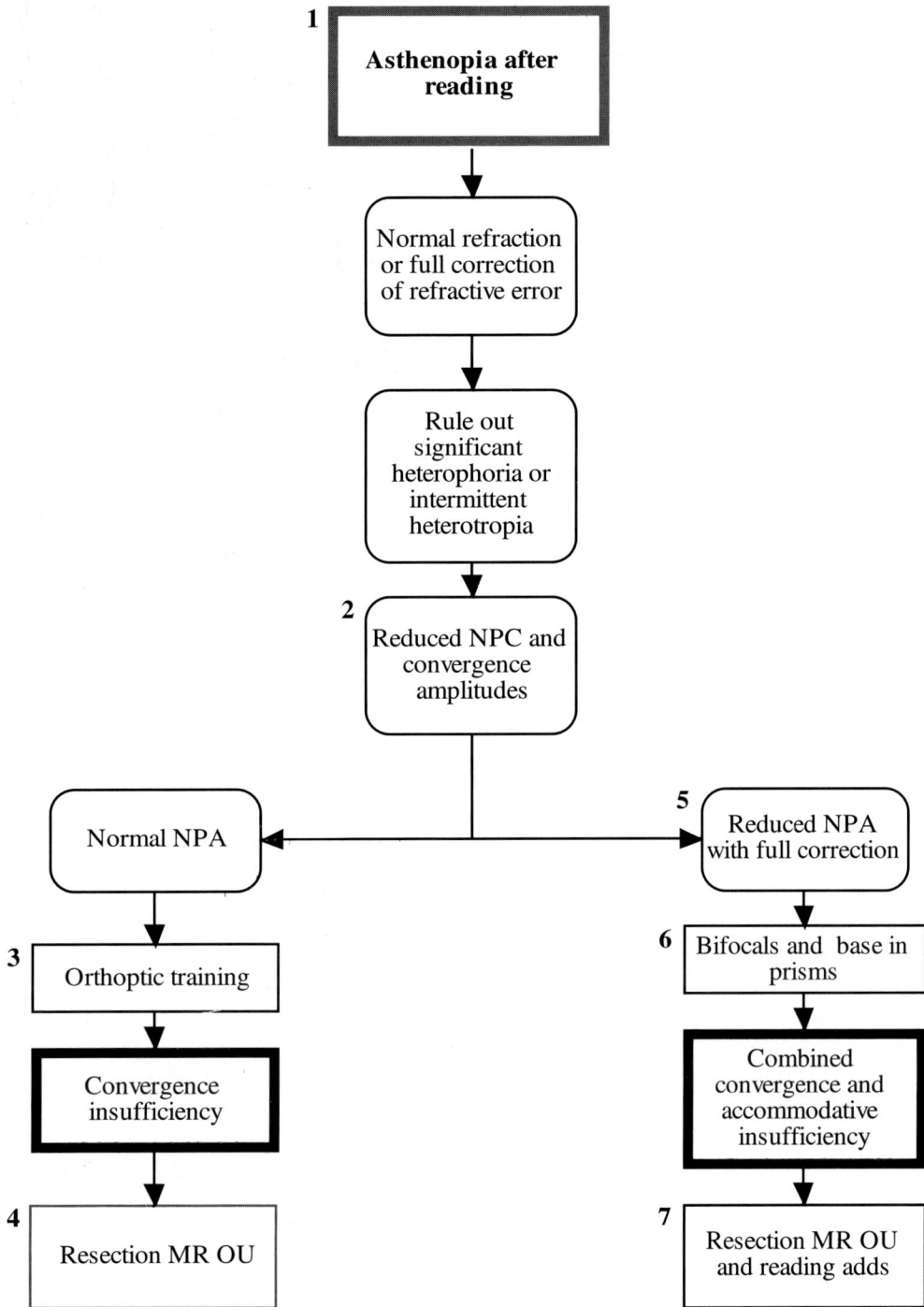

2.48

1 Asthenopia after reading

Normal refraction or full correction of refractive error

Rule out significant heterophoria or intermittent heterotropia

2 Reduced NPC and convergence amplitudes

Normal NPA

5 Reduced NPA with full correction

3 Orthoptic training

Convergence insufficiency

4 Resection MR OU

6 Bifocals and base in prisms

Combined convergence and accommodative insufficiency

7 Resection MR OU and reading adds

2.49   **When to Use Prisms**

(1) Prisms are used for treatment and for diagnostic purposes. Rarely more than 10^Δ per eye are tolerated when incorporated in spectacle lenses. Weight and optical disadvantages preclude prescription of higher powers. Fresnel prisms also cause distortion and decrease of visual acuity in higher powers but are well tolerated in lower powers. They are ideal for short-term use because they are simply added to the present spectacles.

(2) Prisms are indicated to treat diplopia in small-angle strabismus and are well tolerated by most patients. The minimal prismatic correction necessary to maintain comfortable single binocular vision should be prescribed. Incomitant strabismus responds less favorably to prismatic therapy because of different prismatic requirements in different gaze positions. The base of the prism should be placed in the opposite direction as the deviation. For instance, esotropia is corrected with base-out; hypertropia is corrected with base-down.

(3) A vertical and horizontal prismatic correction may be combined in one lens by placing the axis at an oblique angle.

(4) Prisms of sufficient power to shift the neutral point of nystagmus to correct a compensatory head posture are rarely tolerated. However, they may be useful preoperatively for a diagnostic trial.

(5) Base-out prisms incorporated in the distance correction trigger convergence, which may dampen the nystagmus and improve visual acuity at distance.

(6) In adult patients with long-standing strabismus, it is useful to be able to predict whether surgical alignment will cause postoperative diplopia. To accomplish this, the preoperative angle is neutralized with prisms and the patient's response is studied at near and distance fixation. If when the angle is neutralized a diplopia response is paradoxic[57 p.257] and caused by anomalous retinal correspondence, postoperative diplopia is a good possibility but usually is transient. Prism adaptation has been advocated by some to predict the outcome of surgery in acquired esotropia and to modify the amount of surgery accordingly.*

(7) Fresnel prisms are used to neutralize a previous prismatic spectacle correction so that the spectacles may be worn during the early postoperative phase and until the patient is ready for a new permanent prescription.

(8) Absence of diplopia indicates suppression which may protect the patient from diplopia postoperatively.

(9) Fusion and stereopsis after prismatic correction of strabismus is evidence of an excellent functional potential.

---

*Efficacy of prism adaptation in the surgical management of acquired esotropia, Prism Adaptation Study Group, *Arch Ophthalmol* 108(9):1248-1256, 1990.

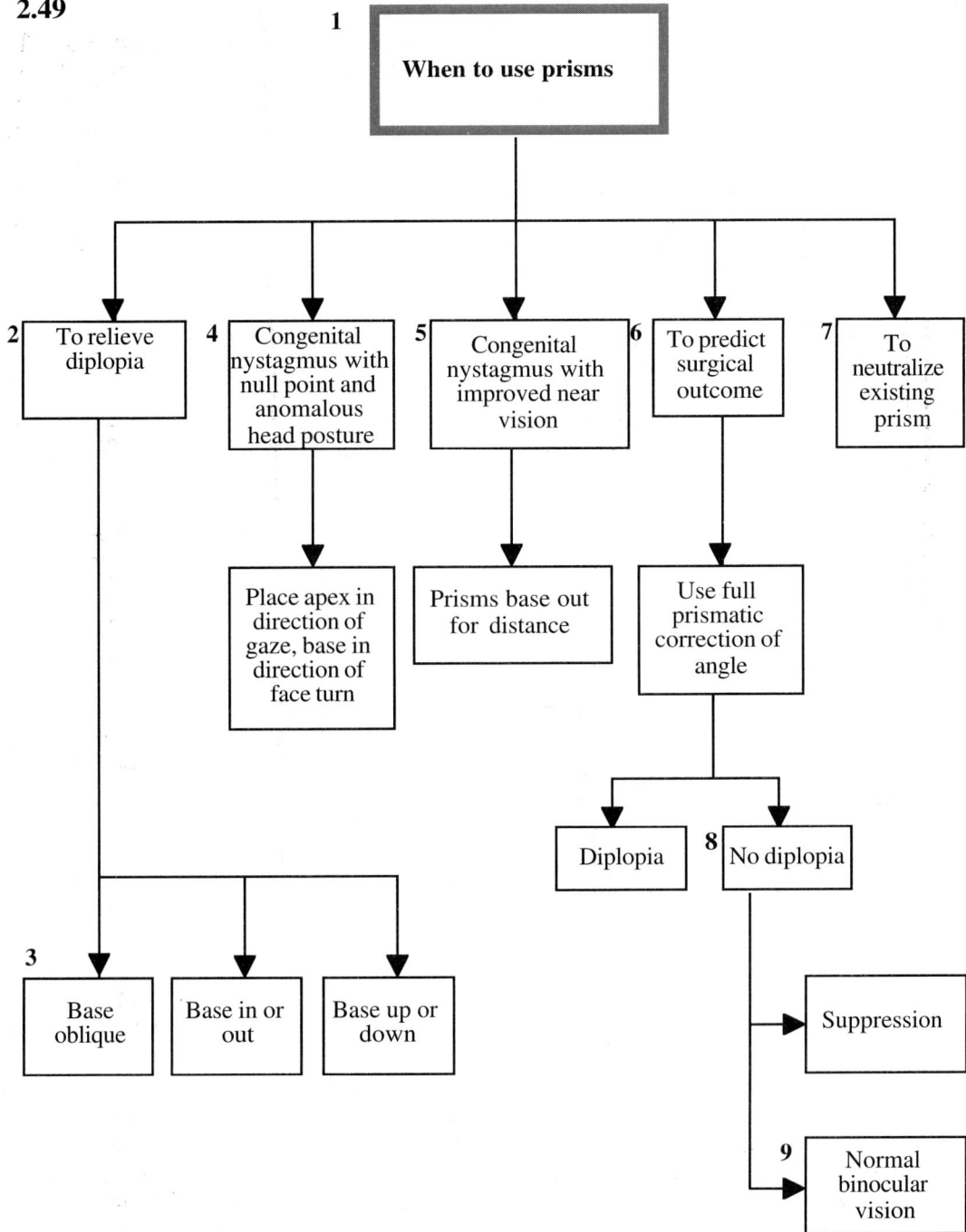

2.49

1 When to use prisms

2 To relieve diplopia

4 Congenital nystagmus with null point and anomalous head posture

5 Congenital nystagmus with improved near vision

6 To predict surgical outcome

7 To neutralize existing prism

Place apex in direction of gaze, base in direction of face turn

Prisms base out for distance

Use full prismatic correction of angle

Diplopia

8 No diplopia

3 Base oblique

Base in or out

Base up or down

Suppression

9 Normal binocular vision

2.50   Duane Syndrome Type I

(1) Duane syndrome type I is the most common of the retraction syndromes. The differential diagnosis between abducens palsy **(see 2.45)** and Duane syndrome type I is not difficult in older children and adults. However, in young children and especially in infants, a Duane syndrome is easily mistaken for a sixth nerve palsy. The consequences of this error are not negligible because the surgical treatment for abducens palsy **(see 2.46)** would be contraindicated in Duane syndrome. Because Duane syndrome is often associated with systemic anomalies, affected children should have or be referred for a complete physical examination.[57 p.398]

(2) The medial rectus muscle may be tight after previous resection, which limits abduction.

(3) Conjunctival scarring involving the temporal aspect of the globe, as occurs after repeated surgeries for pterygium or after removal of a conjunctival lesion, causes retraction of the globe on attempted adduction.

(4) Retraction of the globe, narrowing of the lid fissure on adduction, and widening on attempted abduction are signs that may be difficult to detect in esotropic infants. Limitation of abduction and crossed fixation are frequently present in essential infantile esotropia, a condition that must be distinguished from Duane syndrome type I.

(5) Although numerous surgical approaches have been advocated to improve abduction in eyes with Duane syndrome type I, success is limited in our opinion. Most attempts to improve abduction by surgery on the involved eye result in increased retraction of the globe on adduction.

(6) An esotropia in primary position causes uncrossed diplopia with a compensatory head turn toward the involved side. A recession of the medial rectus muscle improves the head position but, at the same time, may cause limitation of adduction.[23 p.421]

(7) It has been shown by modern imaging techniques that there is little if any vertical movement of the muscle planes of the horizontal rectus muscles in relation to the bony orbit as the eye is elevated or depressed.[5] Therefore, it must be assumed that the globe slips beneath the muscles during vertical eye movements. Co-contraction of the horizontal rectus muscles, as occurs in Duane syndrome on attempted adduction, changes their action to one of elevation or depression, depending on whether the globe is slightly elevated or depressed.[50] When upshoot and downshoot cause cosmetic concern, recession of the horizontal recti[61] is effective **(see 2.17 and 2.18)**. The oblique muscles should *not* be weakened.

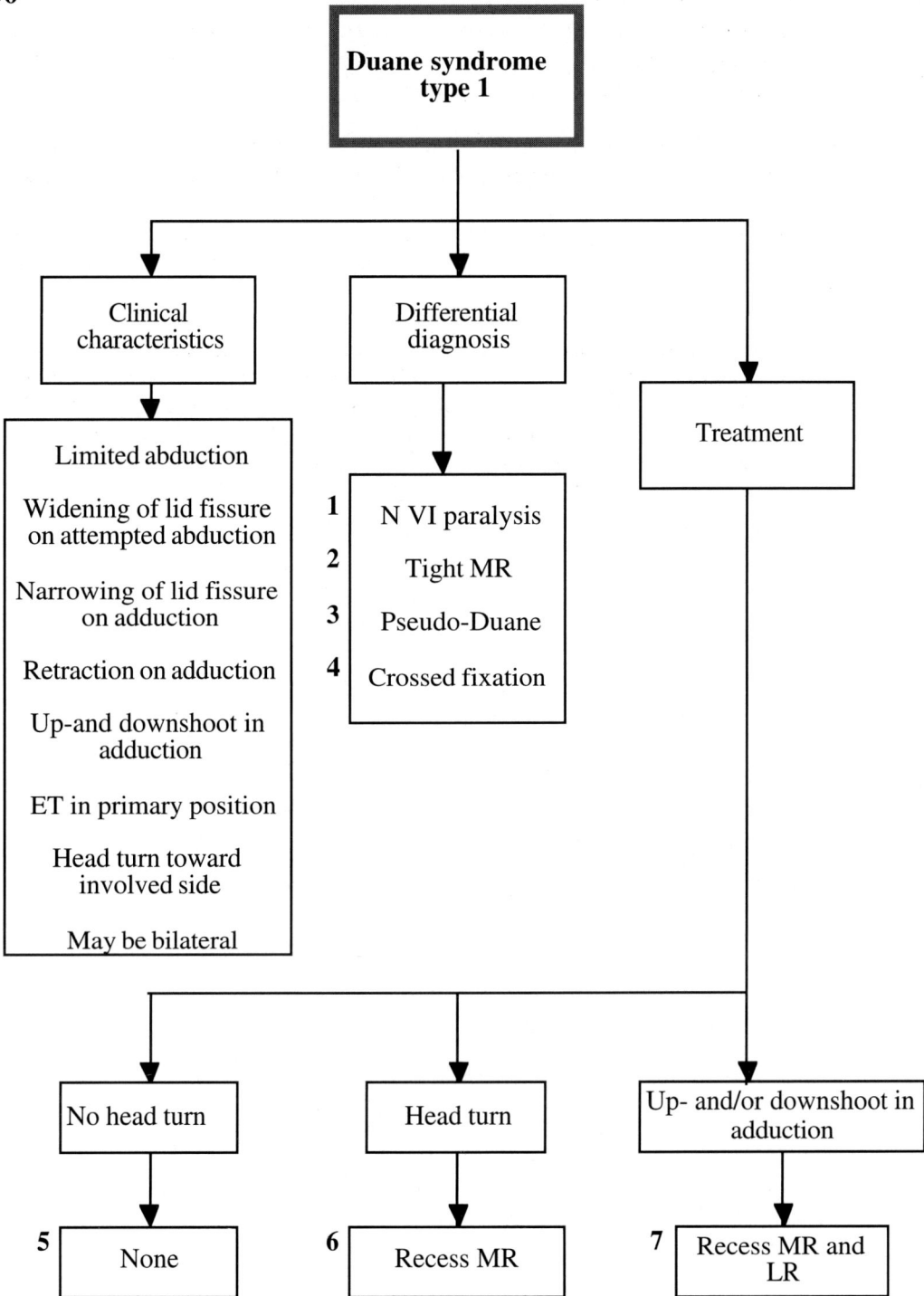

2.50

Duane syndrome
type 1

Clinical
characteristics

Differential
diagnosis

Treatment

Limited abduction

Widening of lid fissure
on attempted abduction

Narrowing of lid fissure
on adduction

Retraction on adduction

Up-and downshoot in
adduction

ET in primary position

Head turn toward
involved side

May be bilateral

1 N VI paralysis

2 Tight MR

3 Pseudo-Duane

4 Crossed fixation

No head turn

Head turn

Up- and/or downshoot in
adduction

5 None

6 Recess MR

7 Recess MR and
LR

2.51   Duane Syndrome Type II

(1) An isolated medial rectus paralysis is rare **(see 2.39)** and must be differentiated from internuclear paralysis **(see 2.28),** which may be associated with abducting nystagmus and normal convergence.

(2) A tight lateral rectus muscle after excessive resection of that muscle causes limitation of adduction and some retraction of the globe on attempted adduction.

(3) Unless there is a manifest deviation in primary position the head position is normal. With exotropia in primary position the face is turned toward the opposite side.

(4) In the presence of exotropia and fixation preference with the noninvolved eye, the ipsilateral lateral rectus muscle is recessed. When the patient fixates with the involved eye, the exotropia (secondary deviation) is usually greater than in the former case. The lateral rectus of the noninvolved eye may have to be recessed and the medial rectus muscle resected.[23 p.463]

(5) **See 2.17 and 2.18.**

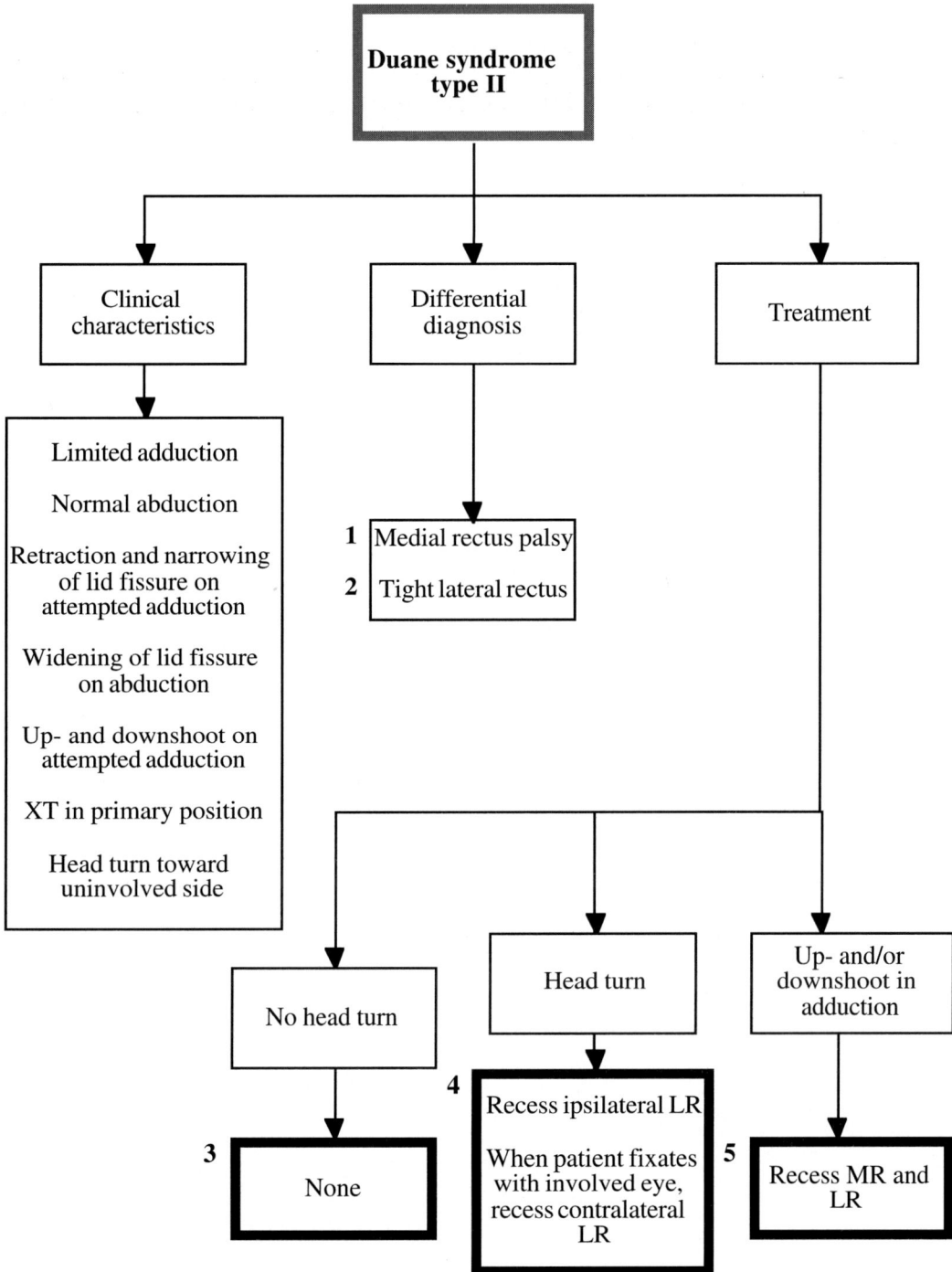

2.51

Duane syndrome
type II

Clinical
characteristics

Differential
diagnosis

Treatment

Limited adduction

Normal abduction

Retraction and narrowing
of lid fissure on
attempted adduction

Widening of lid fissure
on abduction

Up- and downshoot on
attempted adduction

XT in primary position

Head turn toward
uninvolved side

1 Medial rectus palsy

2 Tight lateral rectus

No head turn

Head turn

Up- and/or
downshoot in
adduction

3 None

4 Recess ipsilateral LR

When patient fixates
with involved eye,
recess contralateral
LR

5 Recess MR and
LR

2.52   Duane Syndrome Type III

(1) The differential diagnosis should be easy because no other condition can cause this unique combination of clinical features.

(2) Few cases of Duane type III require surgery. If strabismus is present in primary position, the patient assumes a compensatory head turn. Esotropia in primary position occurs more often than exotropia, in which case the head is turned toward the involved side.

(3) **See 2.17 and 2.18.**

2.52

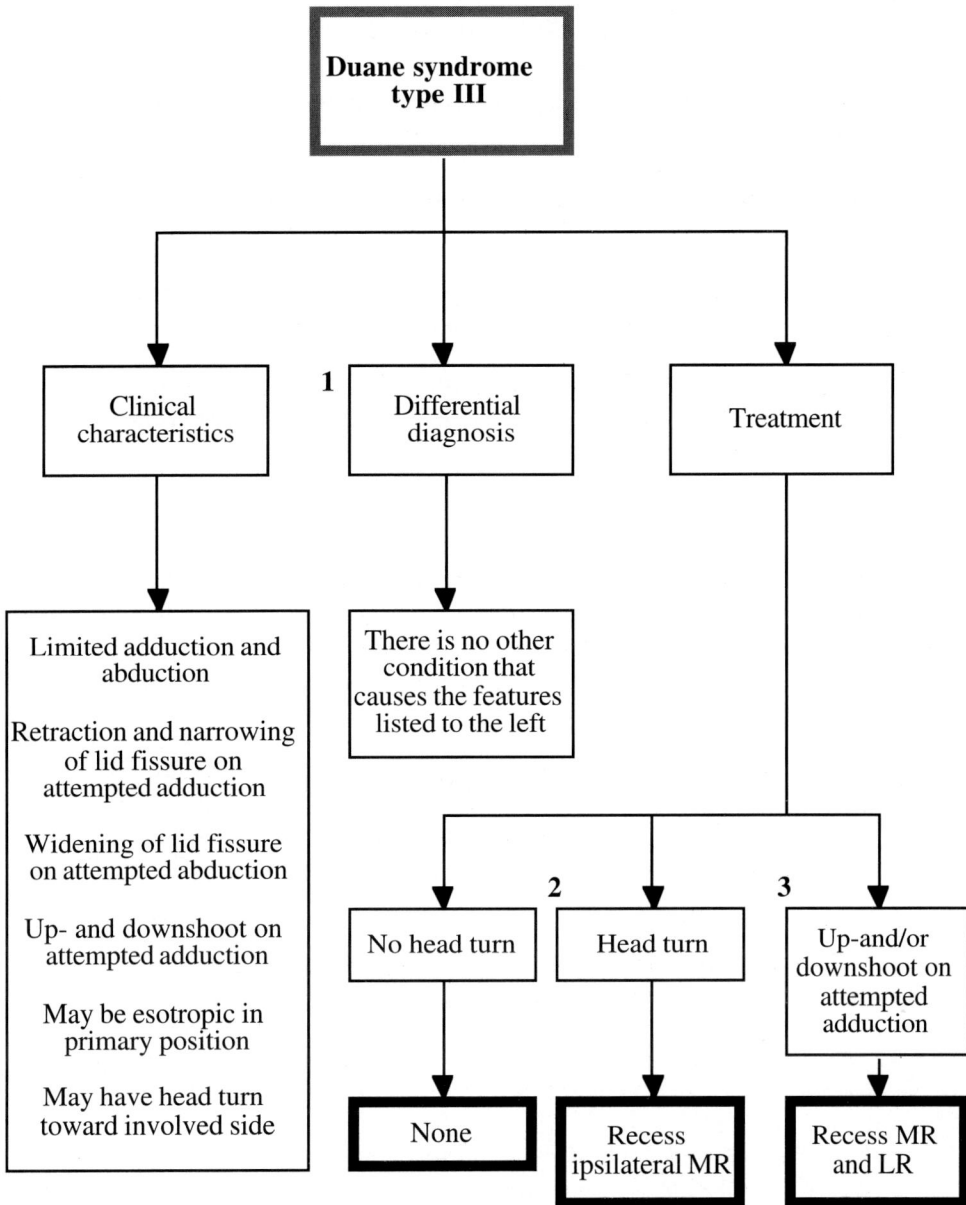

Duane syndrome
type III

Clinical
characteristics

1 Differential
diagnosis

Treatment

Limited adduction and
abduction

Retraction and narrowing
of lid fissure on
attempted adduction

Widening of lid fissure
on attempted abduction

Up- and downshoot on
attempted adduction

May be esotropic in
primary position

May have head turn
toward involved side

There is no other
condition that
causes the features
listed to the left

No head turn

2 Head turn

3 Up-and/or
downshoot on
attempted
adduction

None

Recess
ipsilateral MR

Recess MR
and LR

2.53   Brown Syndrome

(1) The forced duction test is pivotal for the diagnosis of this condition. In children this test cannot be reliably performed in the office and it may not be possible to make the definitive diagnosis until the time of surgery when the patient is under general anesthesia.

(2) In Brown syndrome elevation is severely restricted in adduction. There is less severe or no restriction on elevation from primary position and in abduction. In addition, there is normal action of the contralateral superior rectus muscle. A V pattern and mild overaction of the ipsilateral superior oblique muscle may also be present.[23 p.449; 57 p.404]

(3) In blowout fractures of the orbital floor **(see 2.54)**, restriction of elevation is usually not limited to adduction but exceptions may occur.

(4) In endocrine myopathy **(see 2.55)**, elevation is limited from all gaze positions but exceptions have been observed, especially with myopathy of the inferior oblique muscle.

(5) **See 2.40.**

(6) Most cases of congenital Brown syndrome are caused by thickening or tightness of the superior oblique tendon. Abnormal fibrous attachments to the globe that prevent elevation in adduction have also been described. In some instances, surgical exploration of the superior oblique tendon reveals no obvious abnormalities.

(7) A compensatory head posture to avoid vertical diplopia develops in many patients with Brown syndrome. This usually consists of a variable head tilt and chin elevation that places the involved eye in a position of abduction and depression. Surgery is performed to normalize the head posture.[23 pp.408, 452; 57 p.404]

(8) Superior oblique tenectomy is the most effective procedure in the treatment of Brown syndrome. However, an iatrogenic superior oblique paralysis develops in nearly one half of the patients when followed for 1 year or longer **(see 2.41)**.[54]

(9) Trauma to the trochlea or an inflammatory process in the region of the trochlea may cause an acquired Brown syndrome.[20]

(10) An excessive tuck of the superior oblique tendon causes limitation of elevation in adduction. In most instances, this surgical complication resolves with time. However, in some patients this limitation persists and causes diplopia in upward gaze in which case the tuck may be taken down surgically.

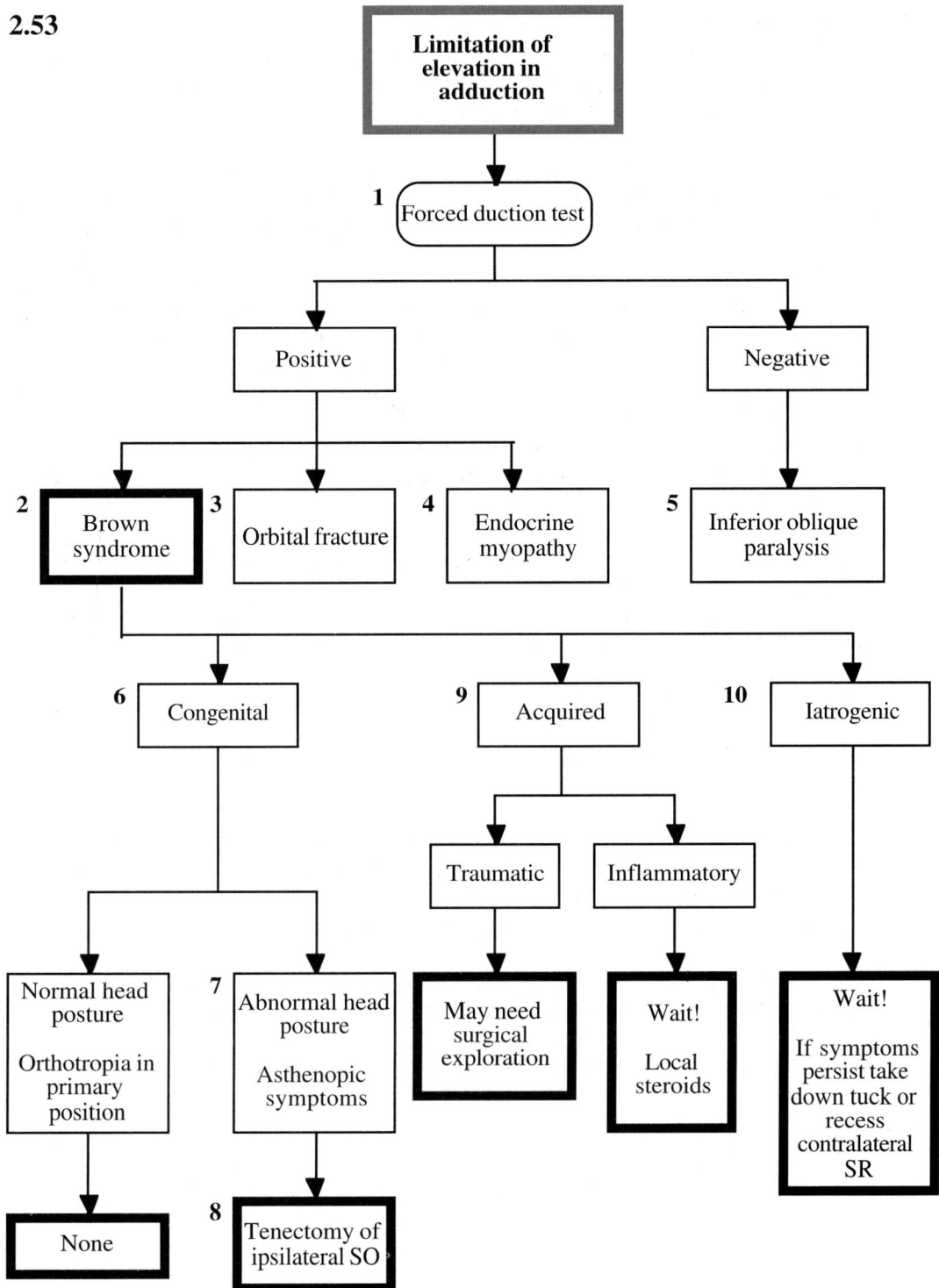

2.53

```
                    ┌─────────────────┐
                    │  Limitation of  │
                    │  elevation in   │
                    │   adduction     │
                    └─────────────────┘
                             │
                             ▼
              1   ┌─────────────────────┐
                  │  Forced duction test │
                  └─────────────────────┘
```

Positive	**Negative**

2 **Brown syndrome**   3 Orbital fracture   4 Endocrine myopathy   5 Inferior oblique paralysis

6 Congenital   9 Acquired   10 Iatrogenic

Traumatic   Inflammatory

Normal head posture

Orthotropia in primary position

7 Abnormal head posture

Asthenopic symptoms

May need surgical exploration

Wait!

Local steroids

Wait!

If symptoms persist take down tuck or recess contralateral SR

None

8 Tenectomy of ipsilateral SO

2.54   Orbital Floor Fracture

(1) Frontal impact to the globe or the orbital rim may cause a blowout fracture of the orbital floor resulting in diplopia. However, other causes and results must be considered in the diagnostic evaluation.[23, p.515; 57 p.415]

(2) It is often overlooked that frontal trauma to the eye may cause injury to the globe in addition to the bony structure of the orbit. A careful and complete ophthalmologic examination is always indicated before other tests are considered.

(3) Increased radiographic density along the orbital floor may simulate clouding of the antrum as seen in blowout fractures but actually may be caused by a submucosal hemorrhage (pseudo-blow out fracture)[16] in patients with an intact orbital floor.

(4) An orbital hemorrhage or orbital swelling during the immediate posttraumatic phase may cause active and passive restriction of ocular motility. This must be distinguished from restriction caused by prolapse of orbital tissue into a fracture site of the orbital floor.

(5) Negative forced ductions do not rule out a floor fracture. Indeed, the defect of the orbital floor may be so large that no restriction exists and the globe can be freely moved in all directions with forceps. Large floor defects are associated with enophthalmos that is noted after the acute swelling has subsided.

(6) In the absence of restricted forced ductions a waiting period is always advisable because diplopia may resolve. However, in the presence of a radiographically proven large defect of the orbital floor, reconstruction of the floor is usually indicated.

(7) A traumatic inferior rectus paralysis (see 2.38) may be caused by direct or indirect injury to the branch of the third nerve supplying that muscle. This paralysis may be only transient and full recovery is possible. If no recovery occurs after a waiting period of 6 months, surgery[66] may be necessary.

(8) Surgical repair should be planned as a team approach with an otolaryngologist or, if other facial bones are injured, a maxillofacial surgeon.

(9) A negative CT scan does not rule out a hairline fracture of the orbital floor.

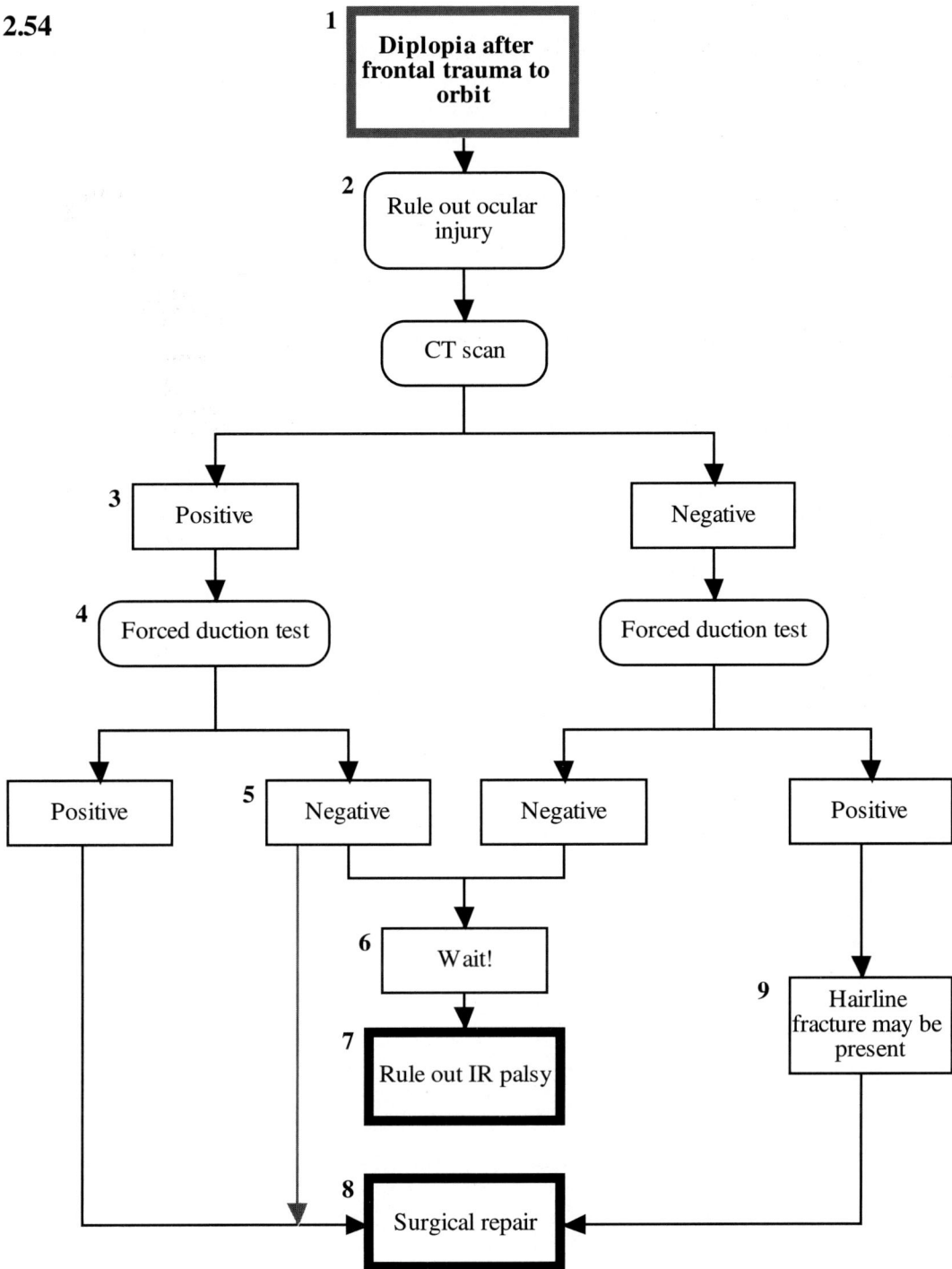

2.54

1 Diplopia after frontal trauma to orbit

2 Rule out ocular injury

CT scan

3 Positive

Negative

4 Forced duction test

Forced duction test

Positive

5 Negative

Negative

Positive

6 Wait!

7 Rule out IR palsy

9 Hairline fracture may be present

8 Surgical repair

2.55   Endocrine Myopathy

(1) Patients with endocrine myopathy may actually be euthyroid, hyperthyroid, or hypothyroid. This should be confirmed by appropriate studies. In any case it is important that normal endocrine balance be achieved before surgical treatment is undertaken.[57 p.410]

(2) Imaging of the orbital contents reveals enlarged extraocular muscles. At times this enlargement reaches grotesque proportions. The inferior and medial rectus muscles are most frequently involved. Neuroimaging of the orbit confirms the diagnosis but is rarely necessary to establish it.

(3) Visual acuity may decrease from pressure on the optic nerve by the engorged extraocular muscles.

(4) Periorbital edema often precedes the development of myopathy.

(5) Intraocular pressure may be elevated as a result of restrictive myopathy especially in upgaze.[23 p.268]

(6) Corticosteroids may be used to decongest the orbit during the acute stage of Graves disease or when vision is threatened by pressure on the optic nerve. However, this therapy has no proven effect on the myopathy.

(7) Orbital decompression is indicated when visual acuity is threatened by orbital congestion, proptosis, or both.

(8) Lengthening of the upper or lower lid may be required after recessing the superior or inferior rectus muscle and may be performed concurrently or, depending on the cosmetic defect, in a second procedure.[23 p.318]

2.55

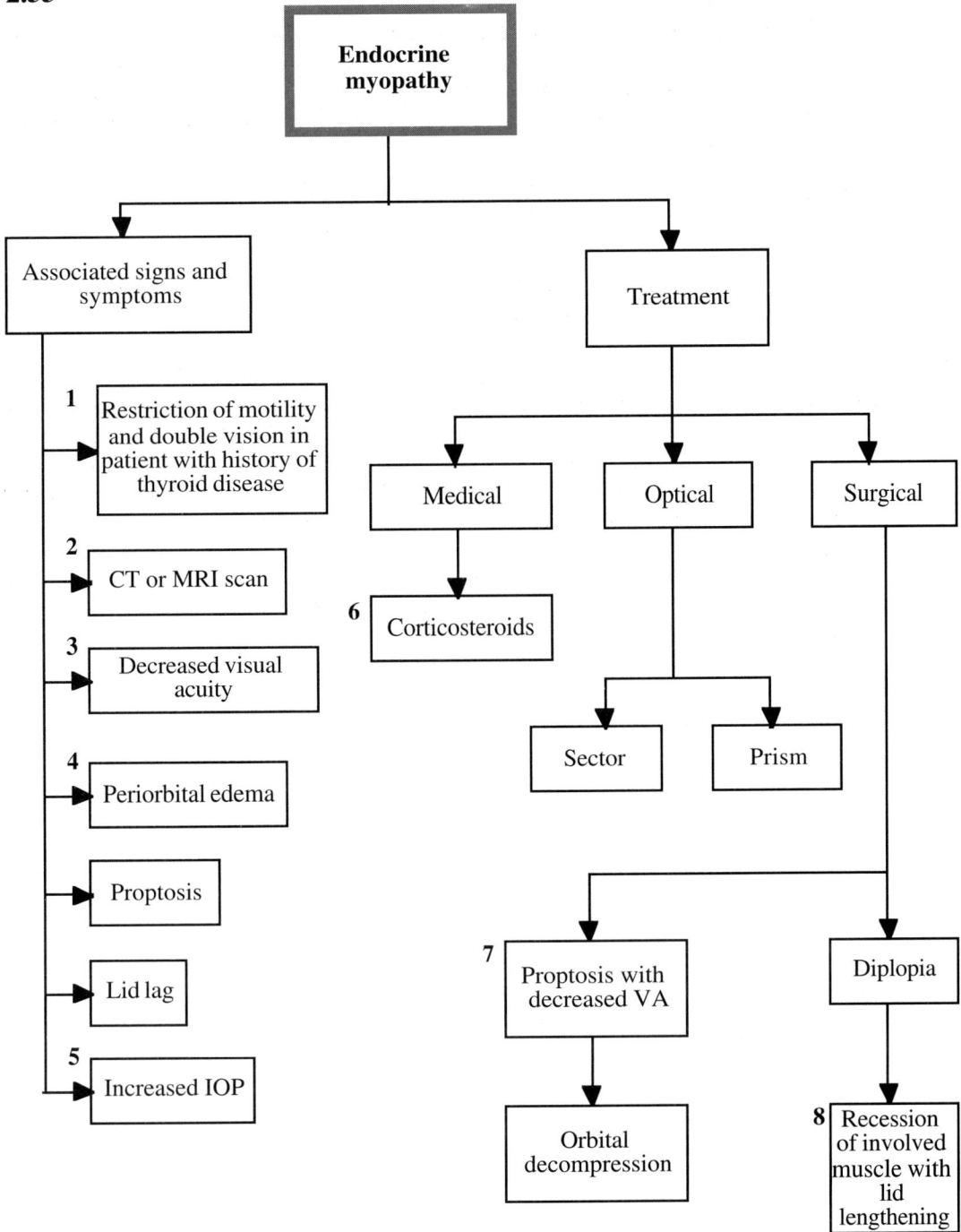

```
                    ┌──────────────────┐
                    │   Endocrine      │
                    │   myopathy       │
                    └──────────────────┘
```

Endocrine myopathy

Associated signs and symptoms

1 Restriction of motility and double vision in patient with history of thyroid disease

2 CT or MRI scan

3 Decreased visual acuity

4 Periorbital edema

Proptosis

Lid lag

5 Increased IOP

Treatment

Medical

6 Corticosteroids

Optical

Sector

Prism

Surgical

7 Proptosis with decreased VA

Orbital decompression

Diplopia

8 Recession of involved muscle with lid lengthening

2.56   Myasthenia Gravis

(1) Myasthenia can affect ocular motility and cause diplopia as a sole symptom of the disease (ocular myasthenia) or can affect both ocular and skeletal muscles. The extraocular muscle weakness may involve any of the extraocular muscles individually or muscle groups may be affected and may mimic supranuclear or internuclear paralyses.[57 p.419]

(2) When myasthenia is suspected, the patient is asked to blink rapidly 20 times. The myasthenic patient demonstrates an increase in ptosis.

(3) Cogan sign is retraction of the upper lid(s) after the patient is asked to look rapidly from down gaze to primary position.

(4) The effect of the Tensilon test is more pronounced on ptosis than on ocular motility. The test is performed by injecting 2 mg of Tensilon intravenously while evaluating the ptosis and/or the limitation of ocular motility. If there is little or no effect, the remaining 8 mg is injected. Atropine should be available for intravenous injection as an antidote. A negative Tensilon test result does not rule out ocular myasthenia; the test may have to be repeated several times.

(5) Surgery is rarely indicated but may have to be considered when there is no improvement from medical therapy and weakness of a particular muscle becomes chronic and does not undergo further changes.

2.56

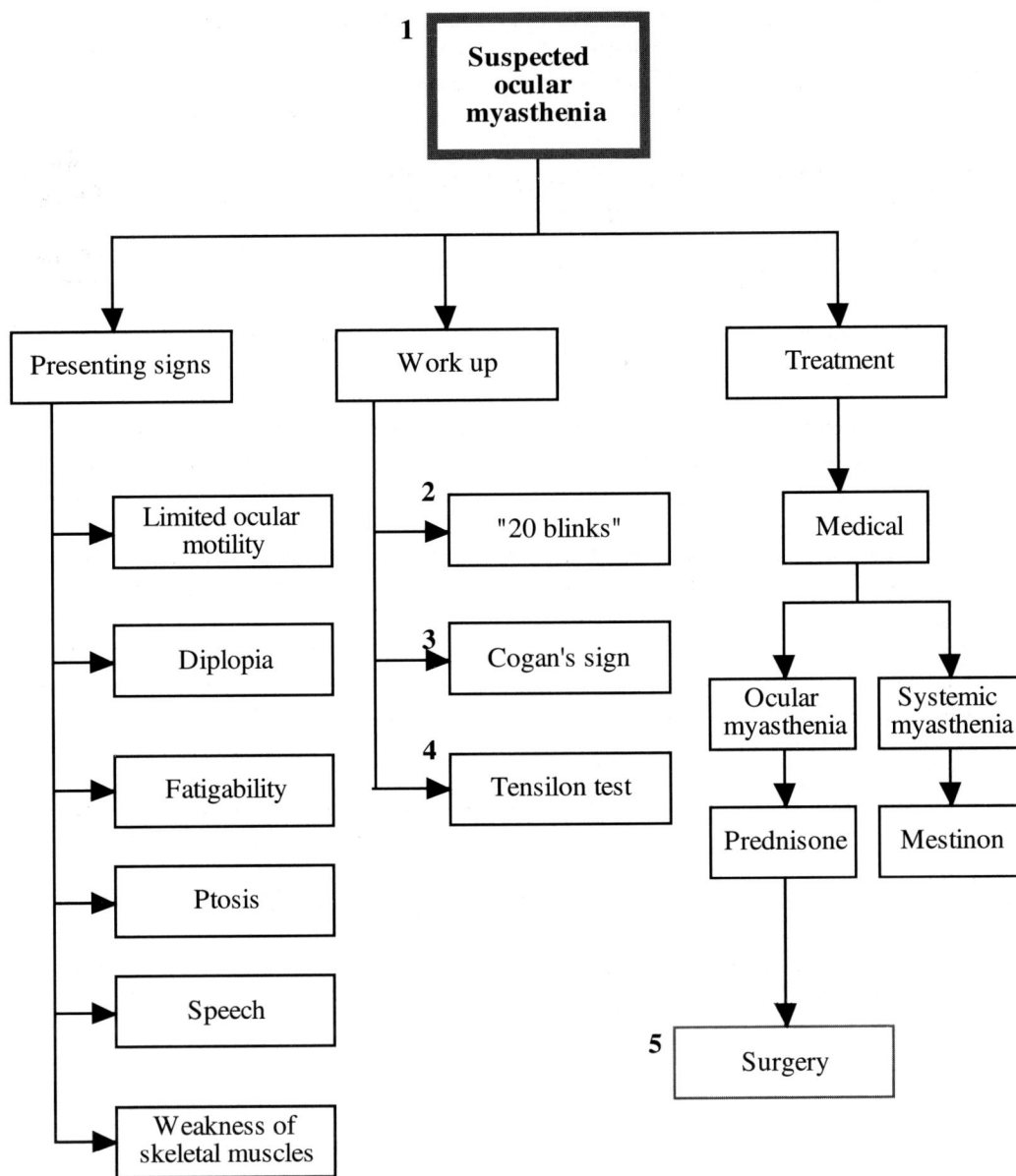

1	**Suspected ocular myasthenia**

Presenting signs → Limited ocular motility, Diplopia, Fatigability, Ptosis, Speech, Weakness of skeletal muscles

Work up → 2 "20 blinks", 3 Cogan's sign, 4 Tensilon test

Treatment → Medical → Ocular myasthenia → Prednisone → 5 Surgery; Systemic myasthenia → Mestinon

2.57   Child With Reading Problems

(1) In an initial discussion the examiner must determine whether the chid has a specific reading problem or a more generalized learning disorder. The child with a typical reading disorder shows a disproportionate defect in reading ability while performing adequately or, at times superiorly, in other academic subjects.

(2) It is important to look at school papers and to review any prior psychometric testing. If psychometric testing has not been done, it should be. These tests of verbal and performance capabilities comprise the IQ or intelligence quotient. A typical pattern is seen in the patient with dyslexia.

(3) Uncorrected hypermetropia or astigmatism may contribute to poor reading performance. In such cases, the appropriate correction should be prescribed.

(4) A rare cause of reading difficulties is premature presbyopia. The near point of accommodation is reduced and prescription of reading glasses or bifocals remedy this problem.

(5) Convergence insufficiency **(see 2.48)** causes asthenopia at near vision and may contribute to poor reading performance. Orthoptic exercises are indicated.

(6) An A pattern exotropia or exophoria or a V pattern esotropia or esophoria **(see 2.23 and 2.24)** may cause diplopia or asthenopia in downward gaze and must be ruled out as a cause for poor reading performance. This is a rare cause of reading difficulty.

(7) Efforts to maintain fusion in the presence of a large heterophoria may decrease reading performance; this may require surgery or orthoptic exercises.

(8) Reading comprehension is tested with paragraph reading and word lists.[24 p.331]

The principal role of the ophthalmologist is to encourage families to pursue traditional educational programs and avoid expensive, time consuming, and ineffective fads.

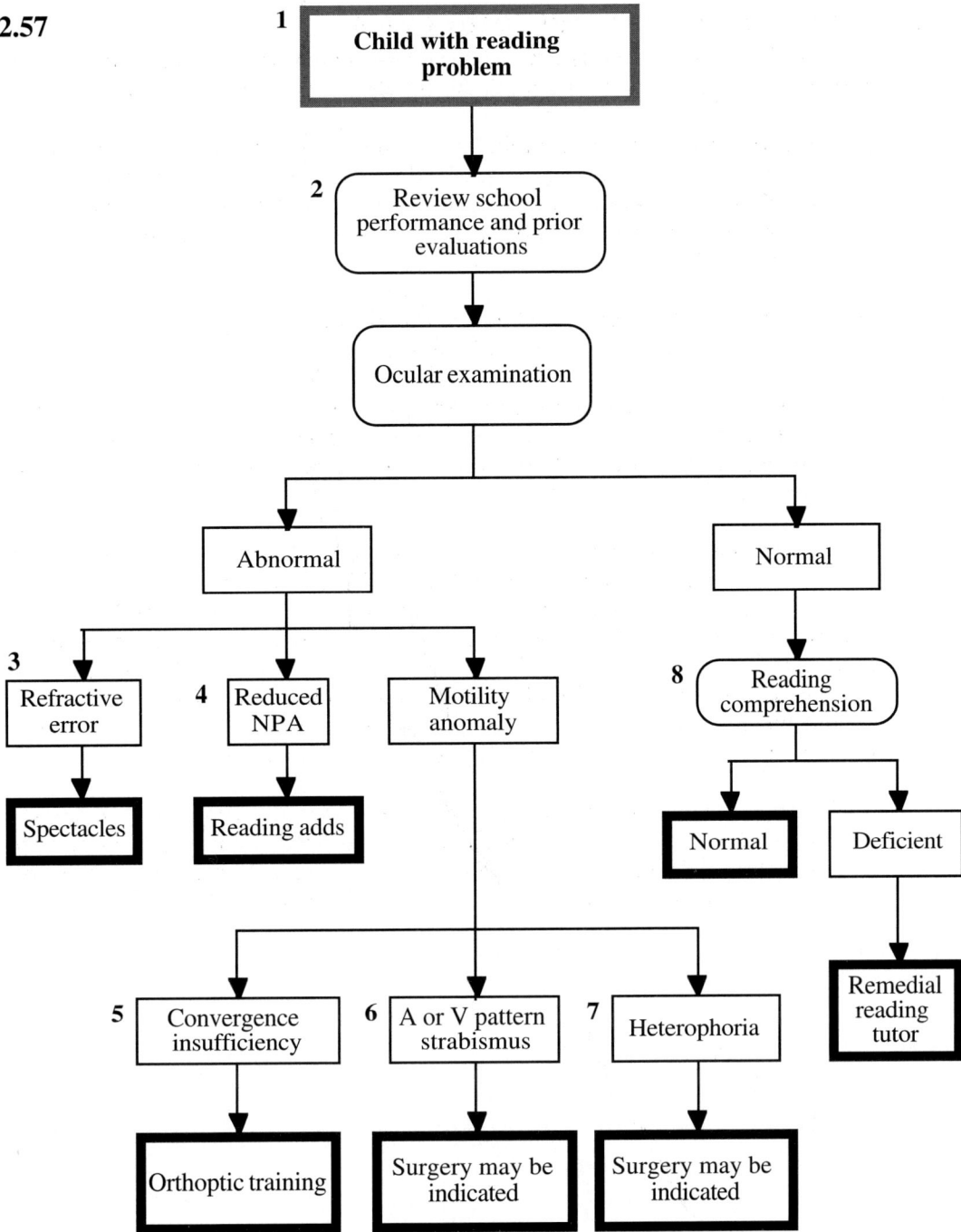

2.57

1 **Child with reading problem**

↓

2 Review school performance and prior evaluations

↓

Ocular examination

Abnormal   Normal

3 Refractive error   **4** Reduced NPA   Motility anomaly   **8** Reading comprehension

↓   ↓   ↓
Spectacles   Reading adds   Normal   Deficient

5 Convergence insufficiency   **6** A or V pattern strabismus   **7** Heterophoria

↓   ↓   ↓   ↓
Orthoptic training   Surgery may be indicated   Surgery may be indicated   Remedial reading tutor

2.58   Muscle Reattachment Techniques

(1) The choice of the muscle reattachment technique is largely determined by the surgeon's preference and is modified by certain patient characteristics.

(2) Anticipated patient noncompliance precludes the use of adjustable sutures. This includes the pediatric age group and certain adults. For instance, patients who show poor cooperation during measurement of the intraocular pressure or performance of the forced duction test are generally poor candidates for postoperative suture adjustment.

(3) In intermittent strabismus the surgical outcome is largely predictable; adjustable sutures offer no particular advantage.

(4) The use of adjustable sutures in patients who show a sensitive oculocardiac reflex during surgery is not recommended. Bradycardia or arrhythmias are difficult to manage in an ophthalmologic office during suture adjustment the morning after surgery.[23 p.274]

(5) The possibility of modifying the eye position postoperatively in the alert patient has its advantages and disadvantages. We use adjustable sutures in about 10% of our adult patients, especially in those with good fusion potential. Disadvantages include late overcorrection and undercorrections, in some cases caused by a slipped muscle, infection, and increased patient discomfort. The use of adjustable sutures remains a highly personal issue among strabismus surgeons. It should be emphasized that the use of adjustable sutures does not make up for deficiencies in diagnosis, the surgical plan, or surgical technique.

(6) Because adequate exposure can be obtained in most instances, reattachment of a recessed muscle at the intended site can be accomplished and is our preferred method. However, "hang loose" sutures are preferred whenever controlled refixation is technically impossible or inadvisable.[23 p.166]

2.58

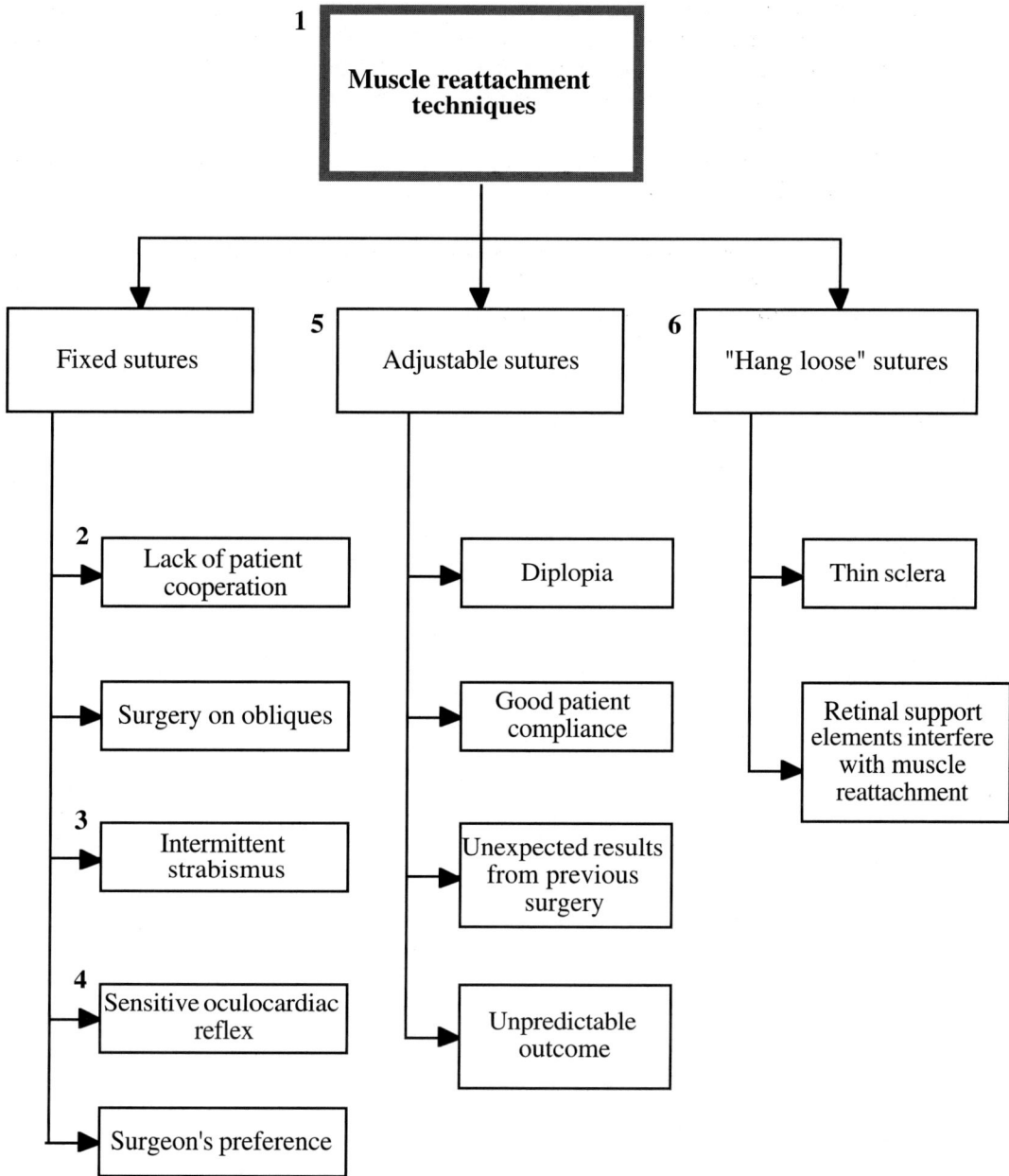

1 **Muscle reattachment techniques**

Fixed sutures

5 Adjustable sutures

6 "Hang loose" sutures

2 Lack of patient cooperation

Surgery on obliques

3 Intermittent strabismus

4 Sensitive oculocardiac reflex

Surgeon's preference

Diplopia

Good patient compliance

Unexpected results from previous surgery

Unpredictable outcome

Thin sclera

Retinal support elements interfere with muscle reattachment

2.59   Advantages of General Versus Local Anesthesia

(1) The decision whether to operate with the patient under general or local anesthesia is made on the basis of several considerations. The morbidity and mortality rate are similar in both. If any patient discomfort is experienced with local anesthesia, it occurs *during* surgery. In contrast, if any patient discomfort is experienced with general anesthesia, it occurs *after* surgery.

(2) Topical anesthesia may be administered with local anesthetic drops alone or subconjunctival injection of an anesthetic agent.[23 p.96; 57 p.491]

(3) Local anesthesia should not be used for any procedure during which an unusual amount of tension on the muscle or rotation of the globe into extreme positions is anticipated because the patient may experience discomfort.

2.59

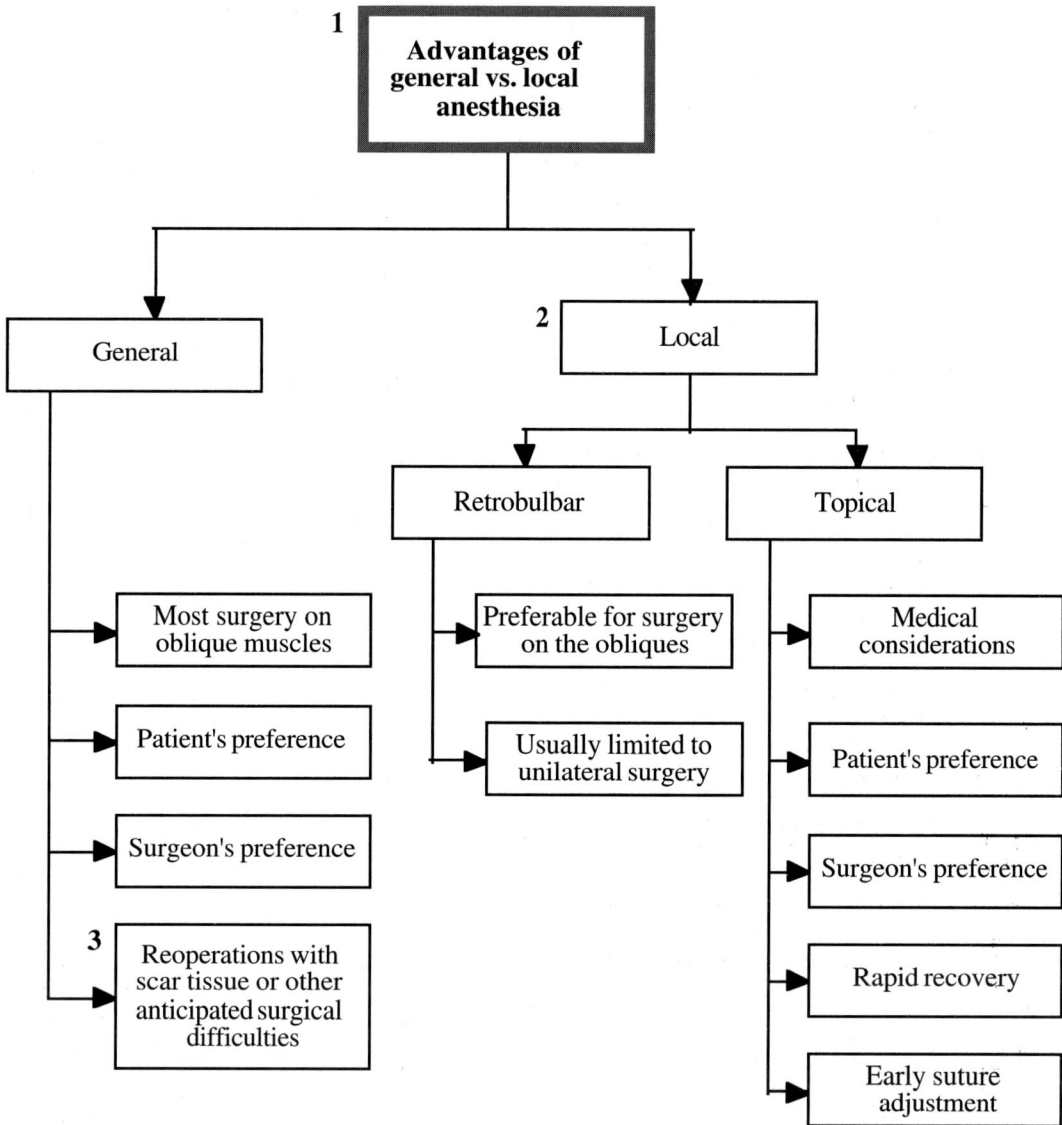

1 **Advantages of general vs. local anesthesia**

General

2 Local

Retrobulbar

Topical

Most surgery on oblique muscles

Patient's preference

Surgeon's preference

3 Reoperations with scar tissue or other anticipated surgical difficulties

Preferable for surgery on the obliques

Usually limited to unilateral surgery

Medical considerations

Patient's preference

Surgeon's preference

Rapid recovery

Early suture adjustment

REFERENCES

1. Archer SM, Sondhi N, Helveston EM: Strabismus in infancy, *Ophthalmology* 96:133, 1989.

2. Bangerter A: *Amblyopiebehandlung*, ed 2, Basel, 1953, S. Karger AG p. 121.

3. Birch EE: Visual acuity testing in infants and young children, *Ophthalmol Clin North Am* 2:369, 1989.

4. Bixenman WW, von Noorden GK: Benign recurrent VI nerve palsy in childhood, *J. Pediatr Ophthalmol Strabismus* 28:29, 1981.

5. Bloom JN, Mardelle PG: A magnetic resonance imaging study of the upshoot-downshoot phenomenon of Duane's retraction syndrome, *Am J Ophthalmol* 111:548, 1991.

6. Burgess D, Roper-Hall G, Burde RM: Binocular diplopia associated with subretinal neovascular membranes, *Acta Ophthalmol (Copenh)* 93:111, 1980.

7. Burian HM: Motility clinic: sudden onset of comitant convergent strabismus, *Am J Ophthalmol* 28:407, 1945.

8. Burian HM, Franceschetti A: Evaluation of diagnostic methods for the classification of exodeviation, *Trans Am Ophthalmol Soc* 68:56, 1970.

9. Burian HM, Miller JE: Comitant convergent strabismus with acute onset, *Am J Ophthalmol* 45:55, 1958.

10. Chamberlain W: Restriction in upward gaze with advancing age, *Trans Am Ophthalmol Soc* 68:234, 1970.

11. Chrousos GA, O'Neill JF, Leuth B, Parks MM: Accommodation deficiency in healthy young individuals, *J Pediatr Ophthalmol Strabismus* 25:176, 1988.

12. Demer JL, von Noorden GK: High myopia as an unusual cause of restrictive motility disturbance, *Surv Ophthalmol* 32:281, 1989.

13. Demer JL, von Noorden GK: Optokinetic asymmetry in esotropia, *J Pediatr Strabismus* 25:286, 1988.

14. Dobson V, Teller D, Lee CP, Wade B: A behavioral method for efficient screening of visual acuity in young infants, *Vision Res* 18:1469, 1978.

15. Duane A: A new classification of the motor anomalies of the eyes based upon physiological principles, together with their symptoms, diagnosis and treatment, *Ann Ophthalmol Otolaryngol* 6:969, 1896.

16. Emery JM, von Noorden GK: Traumatic "pseudoprolapse" of orbital tissues into the maxillary antrum, *Trans Am Acad Ophthalmol Otolaryngol* 79:893, 1975.

17. Fitton MH, Jampolsky A: A case report of spontaneous consecutive esotropia, *Am Orthopt J* 61:86, 1964.

18. Glaser J: *Neuroophthalmology*, Hagerstown, Md. 1978, Harper & Row, p. 271.

19. Guyton DL, von Noorden GK: Sensory adaptations to cyclodeviations. In: Reinecke RD ed: *Strabismus*. New York, 1978, Grune & Stratton, pp. 399-403.

20. Helveston EM: Brown syndrome: anatomic considerations and pathophysiology, *Am Orthopt J* 43:31, 1993.

21. Helveston EM: Cyclic strabismus, *Am Orthopt J* 23:48, 1973.

22. Helveston EM: The origins of congenital esotropia (19th annual Costenbader lecture), *J Pediatr Ophthalmol Strabismus*, 30:215, 1993.

23. Helveston EM: *Surgical management of strabismus. An atlas of strabismus surgery*, ed 4, St. Louis, 1993, CV Mosby.

24. Helveston EM, Ellis FD: *Pediatric ophthalmology practice*, ed 2, St. Louis, Toronto, 1984, CV Mosby.

25. Helveston EM, Ellis FD, Plager DA: Large recessions of the horizontal recti for the treatment of nystagmus, *Ophthalmology* 98:1302, 1991.

26. Helveston EM, Krach D, Plager DA, Ellis, FD: A new classification of superior oblique palsy based on congenital variation in the tendon, *Ophthalmology* 99:1609, 1992.

27. Helveston EM, von Noorden GK: Microtropia, a newly defined entity, *Arch Ophthalmol* 78:272, 1967.

28. Jampolsky A: Management of acquired "adult" muscle palsies. In: Burde RM, ed: *Neuroophthalmology. Transactions of the New Orleans Academy of Ophthalmology*, St. Louis, 1976, CV Mosby, p. 150.

29. Kaufmann H, Kolling G: Operative Therapie bei Nystagmuspatienten mit Binokularfunktion mit und ohne Kopfzwangshaltung, *Ber Deutsch Ophthalmol Ges* 78:815, 1981.

30. Knapp P: Diagnosis and surgical treatment of hypertropia, *Am Orthopt J* 21:29, 1971.

31. Knapp P, Moore S: Diagnosis and surgical options in superior oblique paralysis, *Int Ophthalmol Clin* 16:137, 1976.

32. Knox DL, Clark DB, Schuster FF: Benign sixth nerve palsies in children, *Pediatrics* 40:5460, 1967.

33. Kushner, BJ: Functional amblyopia associated with abnormalities of the optic nerve. *Am J Ophthalmol* 102:683, 1984.

34. Kushner BJ: Functional amblyopia associated with organic disease, *Am J Ophthalmol* 91:39, 1981.

35. Kushner BJ: Successful treatment of functional amblyopia associated with juvenile glaucoma, *Graefes Arch Clin Exp Ophthalmol* 226:150, 1988.

36. Lang J: Microtropia, *Arch Ophthalmol* 81:758, 1969.

37. McDonald M, Dobson V, Sebris S, Baitch L Varner D, Teller D: The acuity card proce-

dure: a rapid test of infant acuity, *Invest Ophthalmol Vis Sci* 26:1158, 1985.

38. Mumma JV: Surgical procedure for congenital absence of the superior oblique, *Arch Ophthalmol* 92:221, 1974.

39. Nixon RB, Helveston EM, Miller K, Archer SM, Ellis FD: Incidence of strabismus in neonates, *Am J Ophthalmol* 100:798, 1985.

40. Norcia AM, Hamer RD, Orel-Bixler D: Temporal tuning of the motion VEP in infants, *Invest Ophthalmol Vis Sci* 31(Suppl):10, 1990.

41. O'Donnell FE, del Monte M, Guyton DL: Simultaneous correction of blepharoptosis and exotropia in aberrant regeneration of the oculomotor nerve by strabismus surgery, *Ophthalmic Surg* 11:695, 1980.

42. Olivier P, von Noorden GK: Excyclotropia of the nonparetic eye in unilateral superior oblique muscle paralysis, *Am J Ophthalmol* 93:30, 1982.

43. Olivier P, von Noorden GK: Results of superior oblique tenectomy in inferior oblique paresis, *Arch Ophthalmol* 100:581, 1982.

44. Parks MM: Isolated cyclovertical muscle palsy, *Arch Ophthalmol* 60:1027, 1958.

45. Pollard ZF: Accommodative esotropia during the first year of life, *Arch Ophthalmol* 23:575, 1976.

46. Ruttum M, von Noorden GK: Adaptation to tilting of the visual environment in cyclotropia, *Am J Ophthalmol* 96:229, 1983.

47. Ruttum M, von Noorden GK: Orbital and facial anthropometry in A and V pattern strabismus. In: Reinecke RD, ed: *Strabismus II*, New York, 1984, Grune & Stratton, p. 363.

48. Scobee RG: *The oculorotary muscles*, ed 2: St. Louis, 1952, CV Mosby, p. 172.

49. Scott AB: Active force tests in lateral rectus paralysis, *Arch Ophthalmol* 85:397, 1971.

50. Scott AB: Strabismus-muscle forces and innervations. In: Lennerstrand G, Bach-y-Rita P, eds: *Basic mechanisms of ocular motility and their clinical implications*, Oxford, 1975, Pergamon Press, p. 181.

51. Scott AB, Magoon EH, McNeer KW, et al: Botulinum treatment of childhood strabismus, *Ophthalmology* 97:1434, 1990.

52. Sidikaro J, von Noorden GK: Observations on sensory heterotropia, *J Pediatr Ophthalmol Strabismus* 19:12, 1982.

53. Souza-Dias C: Surgical management of superior oblique paresis. In: Moore S, Mein J, eds: *Orthoptics: past, present, future*, Miami, 1976, Symposia Specialist, p. 388.

54. Sprunger DT, von Noorden GK, Helveston EM: Surgical results in Brown syndrome, *J Pediatr Ophthalmol Strabismus* 28(3):155, 1990.

55. Sutcliffe J: Torsion spasms and abnormal head postures in children with hiatus hernias, Sandifer's syndrome. *Progr Pediatr Radiol* 2:190, 1969.

56. von Noorden GK: *Atlas of strabismus*, ed 3, St. Louis, 1983, CV Mosby.

57. von Noorden GK: *Binocular vision and ocular motility: theory and management of strabismus*, ed 4, St. Louis, 1990, CV Mosby.

58. von Noorden GK: Idiopathic amblyopia, *Am J Ophthalmol* 100:214, 1985.

59. von Noorden GK: Pathophysiology of amblyopia: diagnostic and therapeutic principles of pleoptics, *Am Orthopt J* 10:7, 1960.

60. von Noorden GK: A reassessment of infantile esotropia. (XLIV Edward Jackson Memorial Lecture), *Am J Ophthalmol* 105:1, 1988.

61. von Noorden GK: Recession of both horizontal recti muscles in Duane's retraction syndrome with elevation and depression of the adducted eye, *Am J Ophthalmol* 11:311, 1992.

62. von Noorden GK: Resection of both medial rectus muscles in organic convergence insufficiency, *Am J Ophthalmol* 81:223, 1975.

63. von Noorden GK, Avilla CW: Accommodative convergence in hypermetropia, *Am J Ophthalmol* 11:287, 1990.

64. von Noorden GK, Brown DJ, Parks M: Associated convergence and accommodative insufficiency, *Doc Ophthalmol* 34:393, 1973.

65. von Noorden GK, Chu MW: Surgical treatment options in cyclotropia, *J Pediatr Ophthalmol Strabismus* 27:291, 1990.

66. von Noorden GK, Hansell R: Clinical characteristics and treatment of isolated inferior rectus paralysis, *Ophthalmology* 98:253, 1991.

67. von Noorden GK, Jenkins R: Horizontal transposition of the vertical rectus muscles in cyclotropia, *J Pediatr Ophthalmol Strabismus* 30:8, 1993.

68. von Noorden GK, Morris J, Edelman P: Efficacy of bifocals in the treatment of accommodative esotropia, *Am J Ophthalmol* 85:830, 1978.

69. von Noorden GK, Munoz M, Wong SY: Compensatory mechanisms in congenital nystagmus, *Am J Ophthalmol* 104:387, 1987.

70. von Noorden GK, Murray EM, Wong SY: Superior oblique paralysis: a review of 270 cases, *Arch Ophthalmol* 104:1771, 1986.

71. von Noorden GK, Sprunger DT: Large rectus muscle recessions for the treatment of congenital nystagmus, *Arch Ophthalmol* 109:221, 1991.

72. Wiggins RE, von Noorden GK: Monocular eye closure in sunlight, *J Pediatr Ophthalmol Strabismus* 27:16, 1990.

73. Wilson ME, McClatchey SK: Dissociated horizontal deviations, *J Pediatr Ophthalmol* 28:90, 1990.
74. Wirth CJ, Hagena FW, Wuelker N, Siebert, WE: Biterminal tenotomy for the treatment of congenital muscular torticollis, *J Bone Joint Surg* [Am] 74:427, 1992.
75. Wright KW, Walonker F, Edelman P: Ten-diopter fixation test for amblyopia, *Arch Ophthalmol* 99:1242, 1981.

Index